FOWLERS AND WELLS'

WATER-CURE LIBRARY.

Embracing

ALL THE MOST POPULAR WORKS

ON THE SUBJECT:

INCLUDING:

INTRODUCTION TO THE WATER-CURE;
HYDROPATHY, OR THE WATER-CURE;
EXPERIENCE IN THE WATER-CURE;
THE CHOLERA, AND BOWEL DISEASES;
WATER AND VEGETABLE DIET;
THE PARENTS' GUIDE;
TOBACCO: ITS NATURE AND EFFECTS;
CURIOSITIES OF COMMON WATER;
WATER-CURE MANUAL;
WATER-CURE IN EVERY DISEASE;
WATER-CURE IN PREGNANCY;
HYDROPATHY FOR THE PEOPLE;
ERRORS IN THE WATER-CURE;
WATER-CURE IN CONSUMPTION.

IN SEVEN VOLUMES.

VOL. I.

HYDROPATHY, OR THE WATER-CURE.

NEW YORK:
FOWLERS AND WELLS, PUBLISHERS,
CLINTON HALL, 129 AND 131 NASSAU STREET.
1850.

HYDROPATHY,

OR

THE WATER-CURE:

ITS

PRINCIPLES, PROCESSES, AND MODES OF TREATMENT.

COMPILED IN PART FROM

THE MOST EMINENT AUTHORS, ANCIENT AND MODERN, ON THE SUBJECT:
TOGETHER WITH AN ACCOUNT OF THE

LATEST METHODS ADOPTED BY PRIESSNITZ.

ILLUSTRATED WITH NUMEROUS CASES OF CURE.

BY JOEL SHEW, M. D.

FOURTH EDITION, IMPROVED AND ENLARGED.

NEW YORK:
FOWLERS AND WELLS, PUBLISHERS,
CLINTON HALL, 129 AND 131 NASSAU STREET.
1850.

BANER & PALMER, STEREOTYPERS,
201 William st. corner Frankfort, N. Y.

PREFACE

TO THE FIRST EDITION.

It will at once be observed, that in the following pages there is no claim to originality. The compiler has for a time had his attention directed to the water-cure, and has with interest witnessed its progress. Having been perfectly convinced of its value, and of its superiority as a system for the treatment of disease, he has been engaged in writing with a view to publicity; but as different works upon the subject have from time to time appeared in Europe—works of merit—some of which are of very recent date, he has thought best to adopt the maxim that "amidst counsellors there is safety," to substitute in a great measure portions of those works in such a way as it is hoped will render the present work one of value. The writings of the several authors will show for themselves. Let it be understood, however, that the compiler does not intend that it shall be inferred that he agrees with *all* that is said.

Various have been the objections urged against hydropathy. By high authority, we have it classed among the various delusions that are, and that have been, and of which it is said, they

> "In turns appear, to make the vulgar stare,
> Till the swoll'n bubble bursts, and all is air."

So it has been ranked in this country; but nearer the retired spot of the "primitive philosopher," Priessnitz, it is different. *There*, in abundance, are to be found the "*hard telling facts*." The actual cures have been performed. *There* has been raised the cry of danger! danger! instead of delusion. As to the dangers in the practice of the water-cure, what are they? Precisely not greater than are to be found elsewhere—not greater than to open a vein or an artery, and to draw out that fluid upon which life so much depends; or to introduce into the stomach, or the circulation, the most virulent and deadly poisons in nature—things of every-day practice. The administration of pure clean water cannot certainly be attended with more danger.

That, by thousands, astounding cures have been performed in the treatment, no one can question. And so was it in tractoration. But there the mistake was as to the *how*. The objector who would class the water-cure with that delusion, has not examined the subject—does not even know what the water-cure is. In the case of tractoration, in which the cures were performed, the subject exercised unbounded faith in the mysterious agency of the tractors. It is true, too, that Priessnitz inspires *his* patients with confidence and courage, and so must any and every practitioner of the healing art, to obtain success. But more: let the objector, professional or non-professional, get a little way into the *secrets* of the water-cure (for to him as yet they are secrets). If he be an invalid, let him awhile leave, of every kind, his vile narcotics and stimulants—in every respect, his hours keep regularly. Let him "daily wash and be clean," and be throughout regular and temperate in his meals, and in all his habits. Let him diminish, if need be, the amount of fluids in the body, by most profuse perspiration; or, by the wet sheet, reduce the temperature of the body, and the velocity of the circulation and heart's action, to any required extent. Let him purify the blood, not by any of the thousand-and-one of the nostrums of the quack, or of the multitudinous forms of drugs innumerable, but by the cleansing effect of Nature's own best pure fluid. Let him, if he can command courage, go to the bath, to the douche; climb among the hills, and breathe freely the pure mountain air of heaven, and all in proportion to his increasing strength; let him be cheerful always; and at evening, according to his inclinations, let him join in some of the social exercises—the music and the dance; and when in time he finds his body has become amazingly strengthened, and his mind active, cheerful, vigorous, and blithesome, and that his old ailments inveterate are cast off, it will be a thing not easy to convince him that *all* is delusion—a work of the imagination. By this time he finds that though he *will*, as if to bring spirits from the "vasty deep," against the effects of the water-cure, it would be willing in vain. There is at least something of physical truth in it. A greater mistake cannot be than to class this with Tractoration, Sir Kenelm Digby's sympathetic powder, or Hahneman's decillionth grain doses of charcoal, flint, silica, or cuttle-fish juice, made too potent by *ten* shakes instead of two. A wider difference cannot be.

The unprofessional manner in which the water-cure is introduced, has been a matter of objection by some. According to Dr. Rush, a medical man should be a student his life long. He should gather information from any and every source—should even lay under contribution the experience of the old woman, whom he might meet in a stage coach or elsewhere, to add to his stock of facts in the healing art. "Life is short, art is long," said Hippocrates, "the old man of Cos."

Should an old woman, or any one, discover a drug of which it should be said, on good authority, that it was capable, in one dose, of producing the most powerful sweating; and in another, of reducing the temperature of the body most efficiently, and of retarding the velocity of the circulation to any required extent, and which consequently could be made to fulfill every intermediate indication, the student-like physician would most certainly set to work and test fairly and fully the power of the old woman's drug. Yet who is there at all willing to do it?

The great physiologist and physician, Magendie, makes the strong assertions, that "the science of medicine is almost the only one characterized by *uncertainty* and *chance*"—that "the existing system of medical study confers trifling good on society"—that "there is scarcely a sound idea on physiology abroad"—that "the plan hitherto pursued in the study of medicine, has been too narrow ever to lead to those happy results that dignify an age by improving the condition of humanity"—and that "the prevalent mode of treating disease, harmonizes admirably with, and is quite as senseless as, the method of reasoning in pathology. The practitioner mixes, combines, and jumbles together vegetable, mineral, and animal substances; administers them right or wrong, without for a moment considering the *cause* of the disease, and without a single clear idea on the why and wherefore of his conduct." Another says, "all things considered, it were better for mankind if not a particle of medicine existed on the face of the earth;" and the learned Hoffman of the seventeenth century said, "avoid medicine and physicians, if you value your health!"

However strong and sweeping these assertions may at first appear, if we carefully examine, we shall find that there is vastly too much of truth in them. The study of the mere relation between symptoms and remedies, without sufficient reference to the removing of the *causes* of disease, has been too much the case in medicine. Hippocrates used but little medicine, and his remedies were few and simple. His principal business was to discover and remove the *causes* of disease.

Medicine has likewise been followed too much as a mere business—a means of livelihood, or a source of emolument. And then again, if we may hazard the opinion, it is too true that the existing system of medicine is often found going in direct opposition to its fundamental principles. This it is claimed cannot in truth be said of hydropathy. The practice in the water-cure is consistent, rational, and explainable.

Let us not be misunderstood in this matter. Far be it from *us* to depreciate, in any way, the value of the profession. It is error, and not men, or any class of men, that we have to contend with. The noble profession of our choice we esteem—a profession, than which there is none of more importance to society and the race. But we could sooner doubt our very existence, than that the healing art comes far short of doing its best work—of conferring its best good upon society. That the profession is a body of worthy and intelligent men, and that of this body are those who are ranked among the highest benefactors of the human family, society fully acknowledges. It is therefore the height of folly for any one to act *against* the profession. The water-cure, and improvements of whatever kind, wherever they may originate, must be introduced to the public generally through this profession.

As if perfection were to be found, and as if *all* medical men, unlike those of other professions, were to be perfect moral beings, we hear in glowing colors, by some, not a little said about the persecutions in medicine. We hear the grave questions, "Who denounced Harvey, the glorious discoverer of the circulation of the blood?" "Who ridiculed vaccination, and persecuted its discoverer, Jenner?" And then, again, when Lady Mary Montague inoculated her child with the matter of small-pox to mitigate the severity of the disorder, it is said that on the part of some there was manifested such an unwillingness to have the experiment succeed, "that she never cared to leave the child alone with them one second, lest in some secret way it should suffer from their interference."

Admit this all true, and more, and we have that which will but poorly compare with the witch manias, and the violent persecutions elsewhere. And be it remembered, too, that among the ignorant traducers of the profession, are to be found those who are ever most ready to lend their names and influence to quackery of every form, but when any thing serious comes upon them, they are equally ready to avail themselves of the gratuitous services of the insulted profession.

The water-cure presupposes that all due attention be given to the removal of the causes of disease—to the prevention as well as the cure. The great ignorance that exists as to the causes of disease, the means of prevention, and the best methods of curing, is an ever fruitful source of quackery of every kind. Teach people to understand the laws of life, health, and disease, and then they are incapable of the imposition of the mercenary and villanous quack. And then, and not till then, will the profession attain its true dignity. And then will the labors of the true physician be rightly valued. Then will the physician's pay be more than now, like that of Boerhaave, when he practiced among his best patients, as he called them—the poor.

The writer has high hopes in reference to what will yet result in this country from the introduction of the water-cure. If he is mistaken in his enthusiasm, in this new world, in the healing art (for Captain Claridge says, Priessnitz, like Columbus, discovered a new world), so it is: he will trust to the intelligence of his country and the profession—to time and mature experience—to convince him of his error. He is young, and can improve. When a better way is shown, he will follow it. But from what he has heard, seen, and *knows*, as yet he *must* be in his humble way an advocate of the water-cure; and, in doing this, he has incomparably more regard for the good which it is destined to bring about in society, than for fame, reputation, or emolument.

As a matter of course, that always convenient word, "quackery," will, by some, be applied to the water-cure treatment. But let it be remembered that it is not Priessnitz, or any one, that such are to contend with, but *the thing itself.* A method of treatment of itself in perfect accordance with the laws of nature. A *natural* remedy, only intensified by *art*. Real quackery will have but little to do with hydropathy. There is in its very nature too much of primitiveness and simplicity—not enough of mysticism—of the wonderful and marvelous. Besides, the practice is too laborious, often severely so, both for patient and practitioner. Let the water-cure be generally understood and practiced, and the very considerable firm of "Messrs. Humbug," professional and non-professional, will turn bankrupt forthwith.

If the water-cure treatment is quackery, we have quackery unique. With his vile preparations, and specifics infallible, the quack may delude the ignorant, and, villain-like, drug mankind to death—employing in every direction his compeers to practice upon his thousands of patients, whom he never sees or cares for if he can but cheat them out of their substance; but to stand by the sufferer in disease, to guide the remaining energies of life in accordance with its own laws, in such a manner as to relieve pain, "remove obstructions, relieve oppression, subdue diseased action," and strengthen and invigorate the system, thus "placing the body under the most favorable circumstances for resisting disease," remains for another besides the *quack* to perform. And this we contend can best be done, when in competent hands, by the primitive natural treatment, the water-cure. Than this to quackery, nothing can be more perfectly, more specifically antipodal.

The simplicity or oneness of the remedy will be with some a matter of objection. It should be understood, that nothing is easier than by the water-cure to produce, to any given extent, directly opposite results; therefore its simplicity is greatly in its favor. Why have drugs been multiplied without number? Precisely because not one of them is to be depended upon. Not so in hydropathy. It is contended that the remedy here *can* be relied upon, and is always, in competent hands, not only safe, but will always do some good—which is not true of drugs.

To the non-professional inquirer, let it be said, no remedy can be powerful for good that may not be made powerful for evil. It may appear a simple thing to "wash and be clean," but even this must be done rightly. Although the "sleeping in wet sheets is by no means the disagreeable thing that it is usually conceived to be," yet it must be done in the right way, or most disastrous may be the consequences. The Russians find their snow bath exceedingly delightful after their sweating, but they know that it can be continued but a few minutes. The Englishman, finding it at once pleasant, remained too long, and thus sacrificed his life to his ignorance.

The water-cure implies temperance in detail. Those who wish to adopt the better plan, prevention rather than cure, may be assured, that in changing habits, mere *feelings* must not be taken as a guide. If they do, a blind leader of the blind it will prove. The invalid mendicant, while asking alms, declared that as long as God should let him live, be would drink every day a dram, because it gave him strength. The minister of the Gospel (not a physiologist) said he would enjoy his tea and coffee and his pipe, even if they *did* cut short his life, rather than be deprived of the good things which God gives us. But whenever the drunkard reforms, however uncomfortable at first he may *feel*, we soon find nature is true to herself. He feels like death, but yet he does not die. Soon like life from the dead he is a new and renovated man.

J. S.

PREFACE

TO THE SECOND EDITION.

The compiler will here state, that since the first edition of Hydropathy, or the Water-Cure, was published, he has had numerous opportunities of testing the efficacy of the new system; and that his former confidence in it is not in the least diminished. That confidence is, if possible, growing more and more strong. The system, consisting, as it does, of an endless variety of applications of water, internal and external, warm, hot, or cold, as the case may require, together with the agencies of air, exercise, diet, clothing, etc., etc., is, if the writer is not altogether mistaken, incomparably more effectual than any other, for speedily relieving pain, subduing inflammations and fevers of every kind, strengthening the body to the greatest possible extent, thus enabling it in the most effectual manner to resist disease. The new system is entirely without parallel—a significant fact, to be pondered by the "scientific" objectors who decry Priessnitz as being an "illiterate hind of the Silesian mountains." Let those improve upon his work who can.

The writer commenced his experiments and investigations in the new system, as indeed he did his first medical studies, with an inflexible determination *to ascertain truth.* Long before he had ever heard of the new system, and both before and after he had commenced the study of the healing art, he was at a loss to know how "setting one poison to catch another" was to be reconciled with reason;—how bleeding a person already nervous and debilitated—a thing often done—was any more rational than the letting down of the strings of a musical instrument whose tones already failed for want of sufficient tension;—how it was reasonable to excite the liver by mercury, causing a certain weakness and derangement of the organ already weakened and deranged—a thing of every-day occurrence in common practice—or how it was possible for a patient in a sinking state to be kept alive, as was so often believed, by alcoholic (poisonous) stimulants. In short, the writer fortunately early learned to distrust the existing symptoms of medicine, and was on the constant look out for something better. He has not been disappointed.

If the old allopathic or common practice of medicine were at this

1*

day wholly set aside, there would immediately be a diminution of disease, suffering, and premature death; and far better still even than now would it be if *all* drug medicines were at once wholly abandoned, and people were compelled, with pure clean water, right food, fresh air, and invigorating exercise, to help themselves as they best could. There would at once be less of sickness and unnatural death. But it is said *quackery* is the cause of the mischief. Is there not quackery "scientific," as well as unscientific? Do not the different sects, even in the established practice, at least *hint* that the other sects kill their patients? "Who shall decide when doctors disagree?"

In the present edition of this work it was thought best to vary to some extent the arrangement and matter from the former edition. Contrary to the ordinary mode, a collection of well-ascertained facts, in the form of cases treated mostly at Graefenberg, are placed first in the volume. First let us have facts—afterward theories. The volume, it is hoped, will not prove uninteresting. J. S.

PREFACE

TO THE THIRD EDITION.

THE following work having passed through two large editions, and the publisher desiring still to continue its sale, the author has deemed best to make numerous alterations and additions in the present issue. This edition will be found to contain about *one third* more matter than the last, while, at the same time, the price remains the same.

There is one feature of the present edition which, it is believed, will render it a much more acceptable one than either of the former. While on a second visit at Graefenberg, in the winter of 1847–8, the author was careful to obtain of Priessnitz his methods of treating the principal diseases to which the human system is subject. These were not trusted to memory, but were written down on the spot. These methods, simple as they may appear, are the results of this great man's experience, gained through many years of persevering toil. His opinions must necessarily have great weight with all who have confidence in the new system of water.

It will doubtless appear evident, from a perusal of the following pages, that the writer has had as an object the production of a work of usefulness, rather than one of brilliant authorship. J. S.

NEW YORK, 1849.

CONTENTS.

CHAPTER I.

THE MORE ANCIENT USES OF WATER.

CHAPTER II.

HYDROPATHY, OR THE MODERN WATER-CURE.

CHAPTER III.

HYDROPATHY, OR THE MODERN WATER-CURE—(CONTINUED.)

CHAPTER IV.

THEORY OF HYDROPATHY—DR. BILLING'S THEORY OF DISEASE.

CHAPTER IX.

PROCESSES OF WATER-CURE—(CONTINUED.)

CHAPTER X.

THE CRISIS OF WATER-CURE.

CHAPTER XI.

DISEASES TO WHICH THE WATER-CURE IS MORE ESPECIALLY ADAPTED.

CHAPTER XII.

GRAEFENBERG CASES OF WATER-CURE.

CHAPTER XIII.

GRAEFENBERG CASES OF WATER-CURE—(CONTINUED.)

CHAPTER XIV.

THE GRAEFENBERG TREATMENT OF DISEASES.

CHAPTER XV.

THE GRAEFENBERG TREATMENT OF DISEASES CONTINUED.

CHAPTER XVI.

TREATMENT OF DISEASES CONTINUED.

CHAPTER XVII.

TREATMENT OF DISEASES CONTINUED.

CHAPTER XVIII.

TREATMENT OF DISEASES CONTINUED.

CHAPTER XIX.

TREATMENT OF DISEASES CONTINUED.

CHAPTER XX.

TREATMENT OF DISEASES CONCLUDED.

APPENDIX.

THE WATER-CURE.

CHAPTER I.

THE MORE ANCIENT USES OF WATER.

Authority of Hippocrates.—Galen.—Celsus.—Boerhaave.—Hoffman.—Hufeland.—Zimmerman.—Hahn.—Father Bernardo.—Hahn the Elder.—Sir John Floyer.—Dr. Ellison—Dr. Baynard.—Dr. Dover.—William Penn.—Indian methods.—Dr. Currie.—Rev John Wesley.

Hippocrates, the great father of medicine, "the old man of Cos," who lived to about ninety years of age, we are told was accustomed to use water in his treatment of many of the most serious diseases. He observed, that it was the general nature of warm water to produce a chill, while cold water produced warmth. His method of effecting a sweat was exceedingly simple, and at the same time most effectual; far more so even than those modes of stimulating and rasping the internal organs by means of drugs. His plan, as we have seen elsewhere, was to pour water over the body, and then to place sufficient warm clothes upon the patient, so that the desired effect was produced. In a work which he wrote on Air, Water, and Situation, when about to speak of water, he says, "Let us see which are good and which bad; it is a point on which health mainly depends." He considered water the best drink. He laid down as an important law, that a bath enfeebles, every time that its heat exceeds that of the body immersed in it. The truth of this Hippocratic precept has often been verified. He said that the affusion of water cures cramp, convulsions, and tetanus; that the gout was to be cured by a large affusion of cold water; for it was certain, holding the foot a long time in it, abates the swelling, redness, and pain.

Galen, who lived in the second century, and who, next to Hippocrates, was called prince of the Greek physicians, said that he had cured many cases of burning continued fever, by giving his patients nothing but cold water to drink, and that not one of his patients died who had recourse to this simple remedy sufficiently early. He had seen many cured of a severe pain in the stomach in a single day, by drinking cold water. He also recommended cold bathing in fevers, and to persons in health, for fleshy ones, and those that use due exercise. According to his directions, the body was to be prepared by exercise in the gymnasium, by friction with coarse cloths, and sometimes by the prior use of the warm bath. The baths were to be taken before eating. After the bath, much friction and rubbing the surface was to be used until the skin was well warmed. He said that the duration of baths is too long, when after coming out of the bath, the body is very pale, and is not soon heated again by friction, and does not recover its natural heat and color thereby. Galen, like Hippocrates, lived to a very great age.

Celsus, a physician and philosopher, styled the Cicero of doctors, employed water for complaints of the head and stomach. He said that nothing is of so much service to the head as cold water. He recommended such as were weak in the head to plunge it into cold running water; and also in cases of weakness of sight, accompanied with a prevalent discharge from the eyes, and in enlargements of the glands. He said that slight cuts or wounds may be healed by applying sponges squeezed out of cold water; but that in whatever way the sponges may be applied, it is only of benefit as long as it retains the moisture.

The illustrious Boerhaave recommended the use of water to render the body firm and strong. Cold water, when limpid, light, and without smell or taste, and obtained from a clear running stream, he declared to be the best drink.

Hoffman, a cotemporary of Boerhaave, and professor of physic at Halle, and physician to the king of Prussia, wrote on the subject of water. He recommended it as the best preventive and cure of a large number of diseases. He said those who drink water, are observed to have much whiter and sounder teeth. They are brisker and more alert in all the actions both of mind and body, than such as use malt liquors. In reference to the use of mineral waters in chronic diseases, he said it was not owing to the light, sparkling air, or to the saline, or other mineral substances combined with the water, so much as to the medicinal properties of common water with which they are mixed, and which is drank in great quantities. "Water proves agreeable to persons of all ages," and "The drinking of water is serviceable in every complexion," are sayings of Hoffman. But his confidence in the power of water is best shown in the following quotation: "If there exists any thing in the world that can be called a *panacea* (a universal remedy) it is pure water; first, because it will disagree with nobody; secondly, because it is the best preservative against disease; thirdly, because it will cure agues and chronic complaints; fourthly, because it responds to all indications." By objectors to the exclusive, or nearly exclusive use of water, it is often said that water is most excellent in its place, and that it is good for a great variety of cases, and has been greatly neglected in the treatment of diseases; but that it *will not* respond to or answer all indications; that is, it cannot be made to answer all the good purposes of medicines. Hoffman, all will agree, is good authority; but the best proof of all, is actual experiment. Priessnitz, during the last twenty years, has cured diseases with greater success than any before him. His only medicine from the beginning of his accidental career, has been *pure clean water.*

Hufeland, who was also a distinguished professor, and editor of a medical journal, mentions the case of a Mr. Theden, veteran surgeon general, who ascribed his long life (more than eighty years) chiefly to the daily use of a large quantity of water, which he drank for upward of forty years. Between his thirtieth and fortieth year, he was a most miserable hypochondriac, oppressed with the deepest melancholy, tormented with a palpitation of the heart, indigestion, etc., and fancied that he could not live six months; but from the time he began this regimen all these symptoms disappeared, and in the latter half of his life, he enjoyed better health than before, and was perfectly free from his hypochondriac affection. He said, "The element of water is the greatest promoter of digestion; an excellent reviver of the stomach, and strengthener of the nerves, and assists all the secretions of the body, and that it purifies, not merely the skin, but freshens and exhilarates both the soul and the body; it strengthens and preserves against the changing influences of air and weather, keeps the solid parts supple and the joints pliable; it preserves the vigor of youth and keeps up the vigor of old age. It is a powerful preventive of bile and putrefaction."

Zimmerman, the author of a well-known work on Solitude, and physician to Frederick the Great, king of Prussia, strongly recommended water. "Water," he said, "does not chill the ardor of genius," and then mentioned the instance of Demosthenes, whose sole drink was water.

Hahn, a German physician of note, wrote a work on the effects of water in 1738. "Water," he says, "does not, as some suppose, weaken the stomach, but on the contrary increases the appetite, as may be seen by the larger quantity of food taken at meals. Those who make this assertion contradict themselves; for a debilitated stomach requires a less, and not a larger quantity of food. Others imagine that by drinking water they lose their color and flesh. Even if such were the case, and they did become a little paler and thinner, such a loss is not to be compared to the general improvement of health which is obtained thereby. It yet remains to be shown, whether a protuberant stomach, with swollen, flabby, puffed-out cheeks, is to be preferred to a more slender shape, and thinner face; or whether the rude country glow of health, with rosy cheeks, is not to be preferred to that pale and sickly hue, so much admired by people of fashion. But water-drinkers generally retain their flesh and healthy color. A few, however, who had swollen, flabby, or spongy flesh, and therefore unhealthy, have in appearance become thinner, and lost their puffiness, having exchanged it for a firm and compact flesh, therefore healthy. Those who, from the use of ardent spirits and thick, glutinous beverages, as beer or brandy, have got reddened, violet, copper-colored faces, have not, by drinking water, become pale, but have exchanged their violet or purple redness for a more natural color. Every man ought, I think, to be satisfied with such a change." This writer says that perspiration, caused by cold water, is more salutary than that by any other known means; and although warm water will produce perspiration, yet it chills the body much more afterward than cold. He mentions that a physician relieved the viceroy of Sicily, Johannes de la Vega, by the use of water, and received from him as a reward, the golden cup out of which water had been drank. He said, that cold water was better to remove impurities from the skin than warm, because warm water dries up the skin, and injures its fine vessels; while cold strengthens it, and renders the body hard and insensible to cold, like that Scythian who went naked about the market-place of Athens, to the great wonder of the people. On being questioned by one of the philosophers how he could go about naked in the cold, asked in reply, why the other did not cover his face up in winter. Upon the Athenian answering that it was accustomed to the cold, the Scythian rejoined, "Then consider my whole body as being all face."

Hahn recommended a woman who had the itch, to get into a tub of water, and remain in it several days, to eat, drink, and sleep therein. This being attended with too much inconvenience, she washed herself several times during the day, and wrapped herself up in wet sheets during the night, and then became cured in a very short time. There was, he says, mixed with this treatment, a little superstition, as it was thought the disorder could only be cured by bathing on Good Friday. Some persons who suffered severely with this disorder, went on a Good Friday, and bathed in their under-clothes, then returned without changing or drying, went to bed, and were entirely cured. A gentleman of his acquaintance had an ulcer on his foot, which he cured by frequently bathing in a pond; and whenever it threatened to reopen, speedily re-established the cure by the same means. A fisherman had a large ulcerated abscess in his thigh, which had continued in spite of every remedy, for the space of two years. The fear that water would aggravate the evil. had caused him to abandon his pursuits, but the prospect of starvation compelled him again to fish. On coming out of the water after two hours, he was agreeably surprised to find the sore much less painful. This induced him to go daily into the river, and in a short time he became perfectly cured. He had ordered his patients to let their sores soak in water, as tanners do their skins, to remove their putridity, for several days and nights. Running streams were more efficacious than washing in tubs, and the more so when the patient wades against the stream, as the water thus enters and cleanses the part more effectually. He had witnessed the good effects of water in St. Anthony's fire, which was removed in the course of a few days, without the slightest injury to the skin; whereas, on the other hand, the application of rose pink and white lead in powder, or of fat and oily pomades and plasters, impede the perspiration, increase the pain, and frequently cause ulcers. Spirituous lotions, in some measure, burn the skin, so that it peels off in large pieces; in like manner, other applications only aggravate the disease, and render it more difficult to cure. In speaking of cancerous ulcers, he says they bear the application of cold water very well. It refreshes and cleanses them, corrects the corrosion and mitigates the pain. He had met with cases where the most bland, innocent, and advisable remedies having proved irritating and painful, the patients had not only obtained great relief, but eventually were cured by cold water. He says, in the acute diseases the fire burns with the greatest violence in the interior of the body, but as may be seen by the thermometer, the skin is also affected in a great degree. Where the fire is, there we must also quench. Cold water, though taken in large quantities, does not relieve the burning skin; but washing the body with cold water, the patient feels immediately refreshed, and scarcely are the sponges applied before instant relief is obtained. So luxurious is the sensation, that many are unwilling that this washing should be discontinued, but like the rustics Latona changed into frogs, would prefer to remain in cold water. Infants who have eruptions on different parts of the body, like to be rubbed with cold water, and are by this simple remedy speedily cured. In exanthematous diseases, as small-pox, measles, scarlet fever, and other rashes, we may freely wash with cold water from the first to the last, during the whole course of the disease, in order to prevent the fever from becoming too violent. The skin is thus rendered more soft, so that the acrid matter can more easily pass through it. In small-pox, the corrosive quality of this acrid matter is rendered milder, so that it does not eat into the skin, leaving scars behind, and very few patients who have been treated in this way, have been marked by the disease. The Africans, he says, wash all their small-pox patients. A captain, having a cargo of slaves, among whom this disease made its appearance, treated them according to the European mode of putting the patients between two mattresses, and otherwise heaping clothes upon them, in order to bring out the disease. In great distress they cried and begged to be allowed to treat themselves according to their own mode. Being permitted, the other slaves tied ropes round the bodies of those that were sick, and dipped them frequently during the day into the sea, drying them afterward in the sun, and in this manner they were cured, and scarcely one died. As in small-pox, it is equally beneficial in measles and other rashes, and of a variety of cases he gave, scarcely any one died of measles, and in small-pox not one fourth of the number die that usually perish under the hot regimen. Out of 156 small-pox patients, which a neighboring physician had treated in this way, only eight died, although the disease raged in a virulent manner. In 1737, during the prevalence of a malignant epidemic, accompanied with *petechiæ* (small flea-bite spots occurring spontaneously, and under such circumstances, that is, in severe fevers, denoting great prostration of strength), very few died who were submitted to this treatment, although they were washed until they became very cool, even during the continued and debilitating sweats.

Speaking of certain late raging epidemics, he had frequently observed that ice, tied up in a cloth, and applied to the head, in case of inflammation of the brain, produced a most visible salutary effect, and in the course of a few hours permanently restored the intellects. He had never known a patient to die in consequence of such treatment.

Again: "Those who are obliged to walk or run a great distance, by which violent or long-continued action the veins of the legs become swollen, and accompanied with great fatigue, will find their pains relieved, and themselves refreshed, by taking a cold foot bath. This is made mention of in the Old Testament, and it was considered an indispensable mark of attention, to present the newly arrived guest with cold water to wash his feet."

Father Bernardo, a Sicilian Capuchin monk, he says, performed many surprising cures in the island of Malta, in the years 1724 and 1725. His practice was to order his patients to drink iced water, and sometimes to take the same as a lavement. He kept them almost fasting for one or two months; and pursued this treatment in winter as well as summer. He cured the Grand Prior Ferretti, aged 92, when at the very point of death, giving him iced water to drink. It is stated that none of his patients perished, either from starvation or otherwise. Thus, by means of ice and cold water, he performed a great number of wonderful cures, in cases which had been given up by physicians, so that he was called "the *water doctor*."

In cases of cramp, contraction, and paralysis, in addition to washing the parts with cold water, it is advisable to wash the head, and particularly the back of the neck; also to use the douche bath to the head, covered with a *sponge cap*, and the parts diseased, either exposed or covered with a cloth. The action of the water is found to produce a warmth in the skin, and penetrating deeper than the cold bath (*i. e.*, producing a more powerful reaction), operates more quickly and effectually. A woman who had for a long time suffered pain in the back, neck, shoulders, and arms, obtaining no relief from the remedies employed, at last applied to me for advice. I ordered a stream of cold water to be poured over the body, in a cool room. I had her wrapped up in sheets dipped in cold water, and which, from time to time, were renewed. She fell into a moderate perspiration, and in a few days was perfectly cured.

The father of Hahn, in his Psychrolusia, laid down the following excellent rules for morning ablutions: "On getting out of the bed in the morning, the face and whole body should be washed with cold water, first with the naked hand, and afterward with a sponge, pressing the water out of the sponge into the eyes and ears; then rubbing the body dry, rinsing out the mouth, and drawing the water through the nostrils, and finishing by taking a hip bath. The trouble thus taken will be amply repaid by the agreeable sensation of warmth and freshness. Sick patients cannot do this; but the attendant should wash them over with a sponge dipped in cold water, and applying bandages, also dipped in cold water, especially to the diseased parts, suffering from heat, pain, swelling, eruptions, etc., not merely once a day, but oftener, as the greater or less intensity of the disease may require."

"A man of seventy-five years of age was seized with a violent fever, and treated in the usual way, according to the hot regimen. A rash made its appearance, while his strength became gradually more and more exhausted. Lying constantly on his back, the skin at the lower part of the spine became inflamed and ulcerated. The patient remained in this state for six weeks, when a hardness and swelling was observed about the knees. The lower extremities had become stiff and immovable, and the muscles shriveled up. The stimulating treatment was now abandoned, and cooling emulsions, and water mixed with the juice of lemons and raspberries, ordered to be drank. Linen rags, dipped in cold water, were frequently applied to the inflamed and ulcerated parts of the back. The same were also applied to the thighs, notwithstanding the rash on the thighs and other parts of the body, and continually renewed, night and day. After a few days, cold foot baths were used, and moist napkins were applied to the feet. This cooling treatment gave immediate relief. The feverish heat left him, and the rash disappeared. He recovered the use of his limbs, and in three weeks was perfectly restored to health, and declared, that after this water treatment, he enjoyed better health than he had done for the last thirty years."

Hahn cured many cases of insanity, by causing the patients to drink largely of cold water. Such as would not drink he chained up, and gave salt herrings to eat. By thus exciting thirst, they were caused largely to drink the water before them. One of them, who ate, for several days in succession, from eight to twelve herrings, and drank eight quarts of water, was cured in three weeks.

Of the earlier English writers upon water, we may notice Sir John Floyer, a practitioner of eminence in his day. His directions for bathing are as follows: "Not to bathe when hot and sweating (meaning, no doubt, the heat and sweating brought on by exercise;) not to stay in the bath over two or three minutes, or as long as the patient can easily bear it, and to go in and out immediately, on the first bathing, after an immersion of the whole body. To use the cold both, before dinner, fasting, or else in the afternoon, toward 4 or 5 o'clock: it is dangerous to go in after great eating or drinking. To use sweating with cold bathing, in palsies and rickets, and several diseases of the nerves with obstructions." He mentions how cold-water sweating was used to diminish the weight of a horse-jockey: "Dip the rider's shirt into cold water, and after it is put on very wet, lap the person in very warm blankets to sweat him very violently, and he will lose a considerable weight." This observation of Sir John Floyer reminds the author of a case he lately had, a clergyman, to whom he is permitted to refer as to the effects of water treatment. By great excess in mental labor, and at the same time, like the generality of mankind, taking too much food, and of improper kinds, he had brought on a complication of difficulties, particularly in the head and nervous system generally. He had also become too fat. During the first week of the treatment, copious sweating, with various other means, being resorted to, he said on weighing that he lost seven pounds. He was at the same time gaining rapidly in strength and improving in every respect.

Washing the feet, this writer says, cures corns, and the hip bath cures hæmorrhoids. His advice upon regimen was very much like that of Priessnitz: "To abstain from excess in animal food, to use much of fruits, and to drink only water: not to use hot things, high sauces, brandy, spirits, fermented liquors, salt meat, spices, tea, coffee, and chocolate; not to wear too warm clothing; flannel renders the person very tender, and subject to the changes of weather, and too much perspiration; not to sit much by the fire, but to take exercise in the open air, riding or walking, and that down beds are very injurious."

This writer mentions the following case: "Mrs. Watts, of Leicester, went to the cold bath at London about Michælmas in 1699. She was troubled with continual vomiting and wandering pains in her limbs and head, convulsive motions or twitchings of the muscles, violent hysterical fits, colic, flatulency, sweatings, loss of appetite, an emaciated state of the body, extreme tenderness, sensibility to slight changes in the weather, chilliness, vapors, and pains, especially in the teeth. Tonics, as bark and iron, emetics and opiates, were tried in vain. Under the advice of Dr. Baynard, she had recourse to the cold bath, and used two-and-twenty baths in the space of a month, dipping herself under water six or seven times every morning, without staying in the water any longer than the time of immersion, and went warm from her bed to the water. By this bathing, the skin became healthy, and she was not subject to colds as before. She recovered her strength and appetite, and became more plump. Her weakening sweats, pains, flatulency, and convulsions, ceased."

Sir John quotes another writer, Dr. Ellison, of Newcastle, showing the results of people going to St. Bede's, Hanwick, or St. Mungo's wells, which were extremely cold springs. "People of all ages resorted to these two wells, for various complaints. Adults remained in a quarter, or near half an hour, the back or other diseased parts being well rubbed all the time. They used no preparative physic. The sick went to bed immediately afterward, and sweat for two hours or more. The healthy went in for pleasure, and immediately on coming out experienced a warmth all over, and were more nimble, and their joints more pliant.

"These springs were very celebrated for the cure of rickets in children. They were dipped in the water quickly, left only long enough for the clothes to become thoroughly wet. The children were then quickly wrapped up in warm blankets, which caused powerful perspiration. After being left a suitable time, the sweating clothes were taken off gradually, so that they cooled by degrees, and then dry clothes substituted. The children were not debarred their usual play; care was taken that their necks were kept warm, to secure them from catching cold."

Dr. Baynard was also a writer upon the effects of water. He is quoted as having said, in view of remarkable cures done by water, which had fallen under his observation, "I always (I thank God) looked upon it as most impious, and one of the worst of wickednesses, in serious things to impose upon the living, but much more to *banter*, and hand down a falsehood to posterity—a fault (I doubt not) too many of our physic observators have been guilty of."

Among other cases of his are the following: "A young man was seized with the rheumatism in every joint, which had become enormously swollen, and had continued for at least six weeks. He was wrapped up in flannel, and unable to move without assistance. He was therefore put in a chair, and thus let down into a bath, and brought up before three minutes were over. He was able immediately to walk up stairs, and in an hour's time walked back to his lodgings. In less than a fortnight his joints were reduced to their natural size. He fully recovered his health, and continued to follow his occupation."

A man with chronic catarrh, by accident fell to the neck into water frozen over. He went home, got warm clothes, slept soundly, and the next day was nearly free from his cough. Sir Henry Covingsby, he said, when a young man, suffered severely from the gout. He is now in his 88th year. He drinks spring water. Formerly his fingers and toes were full of chalk-stones, which had now become entirely dissolved and dissipated, and the joints were reduced to their natural size by the use of the cold bath, which the old knight was positive would cure the gout in every person. He had been under the care of celebrated physicians for a numbness of the lower limbs when 30 years of age. All sense of heat and feeling were lost, so that nettles would not sting him, or clothes make him warm. After some years, he was still worse. Tired in mind, body, and purse, he at last resolved upon another mode of cure. He used all the cold means, and was bled once a month. He went into a cold spring water bath, at all times of the year, but commenced in the summer. The first bath blotched him (that is, brought out an eruption), and so more and more every day, by pimples rising and then dying away. The pores were opened and the natural heat restored. He ever afterward for forty years continued his own doctor.

A learned doctor of laws informed Dr. Baynard, that being light-headed of a fever, and most intensely hot and thirsty, he got from his nurse and rushed into a horse-pond, and stayed for more than half an hour. It brought him presently to his senses, and allayed both his heat and thirst. He went to bed, fell into a profound sleep, and when he awoke (in a great sweat), he found he was quite well, but had afterward some headache, which he thought proceeded from not wetting the head.

Dr. Dover, of Bristol, related a case of a waiter at Oxford, during the small-pox, who went into a great tub of water, and sat there at least two hours, yet recovered and did well. The servant of Sir Thomas Yarborough, during the delirium of small-pox, got from his bed and plunged into a piece of water, but was presently got out. The small-pox seemed to be struck in, but upon his going to bed the disease came out very kindly, and he safely recovered. A countryman, of Harrow-on-the-Hill, suffering from severe rheumatic and spasmodic pains for nearly six months, lost the use of his lower extremities, so that he was unable to stand. He tried various remedies in vain, and had been salivated with mercury. He was entirely cured by cold bathing.

Dr. Baynard said no men live so long and so healthy as the dabblers in cold water. An old fisherman said that little sleep, a cool diet, and thin clothes, were the only means to live healthy and long, and that the *water air* made him eat heartily. He had known many old watermen and fishermen, full or near a hundred; and those who worked at Witney, in Oxfordshire, at the blanket mills, carrying wet blankets in their arms, next their breasts, winter and summer, not only never catch cold, but live to an extreme old age. Dr. Baynard also related an anecdote of a countryman, who, during a discussion as to the best means of getting an appetite, said he had tried the ways proposed, but nothing was like going a-fishing, up to the chin in water for an hour or two; "that will get you a stomach, I'll warrant you; nor am I dry."

Dr. Baynard received a letter from William Penn, as follows: "As I find the Indians upon the continent more incident to fevers than any other distempers, so they rarely fail to cure themselves by great sweating, and immediately plunging themselves into cold water, which they say is the only way not to catch a cold. I once saw an instance of it with divers more in company. Being upon a discovery of the back part of the country, I called upon an Indian of note, whose name was Tennoughan, the captain-general of the clans of Indians of those parts. I found him ill of a fever, his head and limbs much affected with pain, and at the same time his wife preparing a *bagnio* for him. The bagnio resembled a large oven, into which he crept by a door on the one side, while she put several red hot stones in at a small door on the other side thereof, and then fastened the doors as closely from the air as she could. Now while he was sweating in this bagnio, his wife (for they disdain no service) was with an axe cutting her husband a passage into the river (being the winter of 1683, the great frost, and the ice very thick), in order to the immersing himself after he should come out of the bath. In less than half an hour, he was in so great a sweat, that when he came out he was as wet as if he had come out of a river, and the reek or steam of his body so thick, that it was hard to discern any body's face that stood near him. In this condition, stark naked (a body cloth only excepted), he ran to the river, which was about twenty paces, and ducked himself twice or thrice therein, and so returned (passing only through his bagnio, to mitigate the immediate stroke of the cold) to his own house, perhaps twenty paces farther, and, wrapping himself in his woolen mantle, laying down at his length, near a long but gentle fire, in the middle of his wigwam or house, turning himself several times till dry, and then he rose and fell to getting us our dinner, seeming to be as easy and as well in health as at any other time.

"I am well assured that the Indians wash their infants in cold water as soon as born, in all seasons of the year."

An Indian cure for rheumatism is mentioned by a recent writer, in a quotation from Cox's Columbia River. The writer had suffered much annoyance from acute rheumatic attacks in the shoulders and knees; an old Indian proposed to relieve him if he would follow the mode of cure practiced by him in similar cases among the young warriors of his tribe. On inquiring into the method, the Indian replied it merely consisted in getting up early every morning for some weeks and plunging into the river, and leave the rest to him. This was a most chilling proposition, for the river was most firmly frozen, and an opening was to be made in the ice preparatory to each immersion. The Indian was asked if it would not do equally well to have the water taken to the bed-room. But he shook his head and replied that he was surprised that a young white chief, who ought to be wise, would ask so foolish a question. On reflecting, however, that the rheumatism was a stranger among the Indians, and that such numbers of whites were subject to it, and above all that he was 3000 miles from any professional assistance, he determined to adopt the disagreeable expedient the following morning. The Indian first made a hole in the ice, large enough to admit both, upon which he made a signal that all was ready. Enveloped in a large buffalo robe, he proceeded to the spot, threw off the robe, and both jumped into the frigid orifice together. The Indian at once set to rubbing the shoulder, back, and loins, while, meantime, the hair became ornamented with icicles; and while the lower joints were being rubbed, the face, neck, and shoulders became incased with a thin covering of ice. On getting released, a blanket was rolled about the body, and the patient went quickly back to the room, in which a fire had been ordered. In a few minutes, there was a warm glow over the whole body. These ablutions were found so beneficial, they were continued twenty-five days, at the expiration of which, the old Indian was pleased to say that no more was necessary, and that he had done his duty like a wise man. He was never after troubled with a rheumatic pain.

An old Canadian, according to the same writer, who had been laboring many years under a chronic rheumatism, asked the old Indian if he could cure him in the same way. The Indian said it was impossible, but that he would try another process. He accordingly constructed the skeleton of a hut, about four and a half feet high, and three broad, in shape like a bee-hive, which he covered with deer skins. He then heated some stones in an adjoining fire, and having placed the patient inside, in a state of nudity, the hot stones were thrown in, and water poured over them. The entrance was then quickly closed, and the man kept in for some time, until he begged to be released, alleging that he was nearly suffocating. On coming out he was in a state of profuse perspiration. The old Indian ordered him to be immediately enveloped in blankets and conveyed to bed. The operation was repeated several times, and although it did not effect a radical cure, the violence of the pains was so far abated, that the patient could follow his ordinary business, and enjoy his sleep in comparative ease.

These, and like applications in rheumatism, which have been

mentioned, will naturally enough seem to many as extremely hazardous. In the second case of the old Indian, he knew very well that the old Canadian did not need the same treatment as in the other case, nor could he bear it. The old man could have been safely and far more benefited by having had washings and rubbings after his sweatings, and sweating bandages applied to the diseased parts. The writer lately cured a very severe case of rheumatism, so much so, that the man could scarcely move, and was wholly confined to his bed, unless lifted out. He had been well treated, according to the common practice, for nearly three months. The ninth day, he was out walking, with his common-sized boots (his feet having been much swollen), and has been well ever since.

Prof. Elliotson, of the University College, London, in speaking of this disease, says, "With respect to the parts themselves, we shall find it of great use to apply cold water, or cold lotions (cold water is the best), as long as the temperature is higher than it ought to be, and they are comfortable to the patient. There is no danger of applying cold, with these limitations. If the patient should be timid, and yet long for cold evaporating lotions (water is the best lotion), they may be applied tepid, as in the case of gout; but I never saw any injury arise from cold in rheumatism, where the parts were hotter than they should be, and the patient felt hot."

DR. CURRIE'S REPORTS.

One of the very best works ever written on water, is that of James Currie, M.D., F.R.S., of Liverpool, published 1797. His experiments had been more extended, and made with far more scientific precision, than any other before him. They were made with great perseverance, notwithstanding the prejudice and opposition in the use of water, and with a candor that does him great honor.

His work was not intended merely for the profession; for he says, in an introductory communication to the Rt. Hon. Sir Jos. Banks, "He had guarded against the unnecessary use of technical as well as general expressions; that it were better that medicine, like other branches of natural knowledge, were brought from its hiding-place, and exhibited in the simplicity of science, and the nakedness of truth. He had every where endeavored to make his steps so plain that they could be distinctly traced. He hoped that his work would be read by men of general science, and that it would on certain occasions prove useful where medical advice was not at hand."

"Ablution with cold water in fever had been so long employed at the Hospital in Liverpool, and in private practice by his friends and colleagues, Dr. Brandreth and Dr. Gerhard, as well as by himself, that it had become general in Liverpool and the county of Lancaster. He had frequently exhibited the mode of practice by water to those from a distance; but a method so bold and contrary to the common prejudices, made but slow progress. The mode of operation had been misapprehended, and the proper period for using it had not been understood; and on some occasions, it having been resorted to improperly, the consequences had brought it into disrepute."

Dr. Currie commences by giving an account of some cases by his friend, Dr. Wright, known as a medical writer:

"On the 1st of August, 1777 (says Dr. Wright), I embarked in a ship bound to Liverpool, and sailed the same evening from Montego Bay. The master told me he had hired several sailors on the same day we took our departure; one of whom had been at sick quarters on shore, and was now but in a convalescent state. On the 23d of August we were in the latitude of Bermudas, and had had a very heavy gale of wind for three days, when the above-mentioned man relapsed, and had a fever, with symptoms of the greatest malignity. I attended this person often, but could not prevail with him to be removed from a dark and confined situation to a more airy and convenient part of the ship; and as he refused medicines, and even food, he died on the eighth day of his illness.

"By my attention to the sick man I caught the contagion, and began to be indisposed on the 5th of September, and the following is a narrative of my case, extracted from notes daily marked down. I had been many years in Jamaica, but, except being somewhat relaxed by the climate, and fatigue of business, I ailed nothing when I embarked. This circumstance, however, might perhaps dispose me more readily to receive the infection.

"Sept. 5th, 6th, 7th.—Small rigors now and then—a preternatural heat of the skin—a dull pain in the forehead—the pulse small and quick—a loss of appetite, but no sickness at stomach—the tongue white and slimy—little or no thirst—the belly regular

—the urine pale, and rather scanty—in the night restless, with starting and delirium.

"Sept. 8th.—Every symptom aggravated, with pains in the loins and lower limbs, and stiffness in the thighs and hams.

"I took a gentle vomit in the second day of this illness, and next morning a decoction of tamarinds; at bed-time, an opiate, joined with antimonial wine; but this did not procure sleep, or open the pores of the skin. No inflammatory symptoms being present, a drachm of Peruvian bark was taken every hour for six hours successively, and now and then a glass of port wine, but with no apparent benefit. When upon deck, my pains were greatly mitigated, and the colder the air the better. This circumstance, and the failure of every means I had tried, encouraged me to put in practice, on myself, what I had often wished to try on others, in fevers similar to my own.

"Sept. 9th.—Having given the necessary directions, about three o'clock in the afternoon, I stripped off all my clothes, and threw a sea cloak loosely about me till I got upon the deck, when the cloak also was laid aside. Three buckets full of salt water were then thrown at once on me: the shock was great, but I felt immediate relief. The headache and other pains instantly abated, and a fine glow and diaphoresis succeeded. Toward evening, however, the febrile symptoms threatened a return, and I had again recourse to the same method as before, with the same good effect. I now took food with an appetite, and for the first time had a sound night's rest.

"Sept. 10th.—No fever, but a little uneasiness in the hams and thighs—used the cold bath twice.

"Sept. 11th.—Every symptom vanished, but to prevent a relapse, I used the cold bath twice.

"Mr. Thomas Kirk, a young gentleman, passenger in the same ship, fell sick of a fever on the 9th of August. His symptoms were nearly similar to mine, and having taken some medicines without experiencing relief, he was desirous of trying the cold bath, which, with my approbation, he did on the 11th and 12th of September, and by this method was happily restored to health."

The doctor proceeds:

"On the 9th of Dec., 1787, a contagious fever made its appearance in the Liverpool Infirmary. For some time previously the weather had been extremely cold, and the discipline of the house, owing to causes which it is unnecessary to mention, had been much relaxed. The intensity of the cold prevented the necessary degree of ventilation, and the regulations for the preservation of cleanliness had been in some measure neglected. These circumstances operated particularly on one of the wards of the eastern wing, employed as a lock-hospital for females, where the contagion first appeared. The fever spread rapidly, and before its progress could be arrested, sixteen persons were affected, of which two died. Of these sixteen, eight were under my care. On this occasion I used, for the first time, the affusion of cold water, in the manner described by Dr. Wright. It was first tried in two cases only, the one in the second, the other in the fourth day of fever. The effects corresponded exactly with those mentioned to have occurred by him in his own case; and thus encouraged, the remedy was employed in five other cases. It was repeated daily, and of these seven patients, the whole recovered. In the eighth case, the aspersion of cold water seemed too hazardous a practice, and it was not employed. The strength of the patient was much impaired by lues, and at the time of catching the contagion, she labored under ptyalism. I was not then aware that this last circumstance formed no objection against the cold affusion, and, in a situation so critical, it was thought imprudent to use it. The usual remedies were directed for this patient, particularly bark, wine, and opium, but unsuccessfully; she died on the sixteenth day of her disease.

"From this time forth, I have constantly wished to employ the affusion of cold water, in every case of the low contagious fever, in which the strength was not already much exhausted; and I have preserved a register of 153 cases in which the cure was chiefly trusted to this remedy."

Before proceeding to explain particularly the manner in which Dr. Currie used water in fevers, he describes a fever which broke out in the 30th regiment, and the treatment adopted. It commenced about June 1st, 1792.

"Such men as were sent to the guard for misbehavior, were confined in a dark, narrow, and unventilated cell. Several men were put there for drunkenness, and suffered to remain twenty-four hours. The typhus fever made its appearance among these men, and spread rapidly among the rest. The Liverpool Infirmary being full, a temporary hospital was fitted up at the fort. In two low rooms, each about fifteen feet square, were fourteen patients laboring under the fever. One was in the fourteenth day of the disease, two in the twelfth, and the rest from the ninth to the fourth day. In every case there was cough and mucous expectoration. Those who sustained the disease eight days, had *petechiæ* on the skin (spots resembling flea-bites, denoting great prostration). The debility was considerable from the first, and, as Dr. C. says, had been increased in several cases by bleeding, before the nature of the disease was understood. The pulse varied from 130 to 100 degrees. The heat rose from 101 to 105 degrees Fah. There was great pain in the head, and in several instances low delirium.

"Our first care was to clean and ventilate the rooms, which were in a high degree foul and pestilential. Our second was to wash and clean the patients themselves. This was done by pouring sea-water over the naked bodies of those who were not already greatly reduced: the whole heat was steadily above the temperature of health. In those more advanced, whose debility was great, we sponged the whole surface with vinegar, a practice that, in every stage of fever, is most salutary and refreshing.

"Our next care was to stop the progress of the infection. With this view, the guard-house was first attempted to be purified by washing and ventilating, the greatest part of the furniture having been burnt or thrown into the sea. All our precautions and exertions of this kind, however, were ineffectual. The weather was wet and extremely cold for the season. The men on the guard could not be prevailed upon to remain in the open air; and from passing the night in the infected guard-room, several of the privates took the infection. In several of these the fever ran its course, and in others it was immediately arrested by the affusion of sea-water. No means having proved effectual for the purification of the guard-room, it was shut up, and a temporary shed erected in its stead. Still the contagion proceeded. On the morning of the 13th, the whole regiment was drawn up at my request, and the men examined in the ranks. Seventeen were found with the fever upon them. It was not difficult to distinguish them as they stood by their fellows. The countenance was languid—the whole appearance dejected, and the eyes had a dull-red suffusion. These men were carefully separated from the rest, and subjected to the cold affusion, always repeated once and sometimes twice a day. In fifteen of the number, seventeen, the contagion was extinguished: the two went through the regular disease.

"On the same day, the commanding officer, at my request, issued an order for the whole of the remaining part of the regiment to bathe in the sea; and for some time they were regularly mustered and marched down at high water, to plunge into the tide. These means were successful in arresting the epidemic. After the 13th of June no one was attacked. In all, fifty-eight had the disease, of which twenty-two went through the regular course of the fever, and in twenty-six, the disease seemed to be cut short by the cold affusion. Of the thirty-two, two died. Both of these were men whose constitutions were weakened by the climate of the West Indies; both of them had been bled in the early stages of the fever; and the one of them being in the twelfth, and the other in the fourteenth day of the disease, when I first visited them—neither was subjected to the cold affusion."

This fever is generally termed, in popular language, the nervous fever, and when particular symptoms appear, the putrid fever. It is usually caused in situations where there is want of cleanliness, and more especially of ventilation; and when once cured, it is propagated by contagion. This is described by Dr. Currie as the common fever of England. It had usually one exacerbation (augmentation), and one remission or abatement in the twenty-four hours. The exacerbation was usually in the afternoon, and the remission toward morning. According to Dr. C., the safest and most advantageous time for the affusion of cold water, is when the exacerbation is at its height, or immediately after the declination is begun; and this had almost always led him to adopt it from six to nine in the evening; but it is perfectly safe to use it at any time of the day, according to Dr. C., "*when there is no sense of chilliness present; when the heat of the surface is steadily above what is natural, and when there is no general or profuse perspiration.*"*

These rules are really so plain, that it is difficult to see how any one could be at a loss in knowing how to proceed, at least safely, in the affusion of cold water in typhus fever; and yet Dr. C.'s method has been considered as being one which required a great amount of skill to determine when it should be used.

* This rule relating to perspiration, as we have seen elsewhere, relates only to that caused by too much exertion.

Dr. C. afterward says in reference to this fever, when epidemic, "that a great number of cases occurred in which the disease was suddenly cut short by the use of the cold affusion, on the first and second day of the disease. The good results were so uniformly, so precisely similar to what had been related, that a detail of cases would be unnecessary." He says, also, "that when an epidemic is spreading, and the danger is known, patients will take the alarm on the first attack, and the power as well as the utility of such a remedy as the cold affusion, in such situations of general danger, will be easily imagined. It cannot be employed too soon after the first attack, provided the original chill is over, and the hot stage is firmly established."

In cases in which the affusion was not employed till the third day of the fever, he had seen several instances of the same complete solution of the disease. He had even seen this take place when the remedy had been deferred till the fourth day. Some cases are given to show the effect, on the third and fourth days. "Jan. 17th, 1790, A. B., aged 19, a pupil of the Infirmary, caught the infection in attending the fever ward. When I saw him, in seventy-eight hours, the fourth day of the disease, he had all the usual symptoms, headache, thirst, furred tongue, pain in the back and loins, with great debility. Heat 101 degrees, pulse 112 in the minute. A bucketfull of salt water was poured over him, as usual, at noon. His heat sunk to 99 degrees, and his pulse to 98. A profuse perspiration followed, with the cessation of all his feverish symptoms. This intermission continued for several hours, during which he enjoyed some comfortable sleep, but at five in the afternoon, was again seized with feverish rigors, followed by heat, thirst, and headache, as before. An hour afterward, the hot stage was established. Heat 100 degrees, pulse also 100 degrees. The same quantity of cold water was again thrown over him, with similar effects. His pulse fell immediately to 80 the minute, and became more full. The heat became natural. The following night he took twenty drops of laudanum, and slept well. On the 18th, the second day of treatment, at noon the pulse was 96 and soft, skin moist, but a little above the natural heat. The tongue a little furred, and the head ached. He also complained of thirst. The same remedy was again applied. He was greatly refreshed by it. The pulse fell to 90, the skin became cool, the thirst went off, and all the feverish symptoms vanished. On the 19th, the third day of treatment, his pulse was 88, his heat natural, the thirst and headache gone, and appetite improving. The ablution was repeated for the last time at six in the evening. On the 20th, he was farther improved. On the 21st, had some debility. On the 22d, was free from complaint. This patient, during his fever, took no medicine but an effervescing mixture, the dose of laudanum excepted. The affusion was used four times."

Another case we cite: "Feb. 2d, 1792, S. C., a healthy man, 44 years of age, about 72 hours after the attack, came under treatment. Pulse 100 degrees; heat 104 degrees; other symptoms as usual, but the pain in the head and back particularly severe. Two minutes after the affusion, pulse 90 degrees, heat 100 degrees. The patient felt great refreshment, and was entirely relieved of the pain in the head and back. In the evening, however, the exacerbation of the fever was severe, and the headache returned with violence. He passed a restless night. At four in the morning the affusion was repeated by his request. At nine, a gentle perspiration covered the surface of the body, the pulse 84, the tongue moist, the skin cool, and the pains of the head and back entirely gone. In the afternoon the fever returned, though in a less degree. The affusion was repeated the fourth time, with the same happy effects; after which there was no return of the disease.

"Thus it appeared," says Dr. C., "that the cold affusion, used on the third and fourth days of fever, does not immediately produce a solution of the disease, but that it instantly abates it, and by a few repetitions brings it to a happy termination in two or three days."

The cold affusion Dr. C. also used in intermittent fevers, and with signal success, as he had found by many repeated trials. The cold affusion was used in the hot stage of the paroxysms of intermittents, and almost always with the immediate solution of the fit. In general, however, Dr. C. depended also upon other remedies in the intermission between the paroxysms; but in some instances the succeeding paroxysm was wholly prevented by using the cold affusion, about one hour previously to the period of the expected return, and the disease wholly removed by the continuance of the practice.

According to the modern practice by water, nothing is more easy than to break up these intermittents, without the aid of any medicine other than water, together with sweating. Under the restrictions mentioned, Dr. C. always found that in any case, however advanced the stage, that cold affusion moderated the violence of the symptoms and shortened the duration of fever.

Patients are often startled at the thought or proposal of dashing cold water over the naked body. There has been a vast deal of prejudice respecting the use of water in fevers. It has been exceedingly common to deny fever patients the use of water, and this when they most needed it. It should have been understood by all practitioners, that pure cold water is the very best, incomparably the best febrifuge in nature. How often persons given up to die, have been cured by getting at water, when it was supposed that it was the very thing to kill. It is a singular fact, that in the affusion of water, however much patients may have dreaded it, the effects are so grateful and refreshing to the sensations, that they strongly desire to have it repeated.

In these experiments of Dr. Currie, he at first used fresh water, afterward fresh water mixed with vinegar, and at last salt and water, and sometimes the water of the river Mersey, which is salt, containing about 33 per cent. of the mineral. It is now generally well known that a person can endure the effect of salt water much longer than that of fresh, at the same temperature. The reason is plain. The salt produces something of an inflammation of the skin, and where there is such inflammation there is always increased heat. The body is therefore preserved in some degree from the effects of the cold. Some barbers act according to the same principle. They wash the head with stimulating washes and forcibly brush the head, so that a partial inflammation is caused, and the part is thus protected from the action of cold, and the individual is safe; whereas, without such precaution, the taking of a cold would be a sure consequence.

Among other cases, Dr. C. gives an account of the following curious incident: "It occurred," he says, "about three years ago, to Capt. S. of this port, in the Irish Channel. He sprung out of his cabin window in the height of delirium, and was upward of twenty minutes in the water. He was taken up perfectly calm and speedily recovered."

To illustrate the power of the cold affusion in fever, where the ordinary means had failed, we cite another case from Dr. Currie. It was of a boy, 8 years of age, in whom the doctor says he was much interested. "On the 3d day, the pulse rose to 130 and 140 beats in the minute, and his heat to 106 and 107 degrees Fah. His thirst was very great, and delirium commenced on the 2d day and continued without intermission. Various methods had been employed to abate the fever, and particularly to excite perspiration, but unsuccessfully. His heat was not lessened by repeatedly sponging the surface of the body with cold water and vinegar ; and after a copious bleeding, all the symptoms were as alarming as before. It seemed hazardous to repeat this operation. The patient had taken antimonials without any apparent effect, and after watching the state of the thermometer in the arm-pit for more than an hour, though the mercury had sunk a single degree in that interval, it stood at the end of the time, at 106 degrees. In this state of things, we resolved on trying the cold affusion, and every thing being prepared, he was stripped naked, and lifted out of bed. As we were about to throw the water upon him, it was observed that a perspiration had broken out all over him, but the heat being so great, we persisted in our purpose, and four gallons of fresh water, at the temperature of 60 degrees, were thrown upon him. The effects were altogether surprising. On replacing him in bed, the thermometer (the bulb in the arm-pit as before) rose to 98 degrees, and the burning heat of the extremities was converted into a coolness that was rather alarming. The pulse had sunk to 90, but was full and steady. Gentle frictions were applied to the extremities, but not long continued, as the general warmth speedily returned. The heat in the trunk of the body, in about an hour, rose to 100, and the pulse 100. His delirium went entirely off; the fur on his tongue speedily disappeared, and twenty-four hours afterward, he was found free of every complaint but debility."

This case affords something of an exception to the common directions laid down by Dr. C., in reference to performing affusion while there is perspiration. Still the heat was great, and it was for this reason that the application was safe and salutary.

It may be asked, "Did not Dr. Currie find cases of fever that he could not cure by means of water?" There were cases where water, as well as every thing else, failed. At the same time it is important to note, he cured many persons by water, where other means wholly failed, while he did not cure any with drugs, when water had failed.

In all the experiments yet noticed, Dr. C. had not attempted any thing by way of the internal use of water in fevers. The use of cold water internally in burning fevers, was recommended and used by Hippocrates, Galen, Celsus, and most, if not all of the ancient authors, of whom we have any knowledge. But in more modern times, as physicians began to be more speculative, and less practical, it was argued that cold drinks were dangerous. The very learned and celebrated Boerhaave promulgated the doctrine that a lentor, a siziness or glutinous principle in the blood, was the cause of fever. This led him to insist upon warm drinks in fever, as this would be more effectual in diluting this sizy principle in the blood than cold, notwithstanding the precepts of Hippocrates, Hoffman, etc., to the contrary. The prejudice against cold drink in fever, had become very general in the time of Dr. Currie.

The wonderful effects of cold water externally applied very naturally led the discriminating mind of Dr. C. to the consideration of its effects internally. It seemed to be a principle with Dr. C., that he would be satisfied with nothing but actual facts of experiment. Notwithstanding he came to the conclusion, that the same general rules were to be observed, in order to determine when it was safe to use cold water internally, that were to be observed in its use externally; he did not do this by reasoning from analogy alone, but from actual experiment.

Dr. C. says, in reference to cold drink in fevers, "that while the different modes of applying cold water to the surface are employed, it ought also to be poured into the stomach, in large quantities, when the patient's heat will permit it; and the presence of nausea and vomiting is no objection to this practice, if a chilliness of the stomach is not produced."

"The salutary effects of the cold bath, and of cold drink in fever, strongly recommend the adoption of these remedies in the plague. Morendi, a physician at Venice, observes, that some sailors at Constantinople, in the phrensy of the plague, have thrown themselves into the sea; and it is said that, on being taken out, they have recovered.

"Savary, in his letters on Egypt, observes, that if heat were the source of their disorders, the *Said* would be uninhabitable. The burning fever (the Causus of the Greeks) is the only one it gives rise to, and to which the inhabitants are subject. They soon get rid of it by regimen, drinking a great deal of water, and bathing themselves in the river. A captain of a ship (a man of credit) having some sailors on board affected by the plague, caught the infection. 'I felt,' says the captain, 'an excessive heat, which made my blood boil; my head was very soon attacked, and I perceived I had but a few moments to live. I employed the little judgment I had left to make an experiment. I stripped myself quite naked, and laid myself, for the remainder of the night, on the deck; the copious dew that fell pierced me to the very bones; in a few hours it rendered my respiration free, and my head more composed. The agitation of my blood was calmed, and after bathing myself in sea water, I recovered.'"

Dr. Currie also found the use of cold water strikingly successful in small-pox. He says:

"The singular degree of success that on the whole attended the affusion of cold water in typhus, encouraged a trial of this remedy in some other febrile diseases. Of these the small-pox seemed more particularly to invite its use. The great advantage that is experienced in this disease by the admission of cool air, seemed to point out the external use of cold water, which, being a more powerful application, might be more particularly adapted to the more malignant forms of small-pox. The result corresponded entirely with my expectation. Of a number of cases in which I witnessed the happy effects of the affusion of cold water in small-pox, I shall give the following only:

"In the autumn of 1794, J. J., an American gentleman, in the 24th year of his age, and immediately on his landing in Liverpool, was inoculated under my care—the prevalence of the small-pox rendering it imprudent to wait till the usual preparations could be gone through, or indeed till the fatigues of the voyage could be recovered. He sickened on the seventh day, and the eruptive fever was very considerable. He had a rapid and feeble pulse, a fœtid breath, with the pain in the head, back, and loins. His heat rose in a few hours to 107 degrees, and his pulse beat 119 times in the minute. I encouraged him to drink largely of cold water and lemonade, and threw three gallons of cold brine over him. He was in a high degree refreshed by it. The eruptive fever abated in every respect—an incipient delirium subsided, the pulse became slower, the heat was reduced, and tranquil sleep followed. In the course of twenty-four hours, the affusion was repeated three or four different times, at his own desire; a general direction having been given him to call for it as often as the symptoms of fever returned. The eruptions, though more numerous than are usual from inoculation, were of a favorable kind. There was little or no secondary fever, and he recovered rapidly."

In tetanus, or lock-jaw, and other convulsive disorders, Dr. C. found cold water highly useful. The case of Charles Gardner is thus given:

"The head was pulled toward the left shoulder, the left corner of the mouth was thrown upward, the eyes were hollow, the countenance pale and ghastly, the face and neck bedewed with a cold sweat; but his most distressing symptom was a violent pain under the ensiform cartilage, with a sudden interruption of his breathing every fourth or fifth inspiration by a convulsive hickup, accompanied by a violent contraction of the muscles of the abdomen and lower extremities. He felt, on this occasion, as if he had received an unexpected blow on the scrobiculus cordis (pit of the stomach). Before I saw him, he had been bled, and vomited repeatedly, and had used the warm bath, not only without alleviation, but with aggravation of his complaints.

"Opium, mercury, and the cold bath were used in succession. At first, a grain of opium every other hour, afterward, a grain every hour, and at last, two grains every hour; but he grew worse and worse during the two days this course was continued. Being no longer able to swallow the pills, on the night of the 22d February, general convulsions came on once or twice in every hour. The tincture of opium was now directed to be given, and an ounce of the quicksilver ointment to be rubbed in on each thigh. In twenty-four hours he took two ounces and a half of the tincture, without sleep or alleviation of the pain. The dose being increased, in the next twenty-six hours he swallowed *five ounces and a half* of the laudanum. He lay now in a state of torpor. The rigidity of the spasms was indeed much lessened, and the general convulsions nearly gone; but the debility was extreme; a complete hemiplegia had supervened; the eyes were fixed, and the speech faltering and unintelligible. Intermitting the opium, which had relieved the pain, but brought on general paralysis, small doses of camphor were given in a liquid form, and gruel with a small quantity of wine to support the strength. For the next six days he seemed to revive; but on the night of the first of March, he was seized, during sleep, with a convulsion as severe as ever: the jaws were more completely locked than before, deglution was become impossible, and the pain under the ensiform cartilage was so extreme, as to force from the patient the most piercing cries. At this time the effects of the quicksilver ointment were apparent in the fœtor of the breath, and in a considerable salivation.

"All other remedies being in vain, it was now resolved to try the cold bath. Gardner was, therefore, carried to the public salt water bath, then of the temperature of 36 degrees Fah., and thrown headlong into it. The good effects were instantaneous. As he rose from the first plunge, and lay struggling on the surface of the water, supported by two of his fellow-soldiers, we observed that he stretched out his left leg, which had been for some time retracted to the ham: but his head did not immediately recover the same freedom of motion, and therefore he was plunged down and raised to the surface successively for upward of a minute longer, the muscles of the neck relaxing more and more after every plunge. When taken out we felt some alarm; a general tremor was the only indication of life; the pulse and the respiration being nearly, if not entirely, suspended. Warm blankets had, however, been prepared, and a general friction was diligently employed. The respiration and the pulse became regular, the vital heat returned, the muscles continued free of constriction, and the patient fell into a quiet and profound sleep. In this he continued upward of two hours, and when he awaked, to the astonishment of every one, he got up and walked across the room, complaining of nothing but hunger and debility. The convulsive hickup, indeed, returned, but in a slight degree, and gave way to the use of the cold bath, which he continued daily a fortnight longer; and in less than a month, we had the satisfaction of seeing our patient under arms, able for the service of his country."

The doctor continues: "Soon after this I was sent for by a poor woman, who, in consequence of difficult labor, and, as she imagined, of local injury in some part of the uterus, was seized with locked-jaw and other symptoms of tetanus. She was immediately taken to the cold bath, and thrown into it in the same manner of the former patient, and with similar good effects. The spasms disappeared, and though they afterward returned to a slight degree, they gave way entirely to a second immersion."

"In the convulsions of children," says Dr. C., "I have found the cold bath a useful remedy, whether the disorder originated in worms or other causes. I have seldom known it to fail stopping the paroxysms, at least for some time, and thereby giving an opportunity of employing the means fitted to remove the particular irritation."

The following curious narrative is taken from the work of Dr. Currie, and was given on the authority of Dr. Robertson, a surgeon-general of the naval hospital in Barbadoes, and can be relied on as being true. On returning a second time to Barbadoes, Dr. Robertson, according to the request of Dr. Currie, investigated the particulars of the case, which were given in his own words:

"A gentleman of this island, whose name was Weeks, a great votary of Bacchus, was in the practice from fifteen to twenty years, of plunging into cold water when he rose from his bottle, and actually going to sleep in a trough of water, with his head supported on a kind of wooden pillow, made for the purpose, above the surface. When he dined abroad, and had not the convenience of his own trough, he used to strip off his coat, waistcoat, and shirt, and sit exposed in the open air, and in that situation go to sleep, whether it rained or not. And sometimes he went and bathed in the nearest adjoining pond, to which he generally required assistance to be conveyed. The effect of this practice was, that instead of experiencing debility, lassitude, headache, and nausea, he found himself on awaking, cheerful and refreshed, and free from all the effects of intoxication. In the year 1789, dining one day abroad, he got alternately drunk and sober three several times before midnight, each time recovering his sobriety by immersing himself, and sleeping in cold water; and on awaking returning to the company. The last time, after supper, he was so immoderately intoxicated, that he insisted on his companions undressing him, and carrying him themselves to the pond. They carried him accordingly in the chair, and set him up to the chin in water, where he continued upward of an hour, a person supporting him. I had this last circumstance from a gentleman, one of the party, whose veracity may be entirely depended on.

"At home, however, he used, as I have already mentioned, a trough made for the purpose, with a bench in it as a pillow, having been nearly drowned when sleeping in his pond, from the negro, who was appointed to watch him, having himself fallen asleep. In this watery bed he would sleep, one, two, three, or even more hours, experiencing always the greatest refreshment. His wife and family, when they wished him to change his quarters, used to draw out the plug, and let the water run off, when he awoke, and humorously complained of the loss of his bed-clothes. At length this expedient began to lose its effect in rousing him, and one time he continued to sleep in his empty trough. In consequence of this, he was seized with extreme rigors and chills, followed by a fever and attack of rheumatism, which affected him a long time, and made him desist from the practice in future. But to the end of his life he was in the habit of sitting, when intoxicated, with his clothes open, and sometimes quite naked, exposed to the wind and rain. This extraordinary character died of apoplexy, about three weeks ago, aged sixty-three."

TESTIMONY OF THE REV. JOHN WESLEY.

The Rev. John Wesley, well known as a shrewd observer, and an eminently good man, published a work in 1747, on water, which went through thirty-four editions, called "Primitive Physic, or an Easy and Natural Method of curing most Diseases."

After exposing and condemning the prevalent system of drugging and quackery, and the mysteries with which the science of medicine is surrounded, and the interested conduct of medical men, Mr. Wesley gave a long list of diseases (following), for which he recommended the use of water, as the only true and safe remedy.

Mr. Wesley recommended the use of water in the following complaints of children: convulsions; coughs; gravel; inflammations of the ears, navel, and mouth; rickets; cutaneous inflammations; pimples and scabs; suppression of urine; vomiting; want of sleep.

"Water," says Mr. Wesley, "frequently cures every nervous and every paralytic disorder; particularly asthma; agues of every sort; atrophy; blindness; cancer; chin cough; coagulated blood of bruises; complicated disease; consumption; convulsions; convulsive pains; coughs; deafness; dropsy; epilepsy; violent fever; gout (running); hectic fever; hysteric pains; incubus; inflammations; involuntary stools; lameness; leprosy (old); lethargy; loss of speech, taste, appetite, smell; nephritic pains; palpitation of heart; pain in the back, joints, and stomach; rheumatism; rickets; rupture; suffocations; surfeits at the beginning; sciatica; scorbutic pains; swelling in the joints; stone in the kidneys; torpor of the limbs, even when the use of them is lost; tetanus; tympany; vertigo; St. Vitus's dance; vigilia; varicose ulcers; the whites.

"Water prevents the growth of hereditary apoplexies; asthma;

blindness; consumption; deafness; king's evil; melancholy; palsies; rheumatism; stone.

"Water-drinking generally prevents apoplexies; asthma; convulsions; gout; hysteric fits; madness; palsies; stone; trembling. To this, children should be used from their cradles."

Mr. Wesley gives the following prescriptions:

"*For Asthma.*—Take a pint of cold water every morning, washing the head in cold water immediately after, and using the cold bath.

"*Rickets in Children.*—Dip them in cold water every morning.

"*To prevent Apoplexy.*—Use the cold bath, and drink only cold water.

"*Ague.*—Go into a cold bath just before the chill.

"*Cancer in the Breast.*—Use the cold bath. This cured Mrs. Bates, of Leicestershire, of a cancer in the breast, a sciatica, and rheumatism, which she had nearly twenty years. N. B.—Generally, where cold bathing is necessary to cure any disease, water-drinking is so, to prevent a relapse.

"*Hysteric Colic.*—Mrs. Watts, by using the cold bath two-and-twenty times in a month, was entirely cured of a hysteric colic, fits, and convulsive motions, continual sweatings and vomitings, wandering pains in her limbs and head, and total loss of appetite.

"*To prevent the ill effects of Cold.*—The moment a person gets into a house, with his hands and feet quite chilled, let him put them into a vessel of water, as cold as can be got, and hold them there until they begin to glow: this they will do in a minute or two. This method likewise effectually prevents chilblains.

"*Consumption.*—Cold bathing has cured many deep consumptions.

"*Convulsions.*—Use the cold bath."

"Mr. Wesley, in this little work, prescribes for almost every complaint; and the reader of it will be struck with the great similarity of his treatment with that which is recommended in Hydropathy; for in the majority of cases he recommends the use of that element which we are so strongly contending for, namely, cold water."

CHAPTER II.

HYDROPATHY, OR THE MODERN WATER-CURE.

Hydropathy.—Definition of the Term.—Water as a remedial Agent, has been used in all Ages.—Priessnitz's Discoveries the result of Accident.—Curious Anecdotes.—His number of Patients.—Testimony of Dr. Edward Johnson.—Sir Charles Scudamore.—Rev. John Wesley.—R. Beamish, Esq.—Priessnitz's phrenological Developments.—The simplicity of his Theories.—A Remarkable Case of Cure.—A. J. Colvin, Esq.—His excellent Account of Priessnitz's Discoveries.—The Umschlag, or Wet Bandage.—Leintuch, or Wet Sheet.—The Douche.—Sweating Process.—The Plunging Bath.—Abreibung, or Rubbing Wet-Sheet.

The word *Hydropathy*, as used to denote the Water-Cure, has been objected to, as not being etymologically correct in signification. It is derived from two Greek words, together meaning, *water-disease.* It is, however, a term well understood. *Hydro-therapeutics*—which means, *healing with water*—has been substituted, and is decidedly a better term, as far as etymological correctness is concerned. *Hydriatics* has also been used. The best term is the plain English one, the *water-cure.* But whichever term is used, it is not less correct than many others in common use among the best speakers and writers.

That parts of the water-cure have, to some extent, been practiced in the healing art, no one will pretend to deny. As a general thing, water was used to a greater extent as a remedy, in the earlier periods of the history of medicine, than in later times.

Hippocrates, the father of medicine, determined that, in certain kinds of baths, warm water would produce a chill, while cold water would produce a contrary effect. We are also told, that to produce diaphoresis, or sweating, he did not resort to the use of internal remedies, but merely poured warm water over the head and body, and then heaped clothes upon the patient, which would produce the desired effect, without the irritation of the internal organs consequent upon the administration of powerful diaphoretics. This, as will be seen hereafter, somewhat resembled the sweating process of the water-cure. He also recommended the use of water in various ways, and in the most serious diseases. Celsus and Galen also recommended the use of water, both in sickness and health ; and many similar examples might be quoted.

The honor of making certain various discoveries in the application of water to the human body as a remedial agent, is due Vincent Priessnitz, a peasant and native of a small colony called Graefenberg, situated two miles from the town of Freiwaldau, and about half way up one of the mountains of the Sudates in Austrian Silesia, Germany. This has always been his place of residence, and was also that of his father before him.

His discoveries were at first the result of accident. He was, in the common acceptance of the term, " unlearned," having at most only a very limited education, but possessed naturally a strong and observing mind.

He tells us it was in the year 1816, when he crushed one of his fingers, and, as it were, by instinct plunged the injured part into water until it ceased bleeding. He felt the coolness agreeable to the benumbed part, and found that by repeatedly holding it in water, without the least inflammation or suppuration, after secreting only a little white mucous matter, it healed in a very short time. Then he was told, as he says, by some old men of the neighborhood, that they could relate many instances where cold water had been used in similar cases, and had always proved salutary above every other remedy. In the year 1819, he met with the misfortune to break the ribs upon one side, by a loaded wagon. The physician, called from the nearest town, declared the injury incurable thus far: that there would be lumps formed, which, on the least exertion, would cause pain, and thus continue through life. He prescribed some herbs, a decoction of which, in wine, was to be laid upon the injured parts. These fomentations gave him so much pain that he was obliged to tear them off. Recollecting his cured finger, he commenced using swathings of cold water, and thus obtained immediate relief. Then, to press out his ribs to their natural position, he stretched himself, with the abdomen over the edge of a chair, thus leaving the upper part of the body free; and then, by repeatedly holding in the breath, he was able to extend the ribs toward the natural position. He persevered in this way, and with the wet sheets, and in a few days, without having any wound fever, he was able to walk, and finally effected a perfect cure.

Having thus gained a little experience, he afterward, from time to time, found opportunity for performing cures among his neighbors and kinsfolk, until he had finally adopted all the various forms of applying water to the human body, and which has enabled him to practice the healing art with greater success than any other individual that has ever lived in any age.

Gaining thus at first a kind of celebrity among his immediate neighbors, it gradually spread until his house began to be frequented by considerable numbers of sick persons from adjoining parts. And although his cures were often of the most astonishing kind, and generally performed gratuitously, there were not wanting those who were anxious to put an end to the "mischief," as it was called. The laws of the country are particularly severe upon quackery of every form; and no one is allowed to sell medicines of any kind except those who are regularly certificated for that purpose.

One physician alleged that the sponges used by Priessnitz contained some remedial property, which, if true, would have placed him under the jurisdiction of the law. His sponges were accordingly dissected and examined, and of course nothing found.

Another prosecuted him for quackery, pretending that he, and not Priessnitz, had cured a certain miller of the gout. Accordingly both the physician and Priessnitz, together with the miller, were summoned before the court. The miller, in answer to the question, who had relieved him, answered, "Both—the doctor of my money and Priessnitz of my gout." And thus Priessnitz was acquitted from this charge. His government afterward sent a commission of medical inquiry to Graefenberg, and finding that there was no quackery about the establishment, that the only agent used was pure water, with attention to air, exercise, and diet, and that his practice was not only entirely safe, but highly beneficial, he was, on their favorable report, allowed to continue his operations.

He has thus continued to go on, using only the simple agent, pure water, for the treatment of all curable diseases, and the relief of those that are incurable. Persons of all ranks, grades, and professions, have placed themselves under his charge; a large proportion being such as had failed by every attempt to get relief in any other way. At present, says Captain Claridge (1841), there are under his treatment an archduchess, ten princes and princesses, at least one hundred counts and barons, military men of all grades, several medical men, professors, advocates, etc.—in all about five hundred.

At first his numbers were comparatively small. In 1829 the number was only 45. In 1840, it was 1576. Between 1832 and 1842, he had treated in all 7500 patients, and of this number Captain Claridge informs us he lost but 36. This will appear remarkable, when it is remembered how large a proportion of the whole number go there only as a last resort, and whose diseases had withstood every other kind of treatment, and, in many instances, for a great length of time. Since 1840 his numbers have been a little lessened, by the numerous similar establishments that have been formed in different parts. Austria and Prussia have afforded him the largest number.

The water-cure has now stood the test of more than twenty years' experience. Some ten years ago the establishment of Priessnitz was the only one of the kind in existence. Since that time they have increased in all to about one hundred. They are scattered all over Germany, Austria, Prussia, Russia, and Belgium—all have their water-cure establishments. The government of France, like that of Austria, sent an efficient medical officer to the Graefenberg establishment to inquire into its merits, and accordingly they are rapidly multiplying there; and, latterly, England is following the example of her continental neighbors.

Of the correctness of the reports respecting the cures at the Graefenberg establishment, and of the great power of water, there can be no sort of question whatever.

Dr. Edward Johnson, for years a pupil of Sir Astley Cooper, a practitioner of more than twenty years, in which time he has had occasion to write, at different times, as many as twenty thousand prescriptions in a single year, a man well known as an author as well as a practitioner, after remaining at Graefenberg during a whole winter, trying the various processes upon his own person, and after having abundant opportunity of witnessing the cures performed there, says, "Priessnitz in his practice has met with an amount of success perfectly unparalleled in the history of disease and its treatment." And he further says, "I am perfectly convinced that I can cure a greater number of diseases, and in a shorter time, by the hydropathic treatment, than I can by the exhibition of drugs and that there are many diseases which I can thus cure which are wholly incurable by any other known means."

Again: Dr. Johnson says, "There is no well-educated man in England who dare, for his reputation's sake, refuse to admit that a remedy which can produce (at will) the most profuse perspiration, and which can also (at will) lower the temperature, and the velocity of the heart's action, to any given degree, even to the extinction of life—I say there is no well-educated man in England who dare deny that such a remedy *must* possess an immense power over diseases of every kind."

Sir Charles Scudamore, in his valuable work on Hydropathy, says, "The *principles* of the water-cure treatment are founded in truth and nature, and rest, therefore, on an immutable basis. The *practice* may be occasionally abused, and then evil, instead of good, will result. If I could think that such a consequence was necessary, I would not for one moment be its advocate. But convinced, as I am, that we have in our power a new and most efficacious agent for the alleviation of disease in various forms, and in proper hands safe and effectual, I should be no friend to humanity, nor to medical science, if I did not give my testimony in its recommendation."

The Rev. John Wesley, A. M., published a work in 1747, which went through thirty-four editions, called "Primitive Physic, or An Easy and Natural Method of Curing Most Diseases." After deprecating the manner in which drugs were employed in the healing art, he proceeds to speak of the healing virtues of water; and it would seem, by the list of diseases given by him as curable by the use of water, that his observations were strikingly correct as to its powers as a remedy.

Of medicines, he says, "The common method of compounding and decompounding medicines, can never be reconciled to common sense. Experience shows that one thing will cure most disorders, as well as twenty put together. Then why do you add the other nineteen? How often, by thus compounding medicines of opposite qualities, is the virtue of both utterly destroyed? Nay, how often do those joined together destroy life, which, singly, might have preserved it?"

This occasioned that caution of the great Boerhaave against mixing things, without evident necessity, and without full proof of the effect they will produce when joined together, as well as of that they produce when asunder; seeing that several things which, separately taken, are safe and powerful medicines, when compounded, not only lose their former powers, but become a strong and deadly poison.

As to the merits of the discoveries of Priessnitz, there seems to be some difference of opinion, even among those who admit his great and unexampled success in the treatment of disease. Some would appear to inculcate that he is only wisely, ingeniously, and energetically carrying out principles and practices which have been understood and practiced from the time of Hippocrates down.

On this point, Sir Charles Scudamore holds the following language: "I think that some writers on hydropathy have not expressed sufficient praise and acknowledgment to Priessnitz, as the inventor of a treatment constituting a complete, systematic plan. To follow in a path, is always comparatively easy. It is quite true, that parts of the whole plan, and the principles, have been known and practiced since the time of Hippocrates, and by none more ably and scientifically than the late Dr. Currie, of Liverpool. But all that can be quoted from history bears no comparison with the regular and systematic whole which Priessnitz has so happily constructed, and by which he has raised himself an imperishable fame."

Of the abilities of Priessnitz, all are agreed that, for good judgment, clearness, and decision of character, he is peculiar. To the phrenologist, a few admeasurements of his head will be interesting. As given by R. Beamish, Esq., they are as follows:

Circumference across brows	22	inches
Circumference across Causality	21¾	"
Lateral arch from root of nose to occiput	13¾	"
Transverse arch, from ear to ear	14	"
Anterior arch, from ear to ear	12	"
Posterior	11½	"
Anterior lobe	7	"
Height from root of nose to Comparison	3	"

No line divides the perceptions from the reflecting powers, marking rapidity in forming a judgment on what the perceptions take cognizance of. The middle line is well developed, viz.: Individuality, Eventuality, and Comparison. The perceptions are large; so, also, Constructiveness and Acquisitiveness; reflecting organs full. Of the sentiments, Firmness, Benevolence, and Hope, are large; Conscientiousness is full, but Veneration only moderate. Self-esteem and Approbation are large, Concentration full, the domestic groupe moderate, Secretiveness very large, Destructiveness large, Combativeness and Caution moderate. The eyes are small, and are in constant motion; the lips are frequently compressed. The temperament is highly nervous.

Priessnitz, notwithstanding his accumulation of wealth (upward of £50,000), his astonishing success, and the manner in which he is courted and respected by the first nobles of Germany, is said to retain the humility of his former station of life, that of a peasant.

"Some complain that he says too little," says Captain Claridge; "and some who go there merely to learn the treatment, complain that he never explains any thing to them." "It must be evident," he continues, "that a man who has the whole year round from 500 to 600 patients, besides the peasantry of the neighborhood that may require his aid, cannot have much breath to throw away. Let any person speak to him of his own, or of his family's case, and they will find his reply that of a man of profound sense—a reply which he never wishes to retract, and for which he will give his reasons in the most unaffected manner possible. But in respect to the second complaint, it must be avowed that he has no very great regard for medical men, because no one has suffered more from their vindictive feelings than himself; besides, he has ever found it a work of supererogation to endeavor to dispossess them of their prejudices; nor has he time or inclination to enter into disputes upon a mode of treatment which he knows, as directly emanating from nature, to be always true to herself."

As to theories respecting the action of water upon the system, it cannot be expected that Priessnitz would be able to give them in a very scientific form or mode of expression. He deals more in *facts* than in theories.

His assertions are short, comprehensive, and full of meaning. He says that the application of cold water cures diseases by *strengthening the general health and fortifying the system;* and this is precisely in accordance with Liebig, when he says that the *abstraction of heat* cures diseases by *exalting and accelerating the transformation of tissues.* And again, when Priessnitz declares, as he does, that cold water has a tendency to bring "*bad stuff*" out of the system, it is in exact accordance with Liebig's declaration, that it promotes the union of certain matters with oxygen, by which they are *carried out of the system,* and which matters, if not so carried out, become causes of disease. And the same kind of reasoning on the nature of things has taught Priessnitz, as it has Liebig, and all other medical philosophers, that all diseases must be cured by the inherent energies of the living system itself. According to Dr. Gregory, "all remedies are merely to be employed with the view of placing the body under the most favorable circumstances for resisting diseases."

According to Scudamore, he has "one single theory of disease, which serves for all persons and all disorders; that, viz., of the humoral pathology, upon a general principle, not attempting any division of the humors, according to the ancient physicians, but contented to believe that in every disease the blood is more or less charged with morbid matter; and which nature is always ready to throw out of the system, if properly assisted in her efforts. He considers that the use of medicine of every kind is a false interference with nature, and tends to interfere with her efforts; and that, on the other hand, if fortified and assisted by the agency of water, internally and externally, in conjunction with good air, abundant exercise, and the avoidance of hurtful stimulants, she will acknowledge the help given, and will, in a longer or shorter time, throw off disease; usually rendering a proof of such salutary operation, by the production of some kind of crisis."

Respecting this doctrine, the Humoral Pathology, by which all diseases are attributed to a diseased state of the fluids of the body, it may be said physicians are beginning to admit that there is more of truth in it than has generally been admitted.

The simplicity of the remedy in the water-cure is a matter of objection by many, and may be the means of leading those into its practice who are in every way unqualified. The agent being one of great power for good or evil, it will in such hands be liable to the most disastrous consequences. Priessnitz never treats two patients precisely alike. This shows the necessity, not only of understanding all the various applications of water, but also of possessing a thorough knowledge of the human system, both in health and disease.

Priessnitz, by his doings, has proved to the world two things: first, that the water-cure is the most natural and best system of treatment; and second, that he is a man possessing a genius most remarkable. As an example of the power of the remedy, of his skill, and of the necessity of understanding well the treatment, take the following case from Captain Claridge:

A person who had recently lost his wife and two children, was attacked with brain fever. Priessnitz ordered him a tepid bath, in which he sat and was rubbed by two men, who were occasionally changed. The man became so deranged, that it was with difficulty that he could be kept in the bath. In ordinary cases, this disease succumbs to the treatment in two or three hours; but the patient in this case became speechless at the end of this time.

Priessnitz, with that coolness which is so leading a feature in his character, said, "Keep on until he either talks much or goes to sleep." The latter the man at last did, but not until he had been in the bath for nine hours and a half, when he fell asleep from exhaustion at half past ten at night. He was then put to bed, and the next day the fever had left him, and, though weak, he was able to walk about. If, in this case, Priessnitz had become alarmed, after the first two or three hours, and had discontinued the mode of treatment, to try some other experiment, the consequence might have proved fatal.

After the above account had been published in the former editions of this work, our friend, A. J. Colvin, Esq., of Albany, who was himself under treatment at Graefenberg nearly a year, furnished the author the following account of Priessnitz's discoveries, which is the most full and perfect that has ever been given.

"ALBANY, Feb. 1st, 1847.

"DR. SHEW: DEAR SIR—You apprise me of your safe return from Graefenberg, and your intention to publish another work on the water-cure. Anxious to accompany it with a history of the discoveries of Priessnitz, you ask me to furnish mine, which you are pleased to say is probably more accurate than any, or all else. I had intended to prepare my notes for publication, but the length of time which has now elapsed since they were made, will prevent, unless in the shape of detached articles. I with pleasure, therefore, extract what you desire, to print or burn, as you may prefer.

"I was at Graefenberg, you are aware, upward of nine months. I arrived there in the autumn of 1844, in a state of health which might be considered desperate. The water-cure was my last hope for restoration; if that failed me, I had but to look forward to a brief life of misery and the grave.

"I shall never forget my drive up the mountain, from the little village of Freiwaldau to Graefenberg. It was on the morning of the 25th of September, through a driving shower of rain. Although the day was so cold and windy that the teeth chattered in my head, I met on the road numerous persons dressed in light summer clothing, without cravats, the shirt open, and thrown wide over the coat, and the only covering for the head an umbrella. I supposed them the insane of Priessnitz's establishment, but soon ascertained my mistake; for it was the common habit of the patients, while taking exercise, preparatory to the baths.

"I was ushered into the presence of Priessnitz by his secretary, as forlorn and sad a looking object, perhaps, as ever solicited his skill. Priessnitz's dress was of the plainest kind; his coat, a gray frock, loosely and badly cut, pantaloons of the same material, vest double breasted, and buttoned up to the throat; his complexion was fair, and slightly pitted (I afterward heard him say that he had the small-pox before he had a knowledge of the water-cure, or he would not have been marked), hair light, and shortly cut, the forehead expansive and well formed, expressing high perceptive and intellectual power—moral sentiments well developed—eye restless, brilliant, and strikingly penetrating—nose prominent—mouth large and square—lips firmly and handsomely set together—the figure erect and manly—all together, his appearance was impressive. I felt that I was in the presence of no ordinary man. A member of the Aulic Council, who spoke English indifferently, was present, together with several other persons.

"A letter from ex-President Van Buren, which I was careful to have translated into the German, was the means of a ready and favorable introduction. Priessnitz rapidly inquired the history of my malady, passed his hands quickly over mine, said I was curable, and that on the following day he would accompany me to the bath to determine the treatment. * * * *

* * * * * * * *

* * * * * * *

* * * * * * * *

"Having experienced in my own person the efficacy of the practice, and witnessed its extraordinary success in the persons of others, I naturally felt a lively interest to obtain from Priessnitz, not only a connected account of his discoveries, and the mental process by which he arrived at them, but also a sketch of himself and family. I accordingly, a few days before my departure, apprised him of my wishes. So many unfounded and contradictory versions of his discoveries had made their way into books, pamphlets, and newspapers, that he was the more willing to oblige me.

"Vincent Priessnitz, then, was the youngest of six children, and was born on the fourth day of October, 1799, at Graefenberg, the family residence, which has since become so celebrated by his discoveries. Although often stigmatized as an unlettered peasant, and of ignoble parentage, yet his father was a respectable landed proprietor. In virtue of the laws, whereby the real property descends to the youngest son, Priessnitz, on the death of his father in 1838, became possessed of the family estates and residence. He received the rudiments of education at the Catholic school, in the neighboring village of Freiwaldau, and was as well instructed as the majority of farmers' sons in our own country. His mother lost her life in the year 1821, on the same field where himself, not many years before, had received an injury, the cure of which had contributed very greatly to extend his reputation, and lay the foundation of his future system. His only brother, and the eldest born, is a distinguished Catholic priest, and is now at the head of the principal cathedral in one of the neighboring provinces.

"At the age of thirteen, Priessnitz sprained his wrist, which caused much pain and inflammation; he instinctively applied it to the pump. Finding that the water cooled the part, and assuaged the pain, but unable to keep it constantly there, it occurred to him to apply an UMSCHLAG, or WET BANDAGE. He applied one accordingly, which he re-wet as fast as it dried. He found that this was entirely successful in removing the inflammation, and relieving the pain, but that it induced a rash; and as this was a phenomenon new to his youthful mind, as unaccountable, it led to much reflection. Was it favorable, or the reverse, that such a consequence should flow from such a cause? Could it be that his blood was impure? He persevered in the application, and the wrist speedily regained its strength. Shortly after, being in the woods, he crushed his thumb. He again resorted to the umschlag, and with like success: but again the rash made its appearance. He thought his blood must be bad; yet he could not decide without further evidence.

"The success which had attended the application of the umschlag in his own person, filled his mind with delight. He was impatient to see it tried upon others. Whenever, therefore, he heard of a neighbor who had received an injury, or had enlarged or swollen joints or parts, or was afflicted with pain, he urged, and generally prevailed upon him, to use the umschlag: but he remarked that the rash did not uniformly appear; and in such cases the process of healing was rapid, while in those wherein it did appear, the cure was more obstinate.

This convinced him that in one the blood was healthy, while in another it was mixed with peccant matter, and that water possessed the property of extracting that matter. In cases of *chronic ulcers*, and where there was no inflammation, it occurred to him to cover *the wet* umschlag *with a dry one*, for the purpose of creating heat, or a return of inflammatory action, without which, he discovered, a cure could not be effected.

"In the sixteenth year of his age, the accident occurred to which I have alluded, nearly depriving him of life, and the world of the embryo system. Priessnitz was engaged in driving a young horse, with a load of hay, down the mountain. It became necessary to cog the wheels, to prevent the too rapid descent of the cart. He was standing before the horse, holding him by the head, while others were performing the work of chaining; the horse got frightened, and rushed down the hill. Unwilling to allow him to destroy himself, Priessnitz held on, and was dragged down between his feet. While in this position, three of his teeth, two of them upper front teeth, were broken, and his arms and body severely bruised by the horse's hoofs. He could hold out no longer; the cart passed over his body, crushing three of his ribs. He was taken up senseless, and while in this state, the surgeon of Freiwaldau being summoned, probed his wounds, and pronounced them incurable. With a return of consciousness, Priessnitz bethought himself of his never-failing resource. He tore off the bandages of the surgeon, and applied the umschlag. How grateful, and how soothing the application! The inflammation was subdued, the pain alleviated, and he felt persuaded that he should get well. He replaced the broken ribs by pressing his abdomen against the window-sill with all his strength, and inflating the lungs so as to swell out the chest. He then reapplied the umschlag, and finally recovered, although to this day he bears in his side a deep impress of the wheel by which he received the injury.

"The accident, as is usual in country places, created quite an excitement, but the cure far greater. The simplicity of the means, and that a mere stripling had evinced such boldness and fortitude, were matters of astonishment. The reputation of the umschlag was not only increased, it was established.

"From this period, the mind of Priessnitz was directed toward the curative power of cold water. He felt that he had entered upon a mighty field of discovery, and he was resolved to know the extent of it. He now began to use the sponge, in connection with the umschlag, and with such marvelous success, that the peasants believed him a wizard; to test which, he frequently found, in the morning, a broom-stick placed across his door-sill. This credulity, natural, perhaps, to the ignorant, who are prone to attribute to supernatural power every occurrence which passes their comprehension, encouraged him in his experiments.

"What was he to do where disease was general, not local? The umschlag and sponge were found insufficient. Why not envelop the whole body? He was transported with the idea; and the LEINTUCH, or WET-SHEET PACKING, sprung into existence.

"Of all his discoveries, this may be esteemed the most important, considered with reference to the extent and variety of diseases in which it is employed, and would alone have embalmed his memory in the recollections of a grateful posterity. The old and the young, the feeble and the strong, are alike submitted to its soothing and revivifying influence. Priessnitz was elated! And well he might be, for he had made a discovery which entitled him to the homage of the world.

"But he did not stop here. Finding some LOCAL CHRONIC AFFECTIONS resisting as well the leintuch as the umschlag, he conceived the idea of *partial baths*, for a long time continued, to produce perturbation and reaction deep beneath the surface. HENCE THE FOUNDATION OF HEAD, EYE, ARM, SITZ, LEG, AND FOOT BATHS. Still, there was a class of these cases so obstinate as to resist this united treatment. What was to be done? Was there no way in which the water could be here made effective? He had experienced the potency of falling water. Why might it not be the agent which he desired? He erected at once, in one of the beautiful dells of the mountain, a DOUCHE, and the object was attained!

"The SWITZEN, or PACKING IN THE WOOLEN BLANKET, was suggested by observing that perspiration frequently relieved pain, and was efficacious in many diseases, and as, unlike the *vapor* and *hot baths*, it did not accelerate the circulation and debilitate the system; and as sweating in it, after a proper time, would voluntarily terminate, he did not hesitate to give it the preference over all other known modes of promoting perspiration, and adopt it in practice. The patients who were obliged, occasionally, to remain in it some time, on complaining of a sensation of faintness, he relieved, by opening the windows and washing the face. The relief thus afforded, induced him to *sponge* the body, and no ill consequences following, he directed the whole person to be immersed. Hence he was led to the WANNEN BAD, or PLUNGE BATH.

"There was still a class of cases, such as apoplexy, paralysis, tetanus, lock-jaw, hydrophobia, insanity, poisoning, etc., and some cases of determined colds, inflammations, and fevers, to which none of the treatment yet devised, except in some stages, perhaps, the leintuch, was adapted. Here was a trial for the new system. Could it be overcome, the triumph was complete. In all the cases mentioned, a speedy cure was hoped for, in the judgment of Priessnitz, if a marked change could be produced. His genius did not desert him in this extremity. He designed ABGESCHRECTES, or TEPID SHALLOW BATH, to meet the emergency. Containing but a few inches of water, of a temperature of from 60 degrees to 70 degrees Fah., the patient could be kept in it, exposed to active friction, until the object sought for was effected (and he has been known to keep a patient in for nine hours). And here we have the *chef d'œuvre* of Priessnitz's discoveries. It is his favorite resource in these and in all cases of extremity; and it is not too much to say, that without it, many of his most splendid achievements must have been unrecorded.

"The ABREIBUNG, or DRIPPING WET SHEET, was a much later addition to his practice, and was suggested by washing with the hands and a towel. It is used, generally, as preparatory to other and stronger treatment, although it is, in some instances, continued to the termination of the cure.

"After his reputation became somewhat extended, Priessnitz visited patients at their houses; but he remarked that such were not cured as rapidly as those who took the trouble to come to him. Hence he was led to conclude, that to make mankind appreciate a benefit, they must pay for it, either in belief, in trouble, or in pocket; and as he charged nothing for his services, the system would have died a natural death, had he discouraged the idea that there was not something supernatural in it, and permitted it to rest on its simple merits. He also remarked, that as soon as he adopted the plan of calling on the patients, instead of their coming to him, they fell off from hundreds to tens in the year. He therefore declined to go out at all, and refused to prescribe, unless personally solicited at his own residence. *And this was the germ of the present establishment, the fame of which has spread throughout the world.*

"The Medical Faculty were not slow to perceive the tendency of these discoveries to the overthrow of their unprogressive system, which had for centuries, like a pall, covered the earth. As early as 1821, the three practicing physicians of Freiwaldau, Dietrich, the brother-in-law of the Burgomaster, and two brothers by the name of Gunter, formed the nucleus of a plot to destroy him. Every person to whom he had administered was secretly inquired of, whether the *umschlag*, the *sponges*, or the baths, were not medicated, or whether Priessnitz did not make use of some other agent than water, or some herb, or drug, in connection with the water. Could such a fact have been established, the overthrow of Priessnitz had been certain, for in no country are the laws against empiricism more stringent than in Austria. He was thus constantly upon his guard, and his utmost ingenuity and invention were required to make water alone supply the place of every other remedy. Between the years 1821 and 1828, these physicians had him brought several times before the Syndic, or Chief Justice of the town, to answer for unlawful practice; but he was always acquitted. In the year 1828, however, the most determined effort was made to crush him. The country was scoured for witnesses, and a large number were examined, to prove he had done them injury. Not one, however, but acknowledged he had received benefit. One, a miller by occupation, who had been cured of gout, as one of the Gunters declared, by him, on being asked, 'Who had helped him?' replied, 'Both: Gunter helped me out of money, Priessnitz out of my disease.' On being again asked 'What he paid Priessnitz?' he replied, 'Nothing: I still owe him thanks, which I now return him for the first time.' But what availed testimony? The Syndic was in the interests of his persecutors, and Priessnitz was impotent against their wealth and influence. He was declared to be illegally tampering with the public health, and ordered to be arrested. From a sentence so manifestly partial and unjust, Priessnitz appealed to the tribunal of Brunn. This judicature reversed the judgment of the Syndic, and decided, that as it appeared Priessnitz made use of nothing in his practice except water, he was at liberty to pursue it. His persecutions did not terminate here ; the faculty still followed him ; their ancient and cherished system was in danger ; and the arrogant innovator must be silenced. He was complained of before the tribunal of Wiedenau, a neighboring province. His accusers, however, unable to bring any proof other than such as they had before produced, the complaint was dismissed ; but he was forbidden to treat any patients out of his own district. Priessnitz replied, with spirit, that water was free to all, and he would not inquire whence the patients came. But the malevolence of his enemies was sleepless. They resolved that the matter should be brought to the notice of the court at Vienna. For this purpose, the medical faculty there were appealed to. They interfered, and succeeded in bringing the subject before the Emperor Francis. Baron Turckheim, of the Aulic Council, together with a commission of district and staff surgeons, was appointed to proceed to Graefenberg to make investigations, and report the result. They went strongly prejudiced, both against Priessnitz and his system.

"At this time, Priessnitz had at his establishment quite a number of patients, or cure-guests, as they are universally termed at Graefenberg ; and his success in curing disease, which had baffled the arts of the most eminent of the faculty, was decisive.

"The commission examined his *baths*, his *leintuchs*, his *switzens*, analyzed the water, and interrogated the badedieners, or bath-servants and patients. But nothing was elicited to convict the audacious peasant. The bath-tubs were made of wood, the *leintuchs* of linen, the *switzens* of wool, the water was pure and unadulterated, gushing from the thousand springs of the mountain ; and to the interrogatories, the badedieners and patients replied, that no agent except water was employed in the treatment. So favorable were the reports made by the commission, that he was permitted not only to continue his practice, but he was authorized to give certificates of inability for service to military officers, who might place themselves under his care, with the like effect as staff surgeons ; a result of the efforts of his accusers as unexpected as it was galling to them. Instead of his condemnation, which they had confidently anticipated, behold ! he was exalted to an equality with themselves. This was too much for endurance. He must be deprived at least of the countenance of the government. In 1834, therefore, after the death of the Emperor Francis, the head of the Department of Brunn was prevailed upon to withdraw it. Priessnitz was advised strongly to make an appeal to Vienna, but, disgusted with this exhibition of petty envy, he refused. It was not long before the military, numbers of whom from all parts of Europe were now his patients, assailed the invidious interference of the authorities of Brunn. The ambassadors from the different courts at Vienna were induced to interpose, and Priessnitz was restored to the favor of which he had been so unjustly deprived. But it is a significant sign of the apprehensions entertained of the ultimate triumph of the water-cure, that, to this day, all publications in favor of it, and the establishment at Graefenberg, are expressly forbidden in the Austrian dominions, through the influence of the medical fraternity.

"Thus terminated in disaster, after thirteen years of opposition, the attempts to destroy the new system. Henceforth, its disciples have only to be true to it, to witness its final consummation.

"Priessnitz was married in the year 1828, to Miss Sophia Priessnitz, a distant relation, the daughter of the chief justice of the adjacent village of Bochmishdorf. By her he has had eight children, the eldest of which only was a son. This son, while an infant, died from a spasm induced by the administration of a dose of medicine; the mother and friends insisting that water was not calculated for the case. Priessnitz with reluctance yielded to their prejudices. Not anticipating so rapid a termination, he thought he might interpose in time to save, but the fatal dose had sped its errand, and the little sufferer was beyond even the power of water. From that day to this, no medical practitioner has darkened his threshold, except to study his system, or become his patient.

"But I have spun this letter, I fear, to an unreasonable length. In the sincere hope that the blessings of the water-cure may be disseminated, and that it may eventually, as I feel firmly persuaded it should, take the place of all other methods of curing disease,

"I am, with sincere esteem, very truly yours,

"ANDREW J. COLVIN."

CHAPTER III.

HYDROPATHY, OR THE MODERN WATER-CURE—(Continued).*

Why the Profession look unfavorably on the new Mode.—The true medical Philosopher receives Truth from any and every source, however humble.—Cold Water merits at least a fair trial in legitimate Practice.—Distinct Hydropathic Establishments best for giving full effect to the Treatment, but many parts of it may be applied at Patients' own Houses.—What a Water Establishment should be.—Water an old Remedy.—Lanzani's Method.—Sir John Floyer and Dr. Baynard's.—Extracts concerning Life.—Dr. Currie's Practice—Cyclopedia of Practical Medicine.—The ancient Romans.—The modern Russians.—Remarkable revivifying effect of the Cold Plunge Bath after Sweating.—Priessnitz's Mode not only embraces those of previous Authors, but also new and powerful Processes.—Description of Priessnitz.—The Water Process, although simple, may be much varied.—Priessnitz's Mode of commencing with a Patient.—Water drinking.—Exercise, general Routine, Packing, etc.—The various Baths.—Compresses.—Mode of Sweating.—Flannel not to be worn next to the Skin.—Drugs never to be taken at Graefenberg.—True Mode of arriving at the Results of Hydropathy.—Civilized Life, in many respects, productive of Disease.—Advantages of the Hydropathic Diet.—Value of Means applied to the Surface.—Evil Effects of too oft-repeated internal Remedies.—The Hydropathic Treatment as a Counter-irritant.—The Crisis.—Effects of cooling the Body often.—Sympathy of the Surface with internal Parts.—Stimulating effect of the Hydropathic Treatment.—Sedative effect of Cold Water.—Water as a Febrifuge.—Rules of Dr. Currie and Dr. Haen.—Safety of Cold Water in Fevers.—Cold Bathing a Tonic Means.—Erroneous Notions of Medical Men.—Boldness of Hydropathists.—Douche and Shower Baths.—Remarks on the Sweating Process.—Its Safety and Efficiency.—Water as a Purgative and Diuretic.—Tranquillizing Influence of the Hydropathic Treatment.—Remarks on Medical Habits, in reference to Chronic Disease. Ill effects of over-drugging.—Conclusion.

In consequence of the modern water-cure having been originated by a non-medical and uneducated man, and having been subsequently, for the most part, adopted and professed by lay practitioners, or by medical men of somewhat equivocal reputation—and yet more, from the system being held out as a *panacea* or cure for all diseases, with an exclusive scorn of medicinal aid—the medical profession, as a body, have naturally enough, and not inexcusably, treated it with much contempt, not to say aversion, and have

* This very ably written article is quoted from the British and Foreign Medical Review, by John Forbes, M. D., F. R. S., F. G. S. It is proper here to remark, that Priessnitz has quite discontinued the practice of sweating, not resorting to that practice scarce in one case of a hundred. He regards the tonic plan as being more permanent, and better in its effects.

shown a pretty general determination not to admit it into the catalogue of therapeutic means. Exercising a natural influence on the public, medical men have succeeded in communicating to a large portion of the intelligent classes the feelings entertained by themselves. Thus hydropathy has become a tabooed subject, being either entirely excluded from medical journals and books, or only admitted into them for the purpose of being ridiculed or utterly denounced. Indeed, it is regarded almost as a violation of professional etiquette to mention this subject in the language of toleration, much more to speak of it with approbation. Accordingly, we think it not unlikely that some of our brethren, and those even of the most estimable, may regard our present article as a departure from what is medically proper, and will pronounce us almost worthy to have the severe sentence of "water doctor" passed against us. We have, however, been too long accustomed to speak our opinions openly and boldly, when we believed them to be just, whether they were in accordance with the current notions or not, to be deterred, on the present occasion, by any apprehended risk of offending mere professional conventionalism. Whatever we conscientiously believe to be true in medical science, especially if, at the same time, calculated to promote the great end and aim of all professors of the healing art—the increase of the means of lessening the sufferings of mankind—that we shall freely and fearlessly promulgate, careless of personal consequences.

Our purpose, in this article, being carefully and calmly to investigate the real merits of the system now so widely established under the name of hydropathy, we hold ourselves absolved from mixing up this investigation with any considerations whatever respecting the merits or demerits, the objects or motives, of those who practice it. We regret to think that there is, and has been from the beginning, not a little quackery and mystification mixed up with really effective practice, in hydropathic establishments, and that not a few of the conductors of the water establishments have been, and are, very ill qualified to indicate, much less to direct and conduct, any therapeutic processes capable of modifying, in an important degree, the vital conditions and functions of the human body. If it shall appear, however, as we believe it will, on further examination, that the external application of cold water is capable of being beneficially applied, in the cure of diseases, in modes of greater efficacy, and to a much greater extent, than has been hitherto practiced by medical men, there remains only one course for the members of the profession to pursue, viz., *to adopt the improvements*—if such they be—regardless of their origin, or their past or present relations. When the religious reformer proposed to adapt profane airs to church psalmody, saying that he saw no good reason why the devil should have all the good tunes to himself, he is generally supposed to have acted as wisely as he thought shrewdly and spoke quaintly. In like manner, we see no good reason why the doctors of the orthodox or legitimate school should refuse to accept good things, even at the hands of the hydropathists. They have done like things before now, as the pharmacopœia, in more pages than one, can testify ; and we have not heard that there has been any great reason for that they did so. For our own parts, we avow ourselves of such a catholic spirit, and so lowly-minded withal, as to be ready to grasp any proffered good in the way of HEALING, whosoever may be the offerers, and wheresoever they may have found it. Not merely hydropathy, but even mesmerism — yea, stark-naked and rampant quackery itself, may, in this sense, be a welcome knocker at the gate of physic. It is not the demerits of the donor, or the birth-place of the gift, that, in such a case, we are bound to look to ; but simply whether it is qualified to aid us in our glorious and divine mission of soothing the pains of our fellow-men. If it is so qualified, the baseness of its source will be lost in the glory of its use ; and, if aught of its original impurity still attaches to its application in our hands, the fault will be in us, not in it. A saint may sing the devil's tunes without contamination ; a hero may wield the weapon he has wrested from a robber or a murderer ; the medicament or the formula of the most arrant quack may be hallowed in the prescription of the true physician.

It is in this spirit we enter upon an investigation of the claims of hydropathy, as propounded and practiced by Priessnitz and his disciples. And we invite our readers to follow us in a like temper, convinced that they will be benefited by an examination of the subject, whether they adopt our views or not. Some of our views we are sure they must adopt, particularly this : that cold water, applied in the manner of the hydropathists, is a powerful modifier of the condition of the human body, both in health and disease, and, when weighed in the therapeutic balance with other remedies, merits, at least, a fair trial in legitimate practice.

It will be an after consideration in what manner, or under what circumstances, this trial can best be made; and, supposing the result of the trial to be satisfactory, it will be a yet further consideration, and one of great importance, how the remedy shall best be applied in the ordinary practice of medicine. We ourselves believe that distinct bathing establishments will still be found best for giving full effect to the hydropathic system, although we believe, also, that many parts of it may be adopted in ordinary prac tice, at the patients' own homes; and the whole of it certainly be conducted at the water establishments under the authority and general direction of the ordinary medical attendants. If hydropathy is, as we believe, a therapeutic agent of great power and value, it would be worse than absurd to exclude it from legitimate medicine; but, if it is to be adopted by the profession, it can only be adopted in a strictly professional manner. If distinct establishments are found to be requisite for its complete and successful exhibition, the members of the medical profession can, of course, sanction and patronize those only which are conducted by legally qualified and competent practitioners. And they cannot be expected to show any countenance, even to those which, although under the superintendence of legally qualified persons, are conducted on empirical or absurdly exclusive principles. A hydropathic establishment should be simply a great bathing establishment, or water hospital, and should contain the means for using water in all its medicinal forms—hot as well as cold, in the form of vapor as well as liquid, medicated as well as pure. In such a hospital, although drugs would, doubtless, be but in slight requisition, it would be contrary to all rational proceedings to exclude their use entirely. The very fact of a case being sent to such a hospital presupposes the previous failure of drugs, or, at least, presumes their unsuitableness in that particular instance; and they would, for the most part, be dispensed with at the *commencement* of the treatment, at least: but no unprejudiced or competent observer can assert that drugs should be entirely banished from the treatment of any case at all times. The same scientific judgment and the same practical skill that prescribed the water treatment as best calculated to fulfill the indications present at any one time, could alone determine whether, at any one time, medicaments might be proper, either as auxiliaries or substitutes. Nothing but the blindest dogmatism or the wildest empiricism could maintain that, because the water treatment is found useful, all other means must be useless; or, reversely, that, because drugs are often found beneficial, that therefore all other kinds of treatment, hydropathy included, must be injurious. The absolute exclusionist, be he water doctor or drug doctor, is equally unreasonable and equally unjustifiable.

In the composition of the following article, we have derived our materials mainly from the published writings of hydropathists, but also partly from personal observation of the practice of hydropathy itself, and from the reports of patients who had been the subjects of it. We have been careful to select as our authorities the best informed and most impartial of the writers on the subject of the water-cure, and we have used our best endeavors to appropriate what alone seemed trustworthy. It is so extremely difficult for a writer, on any one side of a subject that has become a matter of active controversy, to avoid partiality in relating events and drawing inferences, that we make no apology to our authors for having on many occasions refused their evidence and rejected their conclusions. Many things, however, we have admitted on the authority of the writers alone, when they did not seem to be contradicted by other facts, and were in accordance with the general principles of physiology and therapeutics. We have so far admitted the validity of the maxim—*cuilibet in suâ arte credendum;* and, so qualified, we think the propriety of the admission will not be gainsayed. But we have gone further than this. We have accepted at the hands of our hydropathic authors more than one alleged fact and explanation, even though their validity seems to us questionable. And we have done this because the statements are of a kind justly to challenge attention, and to demand thorough investigation.

On the whole, then, we wish the reader to be prepared to find in the following article, not simply an exposition of the doctrines of hydropathy, as they appear to us well established, but such also as are laid down by the best authorities of the water school; one of our objects in writing it being, not merely to endeavor to ascertain what we consider as truth, for the benefit of our readers, but likewise to incite them to make inquiry and examination for themselves, in order that agencies of such obvious potency on the human frame may no longer be permitted free scope if evil, or no longer be debarred from ordinary medical practice if good.

The internal and external use of water, in the treatment of disease, has been frequently discussed by physicians in all ages, from Hippocrates downward. Their opinions will be found cited in detail by the systematic writers on the subject of baths, and, among others, by Sir John Floyer and Lanzani. To them we refer such as are sufficiently curious to wish for an exact acquaintance with the subject, in its historical relations. For our present purpose, and to render the history of the medical use of water clear to the less minute student, we will group it under a few convenient heads.

1. According to Lanzani,* the true method of using cold water consists almost entirely in its internal administration, in very large doses, in certain stages of certain fevers. His work is most elaborate in every sense ; learned, methodical, and comprehensive. It is divided into two books : the first devoted to an explanation of the causes, symptoms, complications, and nature of fever ; the second, showing that copious imbibition of cold water is the best means of combating the symptoms, on scientific grounds, and consequently the best remedy for fever. This is obviously an argument somewhat theoretical, but it is supported by a chapter of cases, and backed by the opinions of a host of learned doctors, the author's predecessors. The actual value of the work is considerably diminished by its scientific character, because many of the doctrines held in its day have now become obsolete, and tend to encumber and obscure, rather than strengthen and enlighten, the practical facts by which they are accompanied. But the same remark applies to the early advocates of other remedies. Lanzani appears to have had no knowledge of the external use of water, nor of its application to the treatment of chronic diseases. He used it in combination with drugs.

Lanzani may be regarded as the representative of a considerable number of writers and practitioners, both in Italy and elsewhere, among whom water has been employed (internally) as the most effectual febrifuge.

2. About the year 1700, Sir John Floyer and Dr. Baynard employed water very freely as an external application, in the ordinary manner of cold bathing, preceding it by a course of physic, and

* Vero Metodo di servirse dell' Acqua Fredda nelle Febri ed in altri Mali, si interni come esterni. Di Nicolo Lanzani, Medico Napoletano. 2nda edizione. In Napoli, 1723.

accompanying it generally by copious water drinking.* Their practice appears to have been chiefly in chronic diseases, such as rheumatism, gout, paralysis, indigestion, general debility, and various nervous affections, in the whole of which a large amount of success is said to have been attained. The baths at which their cases were treated, were frequently designated by some saint's name. Probably a remnant of superstitious reverence for the saint not only assisted to attract patients to the well, but infused into them a faith in the remedy, which materially promoted their recovery. The practice pursued was simply cold plunging, guarded by certain rules and cautions to prevent accidents.

Sir John Floyer supports his views by the citation of numberless learned authorities, from the Bible to Dr. Mead. He seems to have attached rather an excessive importance to grave precedents, causing his portion of the conjoint work to savor more of the library than the bedside. At any rate, he mingles together practical facts and the opinions of writers in such intricate relations, that it is not always easy to discover on which he relies most confidently for the maintenance of his tenets. Dr. Baynard, on the other hand, deals more in cases, of which he presents an abundant collection. His mode of reasoning is particularly pointed and sagacious. No one can leave the perusal of his work without a strong conviction of his being an honest, shrewd, enterprising, and diligent contributor to medical literature.

These writers mention the occasional practice of persons bathing in their shirts, and wearing them throughout the remainder of the day without drying; they also give an instance or two of cases cured or relieved by the application of a wet towel. The former practice is alluded to as an instance of rashness on the part of patients, and the latter is so rarely mentioned, that in neither can they fairly be said to have anticipated Priessnitz in the systematic employment of the wet sheet or wet compress—although both were actually employed by them. They also speak in very favorable terms of a course of cold preceded by a month's warm bathing, but not in the modern hydropathic method of the cold following immediately upon the warm, or upon sweating, which is a practice they carefully deprecate. They seem to have had but a slight

* Psuchrolousia; or, the History of Cold Bathing, both ancient and modern. By Sir John Floyer, of Litchfield, Knt., and Dr. Edward Baynard, Fellow of the College of Physicians, London. 2d edition. London, 1706.

acquaintance with the use of cold bathing in fever, or acute diseases, though instances of such practice are given.

The following passage from Dr. Baynard, though not strictly a part of our present subject, is a curiosity, and affords a good sample of his peculiar manner. When the period of its publication is considered, it must be regarded, in some of its parts, as a remarkable case of the forestalling of exact experiment by speculative reasoning. Baynard adduces the remarks it contains in support of his hydropathic views; but we need not stay to examine them in that respect. We transcribe portions of the passage:

"I *conceive life to be an actual flame;* as much flame as any culinary flame is, but fed with its peculiar and proper pabulum, made out of the blood and spirits for that purpose; and my reasons are these, viz.: 1. Life is as extinguishable as any flame is, by excluding the air, etc. For hold your handkerchief close to the mouth and nose of any animal that has lungs, and life is put out, the creature is dead in a moment; there is no skin broke, nor bone broke; no wound, nor bruise; there is your whole man, but dead he is. 2d. No flame will burn without aerial nitre, or a *quid aerium,* whatever it be; some will have it a mixed gas of nitre and sulphur, but whatever it be, 'tis a *causa sine quâ non,* something without which no flame will burn; and that the lungs serve to this use, and are air-strainers, is very clear to me, by that experiment of the candle and two puppy dogs, put into a great oven, and stopped close up with a glass door to see through; and in a little time, when they had sucked in some, and the candle wasted the rest of the nitre, the dogs died, and the candle went out with them at the same instant.

"All ustion, as the *quid inflammabile,* wastes, leaves by incineration alkalious and caustical salts, either fixed or volatile, which, from their figure or imbibed fire, become of a pungent, corrosive nature, and fix upon the membranes, being nervous and most exquisite of sense and perception, which, by irritation, cause a light inflammation, which inflammation is called thirst; which salts are melted and washed off by drinking—the grosser by stool with the solid excrements, but those of most solid and subtle particles creep with the chyle into the blood, and have no way out but by the urine. Hence water is the best menstruum to dissolve salts; and that which is most simple and elementary is the best water, as least impregnated; such waters wash off and dissolve their points and angles, by which they prick, sheath, and envelop them in their own pores, and with themselves run off by urine; but if so forced by heat and motion as to disturb them in their passage, the current of urine is checked, and the salts leave their hold of the water, shoot their vortex, and from the channels get into the habit of the body, which, if not dissolved, melted, and thrown off by sweat, they inflame and cause fevers, etc.; nor will they cease their action and inquietude until totally dissolved, or forced back into their common passages, and the salts precipitated and run down by urine. For I look upon the pores and sweat-vents as so many back doors and sally-ports, by which nature drives out the enemy crept into her garrison. The truth is demonstrated in all fevers, where the caustical salts are not washed off, but remain behind on the glands and membranes, forsaken of their dissolving menstruum, the water, etc., *which that ingenious chemist, Mr. George Moult, by chemical analysis, made appear in six quarts of febrile urine, which I sent him, and he found but the thirtieth part of those salts usually found in a sound man's urine,* so that of necessity they must remain behind and be left (like so many French dragoons) to quarter on the blood and spirits at discretion. The history of which is printed in the 'Philosophical Transactions' for some years since.

"Now, that which we call an insensible perspiration, is nothing else but the smoke made from the vital flame, and the pores are the spiramenta through which it passes, and when these are stopped, this smoke is returned and the flame becomes reverberatory, which is sometimes necessary to force an obstruction, for the body has its registers and vent-holes, as well as other furnaces. But to proceed: these salts sometimes crystallize, so that the common menstrua will not touch them, no more than a file will steel or hardened iron, and then it is a true diabetes (and here the physician is at his wit's end, and that no far journey); then hey! for lime-water, quince wine, and other restringents, which, if it were possible, would rather make a coalescence, and tie the knot harder. No; the cure lies in solution by melting down the salts, which must be done by open, raw, and unimpregnated menstrua, such as the Bristol waters are, as most simple, having least contents in them." (pp. 47 et seq.)

3. At about the beginning of the present century, Dr. Currie's practice in fever is well known to have consisted principally of

cold affusion, or immersion, in the early stages of the disease, and in certain acute affections of the nervous system. His work is so well known that it is unnecessary to enter into any detail as to contents.* He seems to have known but little of the application of cold water to the treatment of chronic diseases, as represented by Floyer and Baynard, or not to have employed the copious libations described by Lanzani. He cannot be said to have forestalled Priessnitz in any other respect, than in the prompt and energetic use of cold water in the suppression of acute febrile and nervous affections. He brings a large amount of scientific argument and practical experience to bear out his views. He has also placed in a clear light some points of practice on which important errors previously prevailed, such as the safety of cold applications when the body is heated beyond the natural degree, and the relative value and safety of cold or tepid water, of immersion, affusion, and ablution. On these points his work is of great practical value. We may have occasion to revert to some of them hereafter.

4. The prevalent opinions of medical men in this country, on the general subject of the external use of water, previously to the Priessnitzian era, may be considered to be represented in the article BATHING, in the "Cyclopædia of Practical Medicine," published within the last twenty years. The article in question places bathing in a very subordinate position among means available for the actual cure of disease. In its cold form, it is recommended as a valuable tonic, used with many restrictions, in nervous debility and other analogous states; and, in its warm form, its use is almost limited to the allaying of irritation in certain disorders, the more formidable symptoms of which are to be encountered by other remedies. Other articles in the same work have done justice to Dr. Currie's views. Beyond this, the medical profession have hitherto done little or nothing with bathing as an instrument of cure. We shall hereafter find reason for believing that a vast superfluity of caution has existed in the employment of this remedy, and that some of the supposed cautions have really increased, instead of diminishing the danger, as well as destroyed the efficiency of its application.

The author of the article in the Cyclopædia describes cold bath-

* Medical Reports of the effects of Water, cold and warm, as a Remedy in Fever and other Diseases. By James Currie, M. D., F.R.S., Fellow of the Royal College of Physicians, Edinburgh. 2 vols., 2d edition. London, 1805.

ing as partially or absolutely contraindicated in the following conditions: partially, in infancy and old age; pregnancy; indurations, obstructions, or chronic inflammations of internal parts; acute inflammations of the same; chronic inflammations of mucous membrane: absolutely, during menstruation; in great plethora, or tendency to active hemorrhage, or congestions in important viscera; affections of the heart; loaded state of the bowels; great general debility—though then often advantageous after warm water or vapor bath.

5. The ancient Romans were accustomed to produce perspiration by surrounding the person with heated aqueous vapor, and, while freely perspiring, to plunge into cold water. Interesting remains of baths for this purpose, evidently of Roman architecture, and containing fine specimens of mosaic pavement, may be seen in several parts of England; as, for example, on the margin of the Cranham woods, in the village of Whitcombe, about six miles from Cheltenham; at Bignor, in Sussex, etc. It is also well known to have been a frequent practice of the Roman youth to plunge into the Tiber, when heated by exercise in the Campus Martius.

The modern Russians, also, as is well known, excite perspiration in a similar manner, and then roll themselves in snow. A somewhat similar practice has prevailed among the North American Indians.*

The extraordinary revivifying effect of the cold plunge bath, after the system had been excited by artificial heat, is testified by various evidence of the most unquestionable kind. Numerous travelers have spoken of this very enthusiastically; among others, Stephens, the American (in his "Incidents of Travel"), who took a Russian bath, after a most fatiguing journey, and came out of it, he says, quite a new man. We have had similar information from more than one private source. This practice, however, similar as it is to that of Priessnitz, has never, until his time, been extensively, if at all, employed in Europe as a means of curing disease.

6. In the foregoing synopsis are contained the principal forms in which cold bathing and water drinking have been used in the treatment of disease, before these means were so vigorously adopted by Priessnitz. It will be obvious, that from none of the writers mentioned could he have learned his bold and comprehensive practice. In his method are combined those of Lanzani, Floyer, and Currie,

* Related by William Penn, and described elsewhere.

accompanied by novel and powerful processes, to which those writers were entire strangers. The douche, the wet sheet, the sweating blanket, the cold plunging after sweating, the wet compress, the sitting bath (sitz bath), must be allowed to be, in a great measure, peculiar to the Graefenberg peasant and his disciples. From the same source have proceeded some important precepts on the subject of diet and regimen. Priessnitz, moreover, is distinguished from all the authorities quoted, by his entire abandonment of drugs.

Vincent Priessnitz was originally a small farmer, residing at Graefenberg, near the town of Friewaldau, in Silesia. He is about fifty years of age. The following is a description of him by Sir Charles Scudamore:

"Of Priessnitz himself I shall say a few words, and describe my impressions on first seeing him. His countenance is full of self-possession; rather agreeable; mild, but firm in expression; with an eye of sense, and a pleasing smile. The small-pox, and the loss of some front teeth from an accident, impair his good looks. His manners are sufficiently well-bred. On closer acquaintance, you discover he is quick in perception; is reflective; prompt, however, in decision; simple and clear. He inspires his patients with the most entire confidence, and he exacts implicit obedience."—*A Medical Visit to Graefenberg*, pp. 2, 3.

Other travelers give a similar description of Priessnitz. They all agree in stating that he is a most arbitrary and tyrannical despot, issuing laws as irrevocable as those of the Medes and Persians, commanding obedience with a haughtiness that might well excite admiration and envy even in an autocrat, and exciting as much fear in his patients as is found in the subjects of the Grand Turk himself. He is also represented as remarkably cool and collected in emergencies, ever ready with his remedy on occasions of danger, and possessed of an imperturbable self-reliance. These traits suffice to prove that he is a man of original and powerful mind, exactly adapted to carry out a novel and startling practice. While his firm and decided manner is calculated to secure the confidence of his patients, his coolness and self-reliance enable him easily to bear the responsibility by which such confidence is attended.

His practice originated in a succession of trifling accidents, by which he was led to employ bathing in a neighboring spring, for the relief of disease. It is not necessary to give them in detail.

Success in these first attempts procured him a local renown, and he became the village doctor. From villagers his fame soon spread to patients of a higher rank, and Graefenberg gradually became the resort of the hipped and the halt from all the surrounding district. By these his praises were sung louder and louder, until all the world began to furnish him patients by the hundred. He now possesses an enormous establishment, capable of containing several hundreds of patients, which is almost constantly crowded with ladies and gentlemen of every degree, and from every nation; while his disciples and followers, as is well known, have spread themselves throughout the world, and maintain, in every country, numerous and flourishing establishments formed on the original model of Graefenberg.

His treatment, although apparently constructed of such simple elements, is capable of being varied almost *ad infinitum*, according to the peculiarities of the case or the fancy of the prescriber, and of being rendered so powerful, as often to excite in the patients and spectators apprehensions of danger—and sometimes, no doubt, to produce it in reality. It is scarcely too much to say that he has modified the application of water, and some very few other means, in a manner so ingenious as to render them no imperfect *nominal* substitute, at least, for most of the drugs in the pharmacopœia. He has his stimulant, his sedative, his tonic, his reducing agent, his purgative, his astringent, his diuretic, his styptic, his febrifuge, his diaphoretic, his alterative, his counter-irritant. Combined with these are peculiar regulations as to diet, dress, and regimen. The following is his general mode of proceeding.

In his first interview with the patient, after hearing sufficient to give him a rude insight into the locality and general features of the malady, Priessnitz proceeds to investigate its suitableness to his method of cure. He does this by sprinkling the surface of the body with cold water, or witnessing the taking of a cold bath, and then watching the development of reaction. If this appears in a certain amount of activity, he pronounces the case appropriate to his treatment; if not, he advises the abandonment of all hydropathic intentions. This is a mode of ascertaining the power of the constitution quite original, and it cannot be said to be unscientific. The power of resisting the external application of cold is a most essential conservative property of the animal system, and the degree to which it exists must be regarded as, in some respects, a criterion of the amount of *vis medicatrix* possessed by the patient. We see no very decisive reason for pronouncing it a more fallacious guide than the orthodox custom of feeling the pulse. The only objection to it that occurs to us is, that it may not be always free from hazard.

This point being satisfactorily determined, the patient is straightway admitted into the mysteries of the cure. In the first place, he finds himself restricted to a peculiar diet. Every stimulant is absolutely prohibited, from brandy and claret to mustard and pepper; so, also, are most of the luxuries imported from foreign ports, such as tea, coffee, and every kind of spice. The meals consist of three—breakfast at eight, dinner at one, and supper at seven or eight o'clock. For breakfast, cold milk is the beverage, and bread and butter its only substantial companions. At dinner there is no other restriction than those above named. Supper is a repetition of breakfast, with the occasional addition of preserved fruit or potatoes. Throughout the day, no warm beverages whatever are permitted, and much of the food is brought to table considerably cooled. As some compensation for these manifold deprivations, the patient is allowed to gratify his appetite with every reasonable variety, and a free abundance of substantial and nutritious food. He finds it a maxim that generous diet will promote his recovery, the treatment being responsible for preventing surfeit. He no longer finds an embargo laid on fruit and vegetables, and is not expected to dine seven days in the week off dry bread and mutton chops. So that, on the whole, there is perhaps about an equal amount of indulgence and restriction, as respects diet, to a patient coming to the Graefenberg rules from those of some fashionable physician in London.

In the next place, the majority of patients are directed to enter upon a course of water drinking, the quantity of water varying from five or six to thirty or forty tumblers in the twenty-four hours. A large portion of this is taken before breakfast, the rest at suitable periods after meals, so as not to interfere with digestion, with frequently a glass or two the last thing at night. Exercise is generally advised at the time of water drinking, except when this accompanies some other process of treatment incompatible with it.

A third rule insisted on is, that every patient shall take a large amount of exercise during the day. This is, to some degree, indispensable after the cold baths, as a means of procuring the necessary reaction. Walking in the open air is the mode generally selected, when possible. In case of bad weather, or lameness, other plans are contrived; such as gymnastics, sawing or chopping wood, etc. As a general rule, every patient is required to take a long walk before breakfast. It is a *vexata quæstio*, we believe, among hydropathists, as among doctors, whether the patients should rest or walk immediately after a meal; but the water doctors generally incline to advise very gentle exercise at such times; and, we believe, properly. The well-known experiments on greyhounds, and such other convincing facts, are counterbalanced, to say the least, by the habits of the working-man, who proceeds to his labor as soon as he has swallowed his dinner, and rarely suffers from so doing.

After these preliminaries, and the case being pronounced suitable for the treatment, the next morning witnesses the patient's initiation into more active proceedings. At an early hour of the morning, varying according to the time required for the operation about to be undergone, a bath attendant enters with the formidable machinery for the administration of a rubbing with a wet sheet, a packing in the dry blanket, or a packing in the wet sheet. The first of these processes consists in throwing a wet sheet over the whole person, and applying upon it active friction of a few minutes' duration. A glow is thus excited. The patient then dresses, takes his water, and sets forth upon his morning's walk. The second of the above three operations requires the patient to be enveloped in several blankets, with perhaps the superincumbence of a large feather pillow, until free perspiration is excited, which generally requires a period of about three hours. When the perspiration has continued the prescribed time (from fifteen minutes to an hour, or more), the patient is subjected to some kind of cold bath, either by the wet sheet, as just described, by pouring water over the person from the pails or watering-pots, or by taking a plunge bath. This being followed by friction and water drinking, the morning's proceedings are concluded by exercise. Packing in the wet sheet is similar to the foregoing, with the addition, next the skin, of a sheet wrung out of cold water. It is generally of short duration, as forty-five minutes or an hour, the object being to excite a glow, instead of perspiration. It is followed by cold bathing, as just described. During the packing, in both instances, some glasses of cold water are imbibed through a tube.

At other parts of the day, other portions of the treatment are applied, such as the sitz bath, the douche, the shower bath, head bath, foot bath, etc.

The sitz bath is a tub of cold water, in which the patient sits for a period varying from a few minutes to an hour, or even longer, using constant friction to the abdominal region. The other baths mentioned in this paragraph, need no description. These, as well as the former processes, are sometimes repeated during the day. In certain cases, the day's proceedings commence with some of them, in place of those previously mentioned. A rubbing with the wet sheet is frequently employed before getting into bed at night.

In fever, from whatever source, the patient is enveloped in a succession of wet sheets, renewed as often as they become warm, for a period varying with the intensity of the case—say, from thirty minutes to five or six hours. In other similar cases, cold immersion or affusion is employed with the same view—viz., to reduce the morbid heat of the system.

The *umschlag*, or compress, is an essential and seldom-omitted part of the treatment. It is a cloth well wetted with cold water, applied to the surface nearest to the supposed seat of the disease, securely covered with a dry cloth, and changed as often as it becomes dry during the day. It is sometimes covered with a layer of oiled silk, which, by impeding evaporation, prevents the inconvenience of frequent change. This compress speedily becomes warm, and remains so until dry. It is termed a heating or stimulating bandage. In cases of superficial inflammation, it is more frequently changed, so as to keep cold, whereby its effect is just the reverse, being then a local antiphlogistic.

In some establishments, the sweating has been effected by other means than the simple envelopments of Priessnitz, as by a vapor bath, or a chamber highly heated by a stove. We have heard of a temperature of 180 degrees, and even that of 198 degrees, Fahrenheit, being employed for this purpose. The blankets used by Priessnitz are very bad conductors of caloric, therefore they cause the heat given off by the body to be accumulated around its surface, by the lengthened influence of which the sudorific action is effected. This process differs in no other manner than in degree and rapidity of effect, from exposing the same surface to heat of any other origin. The animal heat, when once evolved, becomes a quality of the surrounding atmosphere. Being kept in contact with the body by blankets, it constitutes an artificial elevation of temperature, and nothing more. Therefore, in cases where active sweating is required, we can suppose no disadvantage to result from using other kinds of artificial heat, and can easily imagine advantages in a higher temperature than that attainable from animal heat alone. But we would limit this remark to dry heat. Aqueous vapor, by a well-known law, impedes evaporation, and would therefore restrict the full completion of the sudorific process. For this reason it is used to prevent plants from parting with their moisture in hot-houses. For the same reason it should *not* be used when the intention is to promote the removal of moisture, or to promote perspiration.

A point uniformly insisted on by Priessnitz is, that his patients should abstain from wearing flannel next the skin. When we consider how generally the use of this article of clothing has been advised by physicians, and adopted by invalids, especially in this country, we can easily conceive that strong prejudices will exist in the minds of patients against relinquishing it. Yet it appears to be almost universally discarded by hydropathists, and, as far as we have learnt, without any mischievous consequence.

Another maxim of Priessnitz is, that his patients are never to take any kind of drug. It should be remarked, that, not being licensed to practice medicine, it would be illegal for him to administer drugs. So that it does not follow, from his disuse of them, that he himself would be opposed to their use *in all cases*, much less that their use is in any way *inconsistent* with his practice. His medical disciples, not being similarly restricted, so far as we can learn, usually employ drugs occasionally, though sparingly.

How are we now to proceed, in order to arrive at a just appreciation of the value of the means thus briefly enumerated? The more usual course would be, to enter upon an examination of the practical results, as published by hydropathic writers. But, in the present inquiry, this plan would scarcely answer; for the means employed are so strange, so much at variance with those by which disease is commonly treated, and not a few of the reporters are so little entitled to claim credit for even a capacity to report medical results truly, that the greater part of our readers would disbelieve the alleged facts, rather than admit the principles they would carry with them. It will be more proper, therefore, to omit matters of evidence for the present, and to see if we can find in hydropathic practice any conformity with the principles on which we should estimate the merits of any other new remedy.

If a new vegetable were imported, or a previously unknown chemical substance discovered, and we were called upon to use it as a medicine, we should first inquire whether it possessed any of those qualities which are regarded as constituting medicinal virtues. We might assume that we are sufficiently acquainted with the characters of most diseases, to pronounce what description of influence would have a counteracting effect upon them. It would then remain to inquire, whether the qualities possessed by the article in question were of a kind to lead us to expect any description of such influence from their operation. If they were not, we should be indisposed to try the remedy until well assured, from abundant and unquestionable practical evidence, of its curative powers. If they were, we should be inclined to give it a trial, even if the proofs of its remedial properties were not unexceptionable. For instance, if the article under consideration merely possessed a nauseous taste, a specific color, or a powerful odor, it would offer little inducement for an experiment of its medical powers, because those qualities are not known to possess any intrinsic influence over any diseased condition. But, if it were a purgative or a sedative, no one could hesitate to recognize it as *à priori* entitled to a trial by physicians; because experience has taught us that, by the means of purging or tranquilizing, certain diseases or morbid symptoms may be cured or relieved. And, since it is the case with many of our present remedies, that with the property we wish to employ is combined another we would gladly avoid (purgatives being debilitating, sedatives narcotic, etc.), and with their amount of usefulness is thus associated a certain tendency to mischief—if the new remedy presented to us appeared to possess the essential quality, and to want the mischievous power of that otherwise used for the same purpose, we should be still more desirous of availing ourselves of it in practice.

If we apply these remarks to Hydropathy, as practiced by Priessnitz, the first inquiry ought to be, Does it furnish the physician with instruments which he, as a skillful workman, can undertake to employ? Does it contain, among its various machinery, any really therapeutic means, any powers capable of carrying out the indications which we regard as palpable in many diseases? Can it evacuate, can it brace, can it tranquilize? We cannot entertain the idea that the professors of hydropathy have hit upon any grand secret concerning the origin or nature of diseases, or the philosophy of their removal. Such a supposition, were it a necessary article of faith in the hydropathic creed, would render us the most obstinate of skeptics. But if the practitioners of this new school profess merely to have introduced more efficient, or less dangerous, means of fulfilling the purposes which all physicians have in view in treating disease, we are willing to give them a patient and impartial hearing. Or, if they profess nothing of the kind, and reject such an idea with contempt—if, nevertheless, their system appear *to us* of the nature we are indicating, we can still entertain it with the hope of discovering something of good in it.

Let us now inquire, then, on physiological and pathological grounds, supported by some personal experience, what appear to be the effects, or among the effects, of a course of water treatment according to the Priessnitzian system.

1. In the first place, we remark the careful withdrawal of all stimulants from internal parts. In this hydropathy is at once distinguished from ordinary practice. The refinement of civilized life, and the complicated affairs of society, prevent the human frame from being treated entirely as a machine. The body is compelled to undergo a usage not always suitable to its welfare, in consequence of its having to minister to the mind. The exhaustion of the latter, from exertion and excitement, is restored by artificial stimuli applied to the former. These are generally directed to parts ill adapted for their reception. Thus, the stomach, constructed to digest simple food, and to admit fluid at the impulse of thirst, becomes the vehicle of conveying to the nervous system alcohol in its various forms, and other similar fluids. These are unnatural to the stomach itself, though grateful to the nerves. Consequently, the mucous lining of the alimentary canal may suffer in the attainment of an object required only by the nervous system. This is, possibly, the very origin of a proportion of those manifold chronic ailments known under the terms dyspepsia, hypochondriasis, bilious affections, etc., and is unquestionably an aggravating cause in many. To the treatment of these affections, the

physician brings his purgatives, his carminatives, his anodynes, his stomachics. But it is to the surface of the same unfortunate membrane that they are all applied; and it frequently results that, when they relieve temporary suffering, they often leave the general health worse than they found it. From this predicament hydropathy professes to be entirely exempt, by abstaining from artificial interference with internal mucous membranes.

2. In the next place, the hydropathists adopt a system of diet, such as other practitioners seldom venture to prescribe. If a person, suffering from constipation, or any of its long train of attendant ills, applies to an ordinary physician, he is probably told scrupulously to avoid fruit, pastry, and all vegetables, except, perhaps, a favorite one, or it may be two. He is also cautioned against the use of veal, pork, beef, and new bread. We have known such a patient ordered to live for months—we might say years—constantly on mutton, and bread never less than five days old. This case is neither singular nor infrequent. What is the consequence of this? The patient is compelled to take aperient pills and draughts every day, or every other day; to stimulate the digestive organs (rendered torpid by the use of so monotonous a regimen) by occasional glasses of sherry or porter; and to compensate the deficient nutrition obtained from so barren a source, by indulgence in strong tea and coffee. Such a patient goes to a hydropathic establishment, and is straightway ushered into a *salle-à-manger*, in which he finds all the variety of food customary at a foreign *table-d'hôte* dinner, and is told to obey the dictates of his appetite. He does so timidly at first, and apprehensive of direful consequences, but he finds, to his astonishment, that he can take the forbidden luxuries of broccoli, turnips, veal, game, puddings, and fruit, with as much impunity as the never-varied mutton and dry bread, to which he was previously restricted. This is an occurrence so frequently experienced, and so universally attested by hydropathists and their patients, that we cannot refuse to admit it as a point attained by *their system*—therein being comprehended the water *and all its accessories and concomitants.*

3. A third important principle of hydropathic treatment is, that almost all its measures are applied to the surface. It is one of the most formidable difficulties with which the ordinary physician has to contend, that nearly all his remedies reach the point to which they are directed, through one channel. If the brain requires to

be placed under the influence of a sedative or a stimulant, if the muscular system demands invigorating by tonics, if the functions of organic life need correction by alteratives, the physician has no means of attaining his object, except by inundating the stomach and bowels with foreign, and frequently to them pernicious, substances. In being thus made the medical doorway to all parts of the system, and so compelled to admit every description of therapeutical applicant, the organ of digestion is contorted to a purpose for which it was never intended. The consequence is, that it has to be consulted before we enter upon the treatment of any case, and it often forbids our availing ourselves of remedies, or plans of action, which are plainly, perhaps urgently, indicated by the condition of other organs, or of the system at large. Thus, to take the three cases above mentioned: how often do we find that one stomach will neither bear ether nor opium; another is injured by steel; and others are intolerant of mercury. The two latter remedies are peculiarly illustrative of these remarks. Iron is employed to raise the tone of the general system, but it occasions constipation by its action on the alimentary canal; therefore, in order to counteract this portion of its effect, it can only be used in conjunction with aloes, or some other purgative, the tendency of which, as respects the system at large, may be exactly the reverse of that of the steel. With mercury the case is just the opposite. We wish to introduce it into the system, but it is purgative as well as alterative and antiphlogistic, and the former quality often renders very difficult our attaining the benefit of the two latter. The physician, then, is frequently placed in the dilemma, either to injure the stomach in an attempt to relieve other parts, or to leave the latter to their fate, because they can only be rescued at the peril of the former. His only mode of escape from this predicament is, to employ a legion of *adjuvantia, dirigentia,* and *corrigentia,* in the multiplicity and confusion of which it is by no means easy to make out so clear a balance of power as shall enable him clearly to foresee which kind of action, in the *mêlée,* will get the uppermost; and, unless he be well skilled in chemistry, he may unconsciously prescribe a dose so scrupulously guarded as to be neutralized and altogether impotent.

Of course we do not conclude that hydropathy has discovered a remedy for this difficulty; but its own plan of proceeding is not similarly embarrassed, because it deals with outward instead of inward parts. Whether it can produce an efficient substitute for steel, mercury, opium, and other remedies, to which we are alluding, is altogether another question, and one which its professors must bestir themselves to solve, by the careful record and honest publication of their successful and unsuccessful cases.

4. Fourthly, hydropathy employs a system of most energetic general and local counter-irritation. It has been held by some medical philosophers, that two kinds of morbid action cannot coexist in the same individual. According to this theory, if we can set up an artificial, but harmless, disease by treatment, its development will be attended by the departure of any other disorder that previously existed. Thus is supposed to be explained the operation of mercury in curing various diseases, the disorder arising from its own action being easily disposed of afterward. We attach no value to this dogma as a dogma, but it serves to embody a large number of well-known facts, and may be as properly appropriated by hydropathists as by other practitioners. By the diligent employment of hydropathic machinery, due regard being had to the constitutional vigor, a condition is often excited, termed by hydropathists *the crisis.* This sometimes consists in the appearance of various cutaneous eruptions; sometimes it is characterized by a series of boils, more or less severe; in other cases its leading feature is disturbance of the function of some internal organ, creating diarrhœa, abnormal urinary discharges, vomiting, etc. In general this effect is trifling, and seldom proceeds to such a degree as to excite alarm, or to give cause for special interference; so that the measures which have led to its appearance are in most cases continued, and in some even increased, until it has run through its course and subsided. This is not always the case. Sometimes it proceeds to a more serious length, and requires careful management to prevent mischief; the boils, in particular, are often very troublesome; even death has, in a certain proportion of instances, ensued, either as an immediate or remote consequence of the so-called crisis.

Whatever the crisis may be—or whether what is so called *be* a crisis in reality—there is no disputing that it results from the operation of a powerful system of counter-irritation—or of irritation at least. It is to this that we now wish to direct attention, because we suspect that in it is contained the true explanation of the good effects of the water-cure in many chronic cases.

5. A fifth physiological feature of the water-cure is the number

of *coolings* to which the body is subjected during the day. The generation of caloric in the animal system has been traced to its real source. It results from the *burning up* of waste matter, which, by accumulation, would become injurious. The oxygen of the atmosphere, admitted into the lungs by inspiration, traverses the various blood-vessels of the body, and, in the minute capillaries, unites with carbonized substances. The union produces the carbonic acid emitted from the lungs in expiration, and is attended with the development of what is called animal heat. It is obvious that lowering the temperature of the body, within certain limits, by awakening an uncomfortable sensation in the nerves, would induce increased activity in this calorific process, in order to maintain or restore the average degree of warmth. This increased activity could only be supported by an additional consumption of carbonized matter. If the carbonized matter were already there, and if its existence constituted the disease, or an important part of it, as is probably sometimes the case, a perfect cure would result from its removal. But supposing there is no such matter present, what then would be the consequence of stimulating this decarbonizing operation? The consequence would certainly be, that the constituents of the tissues themselves would be consumed, in order to supply the pabulum required by the oxygen. This would as certainly excite an effort at restoration, by which the digestive organs would aim to renew to the tissues the amount abstracted by the oxygen. In other words, the appetite would be increased.

Hence it is that more food is required in cold climates than in warm—in winter than in summer. The greater consumption necessary to maintain equal temperature in cold weather, can only be met by increased supply. What, in a vague and general manner, arises from the ordinary progress of the seasons, may be rendered methodical and profitable by the careful interference of art.

It has been urged that the effect here considered would equally result from exposure to cold air, as to cold water. In the words of Mr. Herbert Mayo, "This is not only entertaining, but satisfactory as far as it goes; and admits very well of being popularly and loosely brought forward in favor of cold bathing; but unluckily it is as much or more in favor of our living in Nova Zembla, as of our resorting to Graefenberg."

The same intelligent writer proceeds to notice other modes of exposure to cold, which are found to produce evil instead of good, which are, indeed, familiar as the frequent causes of serious disease, and against which we are of old cautioned:

"Nudus ara, sere nudus—habebis frigora, febrim."

It is singular enough that this very argument, now employed to discountenance the use of cold bathing, is the very strongest theoretical argument in its favor, as was long ago pointed out by that very sarcastic writer, Dr. Baynard, in the following anecdote:

"Here a demi-brained doctor, of more note than nous, asked, in the amazed agony of his half-understanding, how 'twas possible that an external application should affect the bowels, and cure the pain within. 'Why, doctor,' quoth an old woman standing by, 'by the same reason that being wet-shod, or catching cold from without, should give you the gripes and pain within.' "—p. 119.

If a rude exposure of the surface to cold and wet is capable of producing internal disease, there is no doubt that a close relation exists between those agents and the morbid conditions of internal parts. Therefore, if they could, by skillful management, be so applied as to excite the opposite effect from that to which their bad consequences are due, they would then become equally powerful means of removing disease. This is the very thing that Priessnitz and his disciples profess to have done—and to do.

Let us consider a little further the consequence of repeated applications of cold, supposing, for the sake of argument, it is used with due reference to the constitutional powers, so as to create an increased activity of the vital functions. It appears to us that this is exactly the thing needed in the treatment of a great many cases of chronic ailments. It is easy enough to construct methodical catalogues of organic lesions and their symptoms, and to assign, on paper, a "local habitation and a name" for every malady that is to require our treatment. But the truth is, that, practically speaking, there are a vast number of cases in which the symptoms may be said to constitute the only disease that can be detected, and in which they point rather to a general torpidity or derangement of all, or almost all, the vital functions, than to special change or disturbance in any particular organ. Many cases known as indigestion, gout, rheumatism, liver complaints, or nervous affections, come under this description. In a large portion of such cases, and their like, we could conceive the practice of Priessnitz to be peculiarly beneficial, if it consisted in nothing more than the frequent application, and skillful adaptation, of cold water. It was mainly by this means that the cures described by Floyer and Baynard were effected, simple cold bathing having been almost their only instrument.

6. Another physiological feature of hydropathic treatment consists in its creating a large amount of stimulation in the system. This stimulation is of a peculiar kind, and very different from that produced by alcoholic fluids or pharmaceutical stimulants. The difference is in its not awakening abnormal activity, to be succeeded by abnormal depression, in the nerves and organs of circulation, as is done by the stimulants just mentioned. The fall of a heavy douche, the sudden plunging into a cold bath with speedy exit, active friction in a shallow bath, are means of stimulating the system in the manner here intended. The effect, we are told, is manifested in the altered look of the patient after taking the bath, in his freshened cheek, his brightened eye, his elastic step, his cheerful tone. But it is *not* manifested in a quickened pulse, or a heated imagination, nor followed by exhausted energy or lowered spirits. This is the description given by hydropathists (whose practice we are not teaching but describing)—and which we have ourselves heard given by patients. It is also said that drinking, in rapid succession, several glasses of perfectly cold water, has a decidedly stimulating influence on the system. If these descriptions be correct of hydropathic stimulants, that they are powerful as well as innocuous, exciting and not exhausting, they constitute a valuable instrument in the treatment of disease, and deserve the more careful attention of physicians.

We happen to have been acquainted with a case of a lady who was at a hydropathic institution for the treatment of very aggravated chronic rheumatism. Her general powers were much shaken, and she had been unable to walk at all for a period of about four years, before undergoing this system of treatment. After several weeks of sweating and cold plunging, locomotion began gradually to return. The first indication of this was, that she could walk a few steps *immediately after leaving the cold bath.* For a considerable time this continued to be the only occasion of her being able to walk during the day, though she afterward made considerably further progress. We mention this case because we can guarantee its truth, and it always appeared to us a striking and instructive instance of the stimulating property of a cold bath.

7. A still more important and less questionable quality of the water-cure, is its power of lowering the system to any extent, without any of the debilitating means otherwise used for that purpose. In a general inflammatory or febrile condition of the body, a lengthened immersion in cold water, or an envelopment in a succession of wet sheets, would reduce the temperature and force of circulation to the most extreme degree. These means are, to the functions of life, what an extinguisher is to a flame. Their reducing power can be gradually applied up to the point of actual extinction. Any where short of that, withdraw the means, and the flame, whether of oil or of life, gradually resumes its previous brilliancy.

In the treatment of febrile diseases an important indication is to reduce the morbidly increased activity of some of the organic functions, most distinctly manifested in the circulation and the temperature. For this purpose the great instrument heretofore most in use is blood-letting, as being our only certain and expeditious method of reducing the frequency, force, or fullness of the pulse. So that, in order to suppress febrile action, we hazarded occasioning a more or less lingering debility. The *post hoc*, whether *propter hoc* or not, is too frequently a protracted convalescence, during which the patient is in constant danger of relapse. The mortality that occurs during convalescence after fever, from recurrence of the original disease, from some of its numerous sequelæ, or from the accidental inroad of some other disorder, is so considerable as to render this a period of great anxiety to the patient and the physician. It is a question deserving of cautious and dispassionate investigation, whether any portion of the liability to these mishaps is attributable to the bleeding, purging, salivating, and low diet, employed in removing the fever.

In some of the cases of fever described by Currie, we cannot fail to be struck by the rapidity and completeness of the cures effected by cold affusion or immersion, when used sufficiently early. The disease appears to have been suddenly checked or destroyed. In the course of a few hours, or a day or two, a patient threatened with, or laboring under a dangerous fever, was restored to perfect health. No period of debility ensued, no organs were found to have been seriously or permanently injured. The result of his well-known treatment, by cold bathing, of the fever which appeared in the 30th regiment, is thus described:

"These means were successful in arresting the epidemic; after the 13th of June, no person was attacked by it. It extended to fifty-eight persons in all, of which thirty-two went through the regular course of the fever, *and in twenty-six the disease seemed to be cut short by the cold affusion.* Of the thirty-two already mentioned, two died. Both of these were men whose constitutions were weakened by the climate of the West Indies; *both of them had been bled in the early stages of the fever;* and one of them being in the twelfth, the other in the fourteenth day of the disease, when I first visited them, neither of them was subjected to the cold affusion."—*Vol.* i., p. 13.

Again:

"In cases in which the affusion was not employed till the third day of the fever, I have seen several instances of the same complete solution of the disease. I have even seen this take place when the remedy had been deferred till the fourth day; but this is not common."—*Ibid.*, p. 23.

In contemplating these facts, we are driven seriously to ask, not only is not the debility consecutive to fever partly occasioned by the remedies employed in its treatment, but are not its attendant local and organic lesions in a great measure produced by the febrile paroxysm itself? And could they not be avoided by boldly applying a remedy by which this febrile condition would be more speedily subdued? The real nature of fever is, unfortunately, beyond the reach of our present knowledge. We only recognize the disease in its causes, its symptoms, its complications. In them we perceive much to lead us to answer the above questions in the affirmative. It is peculiarly a general disease. Its local characters usually appear subsequently to its general development, and wear much more the aspect of consequences than of causes. Almost any of the local complications of synochus, or typhus, may appear in exanthematous fevers where they cannot be causes.

It appears to us to be a most important subject of inquiry, whether a very serious fallacy does not pervade the medical profession at present, as to the best manner of employing cold water in fever. Dr. Currie says:

"When the affusion of water, cold or tepid, is not employed in fever, benefit may be derived, as has already been mentioned, though in an inferior degree, by sponging or wetting the body with cold or warm vinegar or water. This application is, however, to be regulated, like the others, by the actual state of the patient's heat and of his sensations. *According to my experience, it is not only less effectual, but in many cases less safe; for the system will often bear a sudden, a general, and a stimulating application of cold, when it shrinks from its slow and successive application.*"—*Vol.* i., p. 73.

"It is evident De Haen was not regulated, in his use of external ablution with cold water, by rules similar to those which I have ventured to lay down from several years' experience. Instead of pouring water over the naked body, *he applied sponges soaked in cold water to every part of the surface in succession, for some time together, in my judgment the least efficacious, as well as the most hazardous manner of using the remedy.*" —*Ibid.*, p. 84, *note.*

This is a remark which we suspect to be of very great importance, and to contain the real secret of much of the difference, as to the treatment of fever, between hydropathists and the regular faculty. Modern physicians have professed to regard Dr. Currie as a very high authority on this point, and his work is constantly quoted as the most enlightened guide for the use of water in fever; but the above opinion and precept have been, of late years, entirely disregarded, and the converse has been made the rule of practice. In the article on Bathing in the Cyclopædia formerly referred to, the author says:

"The only cases in which refrigeration is required as a remedy are those in which the animal temperature is elevated above the natural standard; and this happens only *in febrile diseases.* To insure refrigeration, the water should be applied *at first only a little below the temperature of the skin,* its heat being insensibly and gradually reduced, *but never below that of tepid, or at most cool.* The *gentlest mode of applying it is the best, as with a soft sponge;* and the process should be persevered in, without interruption, until the desired effect is produced."—*Art. Bathing, Cyclopædia of Practical Medicine.*

We believe this mode of applying water in the treatment of febrile diseases to be that which has for many years generally prevailed, not from ignorance of the precepts and practice of Dr. Currie, but from a general belief that fever once formed, could not be extinguished by the cold affusion as recommended by him. The hydropathists have renewed his system in its full boldness. It is, therefore, a question of the first interest, on which side does reason preponderate?

On carefully examining the cases of fever reported at length by Currie and Lanzani, it will be seen that their cures were effected by what may be termed a process of reaction. The immediate consequence, in most cases, of the copious libation, "*ultra satietatem*," of the one, and the affusion or immersion of the other, were perspiration and sleep. These constituted the reaction. When exacerbation of the fever ensued, and required a repetition of the remedy, it occurred several hours after the cold application, when the period of reaction had long passed over; and evidently proceeded not from the consequences of the cold treatment, but from the non-removal of the diseased action. The cold appears to have acted in a most decidedly *medical* manner, with a palpable and immediate succession of consequences altogether different from what the gradual coolness of the sponge and tepid water can be expected to produce. If these cases are correctly stated, as they appear to be, it is preposterous to confound the febrile paroxysm with reaction from a cold bath, or to expect any portion of the beneficial effect of cold immersion in fever, from tepid or cool sponging. The two kinds of treatment are in no measure similar.

But it may be supposed there is a danger in the sudden and active employment of the cold bath in fever. We suspect that this is entirely imaginary. Dr. Currie was certainly very bold in its administration, and had extensive experience of its effects. In the second edition of his work he says:

"I have thus related all the instances which have occurred to me since the last edition of this volume (a period of five years of extensive and attentive observation), in which the affusion of water on the surface of the body, cold or tepid, proved either less beneficial in its effects in fever than I had formerly represented it, or entirely unsuccessful. I would add, if any such had occurred, the instances in which this remedy had appeared to be injurious. But experience has suggested to me no instance of the kind, and extensive as my employment of the affusion has been, *I have never heard that it has suggested*, even to the fears or prejudices of others, *a single occasion of imputing injury to the remedy*."—*Vol.* ii., p. 25.

This statement, which does not appear to have been assailed, goes far toward proving the innocence, as his numerous cases do the curative powers of reaction in the treatment of fever. We certainly cannot quarrel with hydropathists for seeking to revive, in its real character, a method supported by so high an authority.

8. It is scarcely necessary to remark that a judicious system of cold bathing is a valuable tonic. This has been always known; but it has not been so widely recognized in practice as in doctrine. It has been thought necessary that cases for cold bathing should be carefully selected; that they should consist only of such patients as have unimpaired constitutions; that certain diseases were absolute contra-indications against the use of this remedy; that it is a treatment requiring unquestionable vigor in the patient, and skill in the physician to employ it without injury. It is scarcely too much to say it has been regarded as a treatment rather for the strong than the weak, and as tending rather to reduce than augment the powers of the system, and yet it is called a tonic. This is an illogical paradox not quite solitary in medical literature. The cold bath seems to be professionally employed to strengthen the body, as temptation is to strengthen virtue, by furnishing an enemy to struggle against. Thus it is considered more as a test than as a source of strength.

The hydropathists have discarded this excessive precaution, and boldly used their remedy as a tonic, wherever a tonic is required. They have administered it to the young and the old, the weak, the bilious, the gouty, the scrofulous, the dyspeptic, and the paralytic. Neither mucous membranes nor mesenteric glands, infantile weakness, nor senile decrepitude, have stood in their way. To almost all cases, all ages, and all constitutions, their method has been applied. Unless it can be shown that this all but universal administration of the system has produced serious evils, we are actually driven to admit that it is in the same proportion safe. And we are bound to admit, though we have known some instances where the practice has been seriously injurious, and have heard of others of a similar kind, that the proportion of bad consequences has not appeared to us greater than in the ordinary modes of treating similar diseases. The practice of the hydropathists is so open, and their disciples so numerous, that the innocence of their proceedings may be said to be established by the absence of evidence to the contrary. We cannot enter any circle of society without encountering some follower of this method, ready to narrate a series of *psuchrolousian* miracles, prepared to defend, and zealous to applaud the Priessnitzian practice; but few or none come forward with satisfactory evidence of any thing like general mischief having resulted from its general practice. Judgment must, therefore, be entered by default against its opponents, and hydropathy is entitled to the verdict of harmlessness, since cause has never been shown to the contrary.

But not only have hydropathists despised the discrimination usually employed in the selection of cases for cold bathing, they have manifested an equal apparent boldness in the manner of using it. In place of the spongings and the dribblings to which ordinary practitioners commonly deem it prudent to limit the use of this remedy, they employ active plunging and powerful douches. Perhaps it is to this that they owe some portion of the impunity with which they appear to have applied it so generally. They assert that the more violent practice is really the more safe, and that the danger to be apprehended is in proportion to the supposed mildness of the process, sponging being less safe than total immersion, and a shower bath more dangerous than a douche. And assuredly theory, in this respect, goes with them to some extent. In the plunge there is a sudden shock, which awakens nervous energy, and leads to speedy and effectual reaction; whereas in sponging, the whole surface is exposed to a gradual and powerful cooling, without the protection of stimulus. In the former, the whole frame is at once covered with water, and shielded from the reducing evaporation which would attend the latter. Moreover, the plunge can be more speedily gone through, and followed up more immediately by exercise. The same distinction may be made between the hydropathic douche and the orthodox shower bath. The force of the latter falls almost exclusively on the head and shoulders, as it merely trickles down the rest of the frame. How different is this from the powerful impulse of the douche upon all the muscular parts!

9. Another conspicuous item in the catalogue of hydropathic machinery is the *sweating process*. On this subject hydropathists are, in some measure, divided. It is said that Priessnitz has considerably modified his views respecting its efficacy and its safety. In the earlier period of his practice he seems to have employed it in nearly all cases. More recently he is said to have discarded it, as a general remedy, in favor of packing in the wet sheet, though still largely applying it in cases to which his matured experience has taught him to regard it as especially beneficial. We wish here

to direct attention to it merely in a physiological and pathological point of view, and need not, therefore, enter into the question as to the relative value of the past and present practice of Priessnitz.

The skin is a part through which nature has arranged that a large amount of matter should be removed from the body during health, and a still larger amount, of different character, in the process of recovery from many diseases. It is well known that a deficient cutaneous excretion is incompatible with perfect health. Perhaps there is scarcely any disease in which the function of the skin is not, to some extent, deranged. To what extent, physicians have not bestowed sufficient pains to learn; nor have they been accustomed to give much attention to this part, in the practical investigation of diseases. Still less has it acquired an important position in the list of parts to which medical treatment is directed. Therefore we possess little information, in medical writers, as to the amount or frequency of cutaneous disturbance in general disease, as to the effect of therapeutic means in correcting such disturbance, or as to the value of the correction in the cure of disease.

According to Priessnitzian writers, in almost all cases of indigestion, gout, rheumatism, nervous affections, indeed of chronic disorders in general, the action of the skin is either deficient or depraved, the part itself being found dry, hard, rough, thick, pale, relaxed, or in some other manner unnatural. They further tell us that a course of perspiration, or of the wet sheet, followed by cold bathing, corrects these signs of disorder, and reduces the part to its normal condition; and that the beneficial influence of the remedy is speedily manifested in the improvement of the case in other respects. But it might be expected that such a course would, at least, reduce the general strength, and require more vigor of constitution than many such patients possess. And yet, if we may believe the hydropathists, or even their patients, a course of active hydropathic sweating is found to strengthen, instead of weakening the system. There is a gain, instead of a loss of weight under its operation. Whether this be attributable to the subsequent cold bathing, to the water drinking, or to the peculiar regimen, may be a matter of question; but the fact would seem to be too notorious to be contradicted. We are told that it is no unfrequent occurrence at hydropathic establishments for the liquid perspiration to be streaming on the floor, having penetrated through the material on which the patient is reclining, as well as the blanket in which he is wrapped! The blanket also, when removed from the person, is dripping with liquid in all directions, as if itself just removed from the bath! On these occasions several pounds of matter must be removed from the body. The patient, dripping and steaming, next hastens into the plunge bath, stays there his appointed time, undergoes the prescribed friction, drinks his water, and finds himself actually invigorated by the strange process he has undergone.

Nay, more; it is placed beyond doubt by experience, that this proceeding may be repeated daily, or even twice a day, for *many months,* without producing any deleterious effect upon the general health! Many cases have occurred in which it has been ascertained that it has been attended with an increase of weight, and that of no slight amount. We know the particulars of one case, in which a gouty gentleman gained seven pounds in a fortnight of such treatment; and of another, in which there was a gain of eight pounds in ten days. We are also acquainted with the case of a lady, who was unable to walk at any other period of the day, except immediately after the sweating process—a sure proof that it did not occasion debility.

The safety of the immediate succession of cold bathing upon copious sweating has been called in question; but the practice of so many hydropathists as there are around us amply establishes this point. On scientific grounds, the question was completely set at rest by Dr. Currie.

An effective and innocuous means of increasing the excretion from the skin being thus found, which appears to combine with its own peculiar action the indirect effect of a tonic, have we not reason to regard it as a promising instrument of cure, in many disordered states of the system? We fully believe that we have. We know the utility of augmenting the secretion of the mucous membranes, the liver, the kidneys; we recognize this in our constant practice. It is by this means that we combat a large proportion of chronic as well as acute maladies. Why should the skin alone be neglected? Physiology teaches us that it is the vehicle for conveying out of the system a large amount of matter, solid as well as liquid; and practical experience exhibits it as the channel through which the *materies morbi* in many instances, and the burden of plethora generally, find their exit. These facts indicate it as a legitimate locality for the same artificial measures which are found serviceable on other secreting organs.

It may be objected to what we are now urging, that profuse perspiration itself characterizes many diseases, of which it is one of the most formidable symptoms. How can sweating cure acute rheumatism, it may be asked, of which it is almost a constant feature? But the same remark applies to other medical phenomena. Excessive purging and increased action of the kidneys are dangerous, frequently mortal symptoms. But does that prevent our employing them as remedies? Do we not, in spite of our frequent experience of their injurious effects, apply them almost constantly to the cure of disease? Are there ten cases out of ten thousand in which some kind of purgatives are not administered? Nay, is not dysentery itself treated by purgative calomel? Let us extend the same tolerance to sweating. It is contrary to all the instruction of experience to confound the consequences of a phenomenon violently excited by morbid causes, with those it induces when seasonably created and carefully managed by skillful treatment.

In many of these cases, the benefit does not appear to result so much from stimulating the function of any particular organ, as from removing a certain portion of matter from the system at large. There is no reason to suppose that exciting the liver, the colon, the duodenum, or the kidneys, for instance, has any special influence over a morbid condition of the brain. We find that drugs which act upon any of these organs, frequently relieve such conditions, and they may often be selected indiscriminately, the one answering much the same purpose as the others. A common antibilious pill, retailed for a penny by a druggist, or a patented nostrum of Cockle or Morrison, will generally do as well as the most elaborate prescription. The particular adaptation seems to depend more on constitutional idiosyncrasy than on any fixed relation of the part diseased with the part treated. The whole of those remedies appear to act in such cases either by a general principle of counter-irritation, or by removing a quantum of fluid or of excretory matter from the circulation, either of which objects might be attained as speedily, as certainly, as extensively, and as safely, by the skin as by any other part.

But the power of the water-cure over excretions is not limited to the skin. It professes to be both a purgative and a diuretic. That it is diuretic, in a certain sense, needs no proof. It is no new discovery, that in proportion to the quantity of fluid imbibed by the mouth will be the quantity emitted by the kidneys. This, though verbally, is not medically a diuretic action. It may consist simply in the mechanical discharge of the fluid imbibed, with no augmentation of the proper functions of the kidneys, as respects the previous condition of the blood-vessels. But it is not perhaps unphilosophical to give hydropathists the benefit of supposing that water drinking may do indirectly what it does not appear to do directly: by its diluting power may it not destroy the influence of any mischievous constituent of the blood, the excess of dilution being immediately repaired by the removal of the water through the kidneys, in company with the deleterious matter dissolved in it? This view might be admitted, if it could be shown practically that drinking water has the same effect on disease as taking diuretics.

The purgative action of hydropathy is less equivocal. It frequently happens, in cases of constipation, that after a few days' or weeks' use of its appliances, the patient is attacked with diarrhœa. This is sometimes troublesome, but we believe seldom dangerous. On its subsiding, the bowels are said to have generally acquired a regular and healthy action, which is thenceforward maintained by persevering in the drinking, bathing, etc. In other cases, a regular action of the bowels comes on in a gradual manner, without the occurrence of diarrhœa, the treatment appearing to influence the bowels through its action on the system at large. In others, and every one has seen examples of this, the mere drinking of a few glasses of water before breakfast is represented as a purgative that may be relied on. In these the daily dose is regulated according to circumstances, being increased when signs of torpidity are observed. We are ourselves acquainted with some persons who regulate this function as accurately by water drinking, as they formerly did by medicinal aperients. There are cases, again, in which the sitz bath, or other external applications of cold water, produce a purgative effect.

It may be asked, Is not this effect too uniform for the purpose of the practical physician? Does it not often result from the mere percolation of water through the mucous lining of the intestinal canal? Is it not, therefore, a mere pouring out of what has been swallowed? Is it not clearly inadequate to excite the particular action of the liver, the pancreas, the lower or upper portion of the intestinal tube? Is it not necessary that we should be able to act on these parts separately, for the effectual cure of disease? These questions, important as they appear, may with equal justice be asked as to the practical proceedings of our profession in general. It is true that, in theory, many nice distinctions are laid down respecting the peculiar operation, as to locality or otherwise, of different cathartics. But are these distinctions generally observed in practice? Did not Abernethy's page 72 contain the curative maxim for all cases? and were not his prescriptions almost always identical? Has not every respectable family doctor his "my pills," carefully prepared from the same ingredients for every difficulty in the bowels? Is not the black draught as universal a purgative as Priessnitz would make cold water? Are not all our moneyed dyspeptics and hypochondriac nabobs sent in a body to mineral springs, because they are purgative, without any preliminary investigation as to their action on the duodenum or the colon, the liver or the pancreas, or as to the expediency of such action in the individual case in question?

11. We observe, also, in the history of hydropathic practice, the development of a peculiar sedative or tranquilizing influence. It is well illustrated in the following passage from Mr. Mayo's preface:

"Through repeated attacks of a sort of rheumatism, my constitution appeared completely broken down. Already crippled in my limbs, *preserving what power of exertion I still retained only through the use of opium,* and my indisposition still increasing, I looked forward to being, before long, worn out with suffering—as to death as a release. I could not bear the fatigue of a land journey, or I should have gone at once to Graefenberg; but Coblentz and Boppard might be reached from London by water—so I went to Marienburg in June, 1842. On arriving there, I was placed on a routine system of sweating and bathing. The immediate effect on my health was strikingly beneficial, *and in a week I was able to relinquish the use of opium.* The rheumatism did not, however, give way proportionably to my general improvement. The pains of the joints were, indeed, heightened."—(p. 1.)

This was a painfully severe case, one in which every conceivable remedy had been previously tried, not excepting repeated change of air, the Bath waters, etc.; yet nothing had succeeded in relieving the system from the necessity of constantly using opium. A "routine system of sweating and bathing" was applied, and in a week the patient was able to relinquish his doses of opium, notwithstanding that the rheumatism did not give way; indeed, the pains in the joints increased. How is this to be explained? Only by supposing that, independent of any curative influence over the actual disease, the water-cure exercised some sort of sedative action on the system at large. Similar instances are said to be familiar at hydropathic establishments. If these accounts may be depended on, hydropathy would appear to contain, in its armamentarium, even an anodyne, and one of great power. Every practitioner knows the difficulty presented in the treatment of chronic cases, by morbid irritability, and painful nervous sensations, which are not only intolerable to the patient himself, but most prejudicial to his recovery; and which can only be relieved, from time to time, by repeated and gradually augmented doses of a drug, whose own effects are almost as pernicious as the symptoms it is used to palliate. This is one instance of a predicament in which the physician is not infrequently placed, when he has most gravely to consider whether there is most mischief in the disease to be combated, or in the only remedy by which it can be encountered. If "a routine system of sweating and bathing" affords a means of extrication from the present instance of this difficulty, this is a strong reason why it should not continue to be obstinately excluded from the well-fenced pale of the medical profession.

12. In addition to the effects already considered, and which have occupied as much as can be spared of our space, the water-cure pretends to the possession of other important powers. Thus, it is said to be a *stomachic*, since it almost invariably increases the appetite. It is a local *calefacient*, in the application of the wet cloth covered by the dry one. It is a *derivative*—cold friction at one part, by exciting increased action there, producing corresponding diminution elsewhere. It is a local as well as general *counter-irritant*, the compress frequently acting, if not like a blister, at least like a mustard poultice. It is essentially *alterative* in the continued removal of old matter by sweating, and its renewal as shown in the maintenance of the same weight.

13. Lastly, our subject brings us to make a few remarks on *medical habits* in reference to chronic cases. In such cases, we have only commenced the treatment, when we have removed the

immediate symptoms; the real difficulty consists in preventing their recurrence.

Accordingly, the patient quits his physician with ample instructions for his future guidance, and with most impressive warnings as to perseverance in their observance. What are these instructions, and to what habits do they lead? Let us take a case of "biliousness," or chronic dyspepsia, and briefly trace the history of its "legitimate" treatment, according to the heroic school of London.

In addition to constipation, the patient, we shall suppose, is affected with acidity, deficient or depraved appetite, foul tongue, oppression after meals, susceptibility to cold, debility, headache, despondency, irritability of temper, inconstancy of purpose, hopelessness of relief, with divers local grievances. A few brisk cathartic doses, combined with mutton diet and a gentle stimulant, empty the bowels, and carry off most of the attendant ills. By continuing this plan for a short time, the patient is what is medically termed cured; but, for future protection, he is furnished with a prescription — say of aloes, colocynth, and calomel, or some such compound, to take *pro re nata;* another of senna and salts to take less frequently, as more urgent symptoms require; a third of calumba, gentian, or cinchona, to take at noon with a glass of sherry. He is told to live on boiled mutton, rice, and dry bread, avoiding fruit and vegetables.

What future, as respects health, has such a person before him? As long as he lives he will be a martyr to the disease, probably in an increasing degree; he must abandon all hope of the action of the bowels ever resuming its normal state; his general strength will gradually diminish; his nervous system will become more and more irritable; his whole comfort and enjoyment will be sacrificed in order to empty the alimentary canal; he will become one of the most pitiable of all sufferers, a "person living by rule;" his health will be supported, as one of our witty doctors remarks, like a shuttlecock between two battledoors, by the alternate impulse of senna and sherry, of calomel and coffee, of jalap and gentian. As long as these instruments are so directed, that their respective influences succeed each other in compensating proportion, all seems, for the time, smooth; but let either overdo or underdo the mark, and every thing breaks down. The game must then be commenced anew, to be continued as long as feather and cork resist the tendency which it has to knock them to pieces.

This is scarcely a caricatured picture of the discipline to which dyspeptic patients are often forced to submit. Every body's experience must furnish abundant proof that the illustration is too close to nature. It is in the latter stages of these affections, when the patients have long been under the influence of therapeutic means, that Priessnitz pronounces them "drug diseases." If, by this term, he means that drugs constitute the whole disease, then he is no doubt wrong; yet, in one point of view, he is right. The original complaint for which the drugs were administered might, very probably, have been one requiring some artificial remedy, and which would have induced more serious consequences, had not some such remedy been employed. But it is quite possible that a persevering use of such remedies may create a train of symptoms, in addition to those which existed before, and induce such a host of wants as may constitute a prominent feature of the case, by the time it is submitted to the curative process of such a practitioner as Priessnitz; therefore his term, drug disease, may not be altogether inapplicable.

But what is often the result of placing the cases now under consideration in a hydropathic establishment? Precisely such as might be expected from the abandonment of a pernicious custom, and the adoption, at the same time, of a more natural mode of life, with healthier and hardier habits; and with the additional mental stimulus of cheerfulness, of faith and hope in the new system, and of unbounded confidence in the new doctor. It is accordingly the general report that, in a large proportion of such cases, the patients are enabled immediately to discontinue the use of purgative medicines; they can bear a mixed animal and vegetable diet, in the ordinary proportion; a regular action of the bowels is shortly acquired, and no further stimulant or pharmaceutical tonic is necessary. When they quit the establishment, formal and complex means being no longer required, we are assured that they are able, for a time, at least, to maintain the ground gained, simply by common-sense diet, drinking a few glasses of water in the morning, taking a daily cold bath, and persevering in their habitual exercise. The country rings with such accounts as these; if they are correct, undoubtedly the patients are in a fair way of recovering their lost health and strength, and are pursuing, subsequently to systematic treatment, a much more rational and scientific course of medical habits, than that enjoined to the dyspeptic disciple of medical orthodoxy.

The questions with which we set out, may now be hypothetically answered: they were, "Does hydropathy furnish the physician with instruments which he, as a skillful workman, can undertake to employ? Does it contain, among its various machinery, any really therapeutic means, any properties capable of carrying out the indications which we regard as palpable in many diseases?" These questions, we think, may be allowed to have been answered in the affirmative, if we may depend on the results of our own limited experience; they must be allowed to be so answered, and unequivocally, if we may admit as perfectly trustworthy the accounts published by the hydropathists themselves, and by those who have subjected themselves to the treatment. On another occasion we may, perhaps, endeavor to sift this evidence in a more rigid manner, in order to ascertain with certainty what in it is true, what false, what doubtful, and what inapplicable. But in any inquiry we may institute, we must continue to examine the water-cure relatively to other modes of practice; this is the only method of arriving at an estimate of its actual value to the practical physician. The imperfections which it shares in common with ordinary treatment, and which are inseparable from all human performances, may be left entirely out of sight; to dwell on them would be uselessly to encumber the question, like inserting a crowd of corresponding items upon both sides of an equation. The philosopher's duty is to remove such superfluities, in order that the real problem may appear in a just and intelligible form.

In conclusion, we will venture to place on record the following, as among the more important impressions which have remained on our mind after a careful examination of the whole subject.

1. We should be glad to see Dr. Currie's practice revived (for the sake of experiment, at least), in all its boldness, for the suppression of the general febrile paroxysm. On carefully looking over the evidence published by Dr. Currie and his contemporaries, it is impossible to deny that they attained a larger amount of success in treating fever by water, than other practitioners have done by other means. We have already pointed out how their practice has been misunderstood by modern writers. But, while we regard this practice as well adapted for treating general fever, we find no proof that it is competent to meet the dangerous local complications with which fever is so often accompanied. These complications may reasonably be expected less frequently, when

the early treatment of fever is rendered more efficacious. But when they do occur, we find nothing in hydropathic writers to show that lancets, leeches, etc., can be dispensed with.

2. In a large proportion of cases of gout and rheumatism, the water-cure seems to be extremely efficacious. After the evidence in its favor, accessible to every body, we think medical men can hardly be justified in omitting—in a certain proportion of cases, at least—a full trial of it. No evidence exists of any special risk from the water practice in such cases.

3. In that very large class of cases of complex disease, usually known under the name of chronic dyspepsia, in which other modes of treatment have failed, or been only partially successful, the practice of Priessnitz is well deserving of trial.

4. In many chronic nervous affections and general debility, we should anticipate great benefits from this system.

5. In chronic diarrhœa, dysentery, and hemorrhoids, the sitz bath appears to be frequently an effectual remedy.

6. We find nothing to forbid a cautious use of drugs in combination with hydropathic measures. On the contrary, we are convinced that a judicious combination of the two is the best means of obtaining the full benefit of each. The water-cure contains no substitute for the lancet, active purging, and many other means necessary for the relief of sudden and dangerous local maladies. The banishment of drugs from his practice was necessary, and perhaps natural, on the part of Priessnitz; the like proceeding on the part of qualified medical men superintending water establishments in this country, evinces ignorance or charlatanry—or both.

7. With careful and discreet management, in the hands of a properly qualified medical practitioner, the water-cure is very rarely attended with danger.

8. Many of the principal advantages of hydropathy may be obtained in a private residence, with the assistance of ordinary movable baths. Therefore, it can easily be brought under the direction of the regular medical practitioner.

9. In many cases, however, it is evident that what may be termed the mere *accessories* of the water-cure, are of extreme importance in bringing about a favorable result; and these accessories are frequently not available—or available in a very inferior degree—in ordinary practice. Among the more important of these accessories we may mention the following as having relation

to most of the chronic cases treated in hydropathic establishments: 1. Relief from mental labors of exhausting or irritating kind, from the anxieties and responsibilities of business, from domestic irritations of various kinds, from mental inaction or ennui, etc.; 2. Change of locality, air, scene, society, diet, etc.; 3. The fresh mental stimulus involved in the almost constant occupation of the patient's time in the performance of the numerous and various dabblings, paddlings, sweatings, washings, drinkings, rubbings, etc., imposed by the water treatment; 4. The frequent and regular bodily exercise taken in the open air, or within doors; 5. The powerful mental stimulus supplied by the confidence generally reposed by the patients in the means employed, and by the consequent hope, alacrity, cheerfulness, etc.; 6. The total abandonment of vinous and other stimulants, and drugs, all of which have, in a large proportion of cases, been tried and found not only useless, but probably productive of disadvantage.

10. A certain and not inconsiderable portion of the benefits derived from hydropathic establishments are, however, attainable without them, by other means, as by traveling, etc., etc. For example, we suspect that many of the most striking results witnessed in such establishments, as in the case of Sir Edward Bulwer Lytton, or Mr. Lane, would have probably been obtained, if the patients had chosen to hire themselves, and had worked as agricultural laborers, in a dry, healthy district, and had lived on agricultural fare, sufficiently nutritious in quantity and kind, for a sufficient length of time.

11. Notwithstanding the success of the founder of hydropathy, its practice by non-professional persons can neither be fully advantageous nor safe. At the same time, it is true that very little experience is necessary to enable an educated medical man to acquire sufficient insight into it for purposes of practice. Many of the best hydropathic physicians have, in the first instance, devoted very few weeks to studying the subject in Germany.

12. Many advantages would result from the subject being taken up by the medical profession. The evils and dangers of quackery would at once be removed from it. Its real merits would soon be known. The tonic portion of its measures might then be employed in conjunction with special remedies of more activity, which, no doubt, would often prove exceedingly beneficial.

13. The benefits ascribed to hydropathy, but arising indirectly from the abandonment of drugs, vinous and other stimulants, etc., may certainly be obtained without sending patients to Graefenberg.

14. Finally, it must always be remembered that the distinction between quacks and respectable practitioners is one, not so much of remedies used, as of skill and honesty in using them. Therefore, let our orthodox brethren be especially anxious to establish and to widen, as far as possible, this distinction between themselves and all spurious pretenders. "*Artem medicam denique videmus, si à naturali philosophia destituatur, empiricorum praxi haud multum præstare. Medicina in philosophia non fundata, res infirma est.*"

CHAPTER IV.

THEORY OF HYDROPATHY—DR. BILLING'S THEORY OF DISEASE.*

Dr. Billing's First Principles of Medicine.—Liebig and Billing.—All Diseases caused by impressions made on the Nervous System.—Congestion and Inflammation.—Tonicity.—The living Body composed of Capillary Vessels.—Functions and Offices of these Vessels.—Action of the Arteries.—Momentum of Blood in inflamed Parts.—Difference between Congestion and Inflammation.—How morbid Growths are Formed.—Irritation.—Nervous Disorders.—There is properly but one Disease and one Cure.—Worms in the Bowels.—The inefficiency of Drugs has multiplied their Number.—The active Bleeding and various Medicines.—Weakness or exhausted Nervous Energy the cause of all Disease.—Illustration of the Hydropathic Treatment.—Operation of Cold Water and Cold Air.—The Cold or Tonic Treatment in Consumption.—The true Principle of treating this Disease.—Various medical Hobbies point to the same End.—Not a single Drug in the whole range of the Pharmacopœia that can be relied on.—Cold Water as a means of unloading and constringing the Capillaries.—Value of cold Applications to the Head.—The general applicability of the Hydropathic Treatment.—Testimony of Analogy and Experience.—Mischief of Drugs.—A Fatal Case from Mercury.—Strychnine and its Effects.—A case of Paralysis.—Hydropathy may be made to do Harm.—Opium and Mercury.—Their Effects.—The Cold Bath and Sweating.—The sudden checking of Perspiration a chimerical Danger.—Facts in Proof of this Statement.

The "First Principles of Medicine," by Dr. Billing, is a work too well known, and too universally esteemed, to need any encomium from me. For years no medical work has issued from the press, which was received by medical critics and the medical profession at large with such universal approbation as this of Dr. Billing. In every medical library it took its place at once, as a

* From Dr. Edward Johnson's "Hydropathy."

standard work, and remains so to the present hour. Though essentially theoretical, yet its theories are every where so completely supported by multiplied practical facts and illustrations—which its author's position as a senior physician to the London Hospital enabled him to accumulate—and the amount of clinical information with which it abounds is so great, the simplicity of its style so felicitous, while the common sense plainness with which the questions are argued is so strong and convincing, that its hypotheses have almost the force of facts.

It will be observed how beautifully Liebig's theory of life (as far as it regards morbid actions), and Billing's theory of disease, reciprocally support *each other,* and *both* the principles of the water-cure.

Dr. Billing's theory is, that "*all*" diseases are caused by impressions made on the nervous centres or their nerves, by which the nervous *influence* (whatever it be) is exhausted or morbidly diminished. That the capillary blood-vessels, which (in health) are always held in a state of *semi-contraction* (*tone*) by virtue of this nervous influence shed upon them by the nerves, become *relaxed and weakened*—(Liebig's diminution of *vital resistance*)—having their *diameters enlarged,* whenever the exhausted nerves fail in supplying them with the quantity of nervous influence necessary to preserve their tone, or state of *semi-contraction upon their contents.* That the weakened, relaxed, and *enlarged* capillaries now admit a *larger* current of blood, whose motion through them becomes *slower.* That they are, in fact, in a state of congestion. And that altered function or functional disease is the result of this altered condition of the capillaries, and altered size and altered velocity of the stream of blood which they carry. When this congestion takes place in the veins, it constitutes simple congestion—when in the arteries, it is accompanied by *degeneration of the arterial coats*—and now takes the name of *inflammation.* This degeneration of the coats of the inflamed arteries is Liebig's *excessive* action of the destructive force of oxygen—the enlarged arteries *now* containing an *excessive* quantity of oxydized blood, while the *resistance* opposed to its influence is (as we have just seen) *diminished.* This degeneration does *not* take place in the veins, observes Dr. Billing. No—because the veins do *not* contain *oxydized* blood.

Man is almost *entirely composed* of capillary vessels. His body may be compared to a sack stuffed with hair, every hair being a tube of a *determinate diameter* (which particular diameter is necessary to the condition of health), and carrying a stream of fluid. which stream must also be of a determinate size. And this bundle of capillary or hair-like tubes is every where permeated by nervous filaments or threads, which shed upon them their electroid influence, whose office it is to *preserve their tone or necessary diameter*—upon the preservation of which their healty functions depend. When any cause deprives them of a due supply of the electroid or nervous influence, by exhausting the nervous system or any part of it, the healthy diameter is lost, becoming *larger*, and they now admit *too large a current* of fluid, and the velocity of its fluxion is *retarded*, producing congestion.

When any cause, as the exhibition of stimulants, elicits from the nerves too great a quantity of nervous influence, *then also* the healthy diameter is lost, but in a contrary direction. The diameter now becomes *too small*—the vessels *contract* too much—and the size of the current of fluid is now too much diminished. This illustration will, I trust, enable the unprofessional reader clearly to understand Dr. Billing's beautiful theory of disease.

Inflammation, then, consists of weakened, relaxed, enlarged arterial capillaries, admitting a too large current of blood, whose progress through them is also retarded, giving rise to congestion or engorgement, degeneration of their coats, and *consequent alteration of their secretions.*

"All the business," says Dr. Billing, "of constant support, and renewal of parts, and supply of secretions, as the growth or repair of bone, muscle, membrane, and other structures, the formation of bile, saliva, mucus, and other secretions, is carried on by the extreme minute branches of the blood-vessels; and while these preserve their proper size and tone, all goes on well; when their action is deranged, disease commences, often prefaced by pain, or other disorders of the nerves." "Some capillaries are too small to admit many of the red particles (oxydized blood-globules), unless when they are *enlarged* by inflammation, as in the eye, which, when inflamed, changes from white to red; besides that, even the red capillaries are so minute, that they are not visible individually to the naked eye, till *enlarged* by inflammation." "During health the capillary arteries go on with their work of nutrition and secretion, the muscles are fed, the mucous surfaces are lubricated just enough to prevent any sensation from the substances which pass along them, the serous surfaces are made sufficiently moist to slide upon each other without sensation, and the skin is kept soft by an insensible vapor. All this time there is another process going on also, which is the removal of superfluous matter by the absorbents: if it were not for these, there would be inconvenient accumulation of what is deposited by the arteries."

"The deposit or precipitation of solid matter by the arteries is not difficult to be understood; and we can, by reference to *chemical action*, account for the removal also of solids; for solids become fluid or gaseous, by what is called spontaneous decomposition" (Liebig calls it *transformation of tissues* by the chemical action of oxygen), "and thus removable by absorbents."

"The action of arteries also is *acknowledged* to be contraction, whether considered muscular or not; but there is some difference of opinion as to the degree of action of the arteries in inflamed parts. It is very common to say, that in inflammation there is an increase of arterial action; but a consideration of the phenomena and of the nature of arterial action will show that in INFLAMED PARTS the CAPILLARY ARTERIES ARE WEAKER in their action; that there is DIMINISHED ARTERIAL ACTION, for the action of arteries is *contraction*. Now the arteries in inflamed parts are *evidently larger* than before—less contracted—that is, acting less."

"It is the opinion of some persons, even at the present day, that the motion of the blood is accelerated in inflamed parts; though the experiments of Parry and others prove the *contrary* to be the case, as *follows* from the capillary arteries being *enlarged*; inasmuch as where fluid passes through a given space, the current beyond that will be slower in proportion to the wideness of the channel, as in a wide part of a river, where the current becomes slower; and the same may be observed by passing water, mixed with grains of amber, through a glass tube with a bulbous enlargement in the middle; the current will slacken in the bulb, and resume its velocity beyond it."

"The difference between congestion and inflammation is, that in congestion there is merely distension of the vessels; in inflammation there is, in addition, alteration of tissue—actual deterioration, more or less, of the structure of the capillaries. * * * * The fault commences in the tissue. As soon as a want of that harmony between the nerves and the capillaries, which is necessary to organization, takes place, their fine tissue begins to compose" (the action of oxygen becomes, according to Liebig, *greater* than the resistance of the vital force—the same sense expressed in different language), "the particles which were held together by this inscrutable agency begin to be precipitated from one another, etc., etc."

"When accidental mechanical injury, or other cause, changes the action of the capillaries, either by a direct impression on themselves, or by primarily injuring their nerves, *the derangement of their action is the commencement* of disease—secretions become altered, checked, or profuse nutrition is either diminished so as to produce emaciation, or there is an excessive deposition—vapory exhalations are diminished to dryness, or increased to fluid—bony matter is deposited in wrong places—or albuminous, fatty, or other particles, so as to constitute tumors—the nerves of parts become morbidly sensible, so as to derange the functions of those parts—portions, on losing their vitality, undergo spontaneous decomposition (destructive action of oxygen, either owing to an unwonted quantity of oxydized blood being carried to the part, or from the diminished resistance of the vital force), and are removed by the absorbents."

"Irritation, continued excitation of the nerves of a healthy part, as just shown, at last produces inflammation, by exhausting that nervous influence which gives the capillaries power; they thus become weakened, allow of over-distension, and the part is in the state of inflammation or congestion." "Thus, in a part inflamed, there is diminution of organic action (contraction), in consequence of which the blood is admitted in excess. As long as the capillaries are supplied with nervous influence, as long as they possess perfect organic action (contraction), they *preserve a due size;* when they lose it, either from the influence not being supplied from the nervous system, or are robbed of it by heat, electricity, cantharides, *or any other cause,* they give way, and admit more blood than before."

Having given this explanation of the nature of inflammation (which is also maintained by many other very able writers, as Professor Macartney, I think, and several others, and proved by the microscopic observations of German experimentalists), he proceeds to show that fever, and that class of diseases called neuroses, or nervous disorders, as chorea, hysteria, tetanus, epilepsy, etc.—all those diseases which are characterized by irritation or morbid sensibility—consist in inflammation, that is, a relaxed, enlarged, and congested condition of the capillary arteries of the nerves—in a word, inflammation of the nerves. Indeed, if Dr. Billing be right in his assertion (and I see not how it can possibly be refuted), that *all diseases have exhausted nervous influence* for their cause, then it follows that all diseases whatever must consist essentially in weakened, enlarged, and congested capillaries, since the relaxation of the capillaries must be the first effect which is produced by exhausting that influence which alone preserves to them their normal size or diameter.

Such being the *one* proximate cause or essential nature of *all* disease, the principal of cure is *one* also. Thus there is (properly) but *one* disease, and *one* cure.

The proximate cause is relaxation and enlargement of the capillaries—the indication of cure, therefore, is to *constringe the capillaries*, to cause them to *contract and resume* their healthy dimensions.

Dr. Billing having established this position by a multitude of illustrations and practical facts well known to medical men, together with illustrative cases of particular diseases, as rheumatism, palsy, dropsy, consumption, skin diseases, hysteria, nervous affections, locked-jaw, gout, etc., etc., then proceeds to show that all medicines, numerous as they are, together with bleeding, produce their good effects on disease *by* the power, and *in proportion* to the power, which they possess, directly or indirectly, of causing the *relaxed* capillaries to *contract and resume* their healthy dimensions.

He reduces all medicines whatever to no more than *four*—sedatives, tonics, narcotics, stimulants.

Sedatives, direct and indirect, among which are included purgatives, emetics, and bleeding, are such as "diminish the action of the heart and other organs, by repressing the nervous influence," thus lessening the velocity with which the capillaries are supplied with blood by the injecting force of the heart; and such as, by *emptying* the capillaries, facilitate their contraction by removing or lessening the resistance offered to their contracting sides by the contained blood.

Tonics are such as, being circulated *in* the blood *through* the capillaries, have the direct effect of constringing them, or causing them to contract upon their contents, and thus to force or *squeeze* the fluid onward.

Stimulants are such as elicit from the nerves a temporary, forced, and more than ordinary quantity of nervous influence, causing a corresponding degree of capillary contraction. But the effect of these last remedies is but temporary, since all forced excitement of the nervous centres must ever be followed by a corresponding degree of exhaustion.

Narcotics are such as, by dulling the sensibility of the nervous system, procure sleep, and thus afford an opportunity to the inherent curative power, or vis medicatrix naturæ, to restore the tone, or normal degree of contraction, of the capillaries.

Thus, then, however numerous be the *forms or symptoms* of disease, there is, de facto, but *one disease.* And, however numerous may be the means and appliances of the healing art, there is in fact but *one intention* to be fulfilled—the restoration of the capillaries to their normal dimensions by *constringing their coats.*

I was once asked by a physician, for whose talents I entertain the highest respect, how I reconciled with this theory *that disease* called worms in the bowels. But to this I replied, that a worm in the bowels, UNTIL IT HAS PRODUCED IRRITATION, is no more a disease than a fly on the hand, or a flea on the back—and when that irritation has been produced, then it is that IRRITATION which constitutes the disease, of which the worm was the REMOTE CAUSE, as a musquito is the remote cause of the inflammation which its bite produces; and we have already seen that irritation (which Dr. Billing with much more propriety calls morbid sensibility) consists in inflammation of the capillaries of the nerves. But no one would think of calling a musquito a *disease!*

It is the *inefficiency* of drugs which has multiplied their number. Two, or two thousand, are required, because there is *not one* which can be depended on. If *one* could be discovered which would always effectually produce the necessary degree of *capillary contraction, then* that *one* would be *sufficient.*

"In some cases of disease," says Dr. Billing, "when the secretions of the skin and kidneys are deficient, we renew them by bleeding, digitalis, antimony, etc., which lower the force of the pulse, thereby *diminishing the distension of the capillaries,* in conformity with the above statement."

"Medicines, such as mercury, iodine, etc., have an effect on the arteries themselves, directly or through the nerves, so as to *make the inflamed capillaries* CONTRACT independently of the considera-tion of the vis à tergo (state of the heart's action), or quantity of circulating fluid."

"Inflammation is always the *same debility* of capillaries."

"We see that solutions of metallic salts, such as nitrate of silver, tartar emetic, acetate of lead, bichloride of mercury, etc., and some acrid vegetables, such as mezereon, etc., act on the capillaries as ASTRINGENTS."

"We know that substances applied to the primæ viæ, or skin, are absorbed and carried into the circulation, and we judge that in this way these metallic salts, oxydes, etc., are carried to the capillaries of diseased parts, and strengthen and cure."

"All organic action is contraction." All organic or animal strength, therefore, depends upon the power of the different parts of the body to contract. And, for the same reason, all animal weakness depends upon a loss, more or less, of the power of contraction. And again, for the same reason, all remedies which strengthen can only do so by increasing the power of contraction.*

"Mercury and iodine remove morbid growths by starving them, which they effect by contracting the capillaries."

"I therefore consider mercury neither stimulant nor sedative, but tonic; that is, by its specific action on the capillaries, whether directly on their tissue, or through the medium of their nerves, it causes them to contract."

"When introduced into the system, it (mercury) circulates through the capillaries, and gives them tone to contract. Liquor arsenicalis (solution of arsenic), nitrate of silver, the sulphates of copper and iron, mezereon, dulcamara, calchicum, etc., have a similar action. This is also the rationale of the mode of operation of the so-called alteratives, and of what is called stimulating the secretions of the internal organs. When their capillaries are weak, they have their tone restored by mercury, and the secretions are thus renewed; but it should not be forgotten that mercury, like some other tonics, in excess becomes poisonous, and may cause inflammation in other parts, as it does in the gums, on the principle adduced before, that one degree of contraction of the capillaries is

* See this same argument enforced under the head of contracting, in my work on "Life, Health, and Disease."

necessary to reduce inflammation, while a still further degree will stop nutrition and bring on wasting and disease."

"And to this influence (constringing the capillaries) I attribute the universal efficacy of antimony as an antiphlogistic remedy, it being doubly valuable in acute cases, from its sedative effects on the heart and pulse, combined with its locally *tonic or astringent effects on the capillaries* of inflamed or congested parts, as well as on those of all the secreting structures.

"I think from the various statements already made, it may be deduced, that the diseases of morbid sensibility, were it proved that they depend upon inflammation" (and Dr. Billing has endeavored to show that they *do*), "*are not curable by common depletion:* the medullary tissue is too fine to be affected by the force of the circulation, or relieved by taking off the vis à tergo, by bleeding, digitalis, etc. ; hence neuralgia, tetanus, hydrophobia, chorea, hysteria, etc., must be reached through the circulation, by what have been called tonics, iron, bark, arsenic, etc."—and we have seen that these operate only by *constringing the capillaries.*

"Inflammation is that which destroys the life of the part, whereupon the separation of the dead portion takes place :" this is nothing more than Liebig's theory of the destructive force of oxygen, told in other and more general terms.

But it is not necessary further to multiply quotations from Dr. Billing's first principles. The whole scope and tendency of that work is to prove the position that there is but *one* immediate cause of disease, viz., *weakness*, or exhausted nervous energy—*but one disease*, viz., a *relaxed* and *congested condition of the vital capillaries*—and *but one remedy*, viz., the restoration of the capillaries to their normal or natural dimensions.

It is true Dr. Billing admits of *four* different kinds of remedies, but we have already seen that these are but four different instruments for enabling us to produce one grand effect, and this is, in every case, the restoration of the capillaries to their healthy size. Even narcotics, given to procure sleep, would be of but little service if they did not more than this; for the pain or other disease would return on waking. But they do, indirectly, more than this; for, by procuring sleep, they give time and opportunity to the inherent powers of the system to restore the capillaries to their healthy standard degree of semi-contraction—in one word, to recover their tone.

Now how does all this bear upon the hydropathic treatment of disease? In what manner does Dr. Billing's theory of disease support, and justify, and recommend that treatment? It bears upon it immediately, and in the strongest and most conclusive manner. According to Dr. Billing's theory, the great object is, in all cases, to unload the engorged capillaries, and to constringe their coats. What are the two main features of the hydropathic treatment? Profuse sweating, and the application (partial or general, as circumstances may require) of cold—that is, profuse sweating to unload the capillaries, and the application of cold to constringe their coats; for I suppose it will not be denied by any one for a moment, that cold possesses this power of constringing the living fibre in a most remarkable degree. Both surgery and medicine are perpetually compelled to resort to cold water and even ice for this express purpose, as, for instance, in hæmorrhages, the reduction of strangulated hernia, etc. The efficacy of cold wet cloths, applied either in the inside of the thighs, or to the back, in bleeding from the nose, is sufficiently well known, and even proverbial. That feeling of creeping, chilliness, and even shivering, which is produced by the application of cold, is a very common and well-marked proof of the very powerful influence of cold in constringing the capillary vessels.

The mode of operation of the hydropathic treatment may be illustrated by what is done in the dropsy of the belly. The surgeon first *taps the belly,* and draws off the water. *Then* he applies around it a bandage, in order to support its loose and flaccid sides, and assist it in *recovering its natural dimensions.* This is precisely what the hydropathic treatment does in ordinary diseases —inflammations, fevers, the neuroses, etc., etc.,—it *taps the capillaries* (by sweating), and then *supports and constringes their sides,* by the cold bath.

Dr. Billing himself seems fully aware of the value of cold water and cold air, as a remedy. At page 23, after describing inflammation to consist of weakened, relaxed, and congested capillaries, he says: "The way to diminish the inflammation is by increasing the action (contraction) of the arteries, as by cold or astringents, which make the arteries contract, that is, increase their action."

"When the congestion or inflammation subsides without solution of continuity, it is called resolution; and it is very intelligible how cold and astringents promote this desirable termination." Again:

"A still farther proof that they (the capillaries) are in a state of morbid congestion, is the effect of cold to the loins, in renewing the secretions; AND THE CONSTRINGING EFFECT OF COLD WATER, or cool air, in promoting the secretion of insensible perspiration, and thereby softening the congested skin, in scarlatina."

"By studying the operations of nature,* we are led to imitate by analogy. Independently of the regulation of temperature, the usual benefit derived from a poultice is that of preventing premature scabbing, by the soft moisture assisting the pus to protect the granulations. The German water-dressing has much the advantage over the poultice." And again: "Cold will cause the vessels to shrink." The effect of cold water in constringing the capillaries, that is, in causing them to shrink, may at any time be witnessed by plunging the hand, when hot, into cold water. When a person has been heated by exercise, the veins on the back of the hand will be observed, in most persons, to be very enlarged: and in delicate, thin, and weakly persons, they are almost always so toward evening. Whenever these veins are in this condition, if the hand be plunged into cold water, and held there for a short time, they will be found greatly diminished in size when the hand is withdrawn.

"But often," says Dr. Billing, "the case is more obstinate, and a torpid, congested, or perhaps we should say subacutely inflamed state of the liver, requires not merely repeated doses of calomel or other materials, but leeches and poultices, or cold wet cloths, to the epigastrium" (region of stomach). And here, in a note, he observes, "the application of cold is, I think, not sufficiently often used in inflammation of the viscera of the chest and abdomen when the surface becomes decidedly hot."

Speaking of consumption, he says: "Some years ago, a gentleman of the name of Stewart adopted a rational mode of treatment, with which he had considerable success; but, because he could not work miracles, his plan was unjustly depreciated. His method was entirely tonic, and especially the cautious use of cold and tepid ablutions of the skin—a modification of cold bathing—a remedy that is found so universally beneficial in promoting the resolution of strumous (scrofulous) tumors.

* It is this "*studying the operations of nature*" to which the late Sir A. Cooper was so largely indebted for his extraordinary success in *surgical* practice.

"One thing of which I am convinced is, that the true principle of treating consumption is to support the patient's strength to the utmost"—and it must be remembered that the grand aim and principal effect of the water-cure is to strengthen the system, thereby giving the inherent curative power the fairest opportunity of doing its own work. .

Again: "Schwann (Muller's Handbuch der Physiologie, Coblenz, 1833), by experiment on the mesenteric arteries of small living animals, has demonstrated that I was right as to the modus operandi of cold as a remedial agent in inflammation"—viz., that it acts by constringing the capillaries.

With regard to the oneness of the effect to be produced, in treating diseases, notwithstanding the hosts of different drugs and chemicals with which our national pharmacopœia groans, Dr. Billing has the following observations: "I have explained how some medicines become useful in such a variety of diseases as almost to realize the dreams of the ancients and alchemists respecting a panakeia, or an elixir vitæ; and thus why one empirical remedy, antimony, held the reins of the 'currus triumphalis' until superceded by the more modern blue pill. I have shown that tonics are not stimulants; and why they may be combined advantageously with sedatives, with stimulants, or with narcotics (the ultimate effect of all being the same); how stimulants are tonic; how sedatives are tonic; how narcotics are tonic. I have shown how every medical man has his hobby to carry him to the same point, which, though he thinks it very different from his neighbor's, is as like it as one four-legged jade is to another; how one man thinks he has made a discovery that he can cure cholera with sugar of lead, and that there is nothing equal to it; while tartar emetic, calomel, Epsom or Glauber's salts, or common salt, or mustard, or lemonade, or vinegar and water, etc., etc., will do the same thing; though none of them more quickly carry off the vomiting and purging than two of these hobbies in double harness—tartar emetic with some neutral salt, I care little which."

Thus, then, it will be perceived that the reason why we have such a multiplicity of effects to be produced, is because there is not one out of all our drugs which can be relied on, at all times, for producing the one effect desired. That one effect is the constringing of the capillaries to their normal diameters, when they have become weakened, enlarged, and congested—and in producing this effect cold water never fails.

These last observations of Dr. Billing (and indeed his whole theory) are a complete answer to those who object to the water-cure on account of its apparent oneness and simplicity, since he shows that there is but one proximate cause of all diseases, and that but one remedy is necessary; and that the great multitude of drugs has only arisen from the inefficiency of any one of them, at all times, to produce the desired effect. According to Dr. Billing, there is scarcely any one drug which would not alone be sufficient to cure almost any disease, provided that one could always be relied on to empty and constringe the capillaries. And he clearly states that different drugs are only so many different means by which different practitioners produce the same effects.

Now, then, if it be true that the one great effect to be brought about in the treatment of all diseases be to unload and constringe the capillaries, how can this be better achieved than by profuse perspiration and the cold bath? The hydropathic treatment, which unloads the capillaries by sweating, and constringes them by cold, is clearly an efficient substitute for bleeding, purging, vomiting, uva ursi, digitalis, antimony, mercury, arsenic, nitrate of silver, sulphate of copper, iodine, iron, and multitudes of other remedies, enumerated by Dr. Billing as being beneficial merely by their powers of unloading and constringing the capillaries.

"In fact," says Dr. Billing, "experience proves that cold to the head, with moderate saline and other sedative medicine, will cure typhus, or prevent the typhous state from occurring in synocha; whereas when wine, with or without opiates, is employed, the disease frequently proves fatal. I had one very useful opportunity of seeing the contrast of the different modes of practice during the fever which prevailed in Italy, 1817, the proportionate mortality being very much greater in a hospital where the stimulant practice prevailed, than in that under the direction of Dr. Aglietti, in Venice, who (I suppose out of compliment) called his manner of practice the English, consisting of contra-stimulants (sedative evacuants), antimony, salts, purgatives, etc., internally, with the external application of cold water and free ventilation."

Such are the opinions of Dr. Billing with regard to the nature of disease, and with regard also to the modus operandi of all medicines whatever, in curing it, viz., by emptying, constringing, and strengthening the weakened, relaxed, and gorged capillary arteries. And if these opinions be true, the hydropathic treatment is obviously and even glaringly a remedy of almost universal application—if not to cure, at least to relieve—since its two grand features are those of sweating, and then of constringing, strengthening, and giving tone to the whole capillary system. And yet, opposed as this treatment is, without consideration, by the great body of medical men, if I were to repeat all the laudations bestowed on Dr. Billing's book, both by the medical press and private individual practitioners, they would fill a volume.

But it requires very close attention, habits of reflection, and a perfect freedom from all prejudice, in order to discover how completely principles sometimes agree even where the practice is exceedingly different. And indeed to illustrate the truth is one of the objects of Dr. Billing's work—to show how the different hobbies of different medical men are all carrying their unconscious masters to one and the same point—capillary contraction. And when we recollect that all the functions of life are performed in and by these same capillaries, we ought not to be at all surprised to find that it is upon these that all causes of disease produce their first impressions; these are the organs whose actions first become deranged; and that it is upon these that all remedial agents must be made to operate, in the treatment and cure of all disorders.

Such are the views and opinions of Dr. Billing. And it must be remembered that Dr. Billing is no obscure physician—all theory and no practice—but that he has been for years, and is still, senior physician to one of the largest hospitals in England, viz., the London—enjoying a field for practical observation and experiment which can fall to the lot of but few.

I will make only one more quotation—its object is still farther to show that the simplicity and apparent oneness of the hydropathic treatment is no argument against it, disease itself being more simple and more unique than is generally supposed. Thus Dr. Billing cures ague, blue cholera, and influenza, on the same principles, and with the same remedies—Epsom salts, antimony, and sometimes bleeding. Yet there can scarcely be three diseases more apparently dissimilar—and certainly no three diseases can differ more as to severity and the degree of danger. "There is," says Dr. Billing, "but one simple fever, and which is exanthematous (eruptive), petechial, though the rash may never be sensibly developed, as in scarlatina maligna; and it is continued, synochous (synocha, συνεχω), whether with high or low pulse, high or low temperature; and that, when the sensorium is oppressed in addition, it is typhous." This whole passage is printed, in Dr. Billing's book, in italics. It is surprising to me how Dr. James Johnson could speak in such high terms of praise concerning Dr. Billing's views of disease, and of the modus operandi of all remedial treatment, and yet that he should write disparagingly concerning hydropathy, since the whole of Dr. Billing's work is, de facto, one long argument in its favor.

Thus I have shown that the principles of hydropathy are in strict harmony with the opinions held, and the doctrines publicly taught, by two of the most celebrated and scientific men (each in his own department), with regard to the nature of life, health, and disease, and the true end and object of all remedial treatment, viz., Liebig and Billing—the two Atridæ of medical science—the Agamemnon and Menelaus—the δυω κοσμητορε λαῶν—of the medical profession.

I will now quit the more particular arguments of science, and endeavor to show that all general reasoning—all analogy—all the deductions of experience—also unite to add their testimony to that already given.

With regard to any danger to be apprehended from the hydropathic treatment, it only differs from ordinary practice just thus much. In ordinary practice, even in the most skillful hands, there is always more or less danger in the administration of the most common and useful drugs, for all these are poisons of the most virulent kind, as mercury, arsenic, prussic acid, opium, oil of vitriol, aqua fortis, lunar caustic, iodyne, strychnine (nux vomica), copperas, etc., etc., all medicines daily and hourly administered internally, whereas in the practice of hydropathy there is never any danger at all—provided always it be practiced by competent persons.

It is evident to the most ordinary understanding that such virulent poisons as those mentioned above, and which are in hourly use, cannot be introduced into the human stomach, even in minute doses, without always doing a certain amount of mischief—and indeed this is admitted on all hands—and that even minute doses may, and often *do*, in delicate habits, or from some peculiar diathesis, produce very powerful and dangerous effects. A case in point occurred, some time since, in one of our hospitals. A woman had been taking mercury—and one day, while sitting up in bed, eating some broth, her head fell suddenly forward, and she died instantly. A post-mortem examination explained the mystery. The atlas—a pivot which supports the head, and on which it turns—had been eaten away by the mercury until it became too weak to support the weight of the head. It snapped while bending over her broth, the neck became bent double, and instant death ensued, the inevitable consequence of compression of the spinal cord by the doubling of the neck.

Strychnine, according to Andral, produces *softness of the brain.* A young lady, having paralysis of the lower extremities, after trying many remedies, was recommended by her physician to rub in strychnine. After a time she went to a watering place, and there died. Dr. Pereira, of the London Hospital, commenting on this case in his lectures, declared that he had no doubt that this young lady's death was hastened by the strychnine.

In a case of paralysis at the Dreadnought Hospital, strychnine was exhibited, at first in doses of one sixteenth of a grain three times a day, then one eighth, then one fourth, then one half, all without any *apparent* effect. But one night the surgeon was suddenly called to the man, who was said to be in a fit. It was a first attack of tetanus, or cramp. This first attack was almost succeeded by a second, which killed him. There can be no doubt that it was the strychnine which destroyed him.

That hydropathy can kill—and that it may kill, in the hands of the ignorant practitioner—is perfectly true. It would not be worth two straws if it could not. For that which, *when abused,* can do no harm, cannot be capable of much good when *properly used.* Such a remedy is mere "chip in porridge." But where hydropathy has destroyed a single victim, the practice of medicine has slain its tens of millions—a position so notoriously true that I scarcely think any medical man of character will be found to question it. And the danger to be dreaded from the use of deadly drugs is greatly augmented by the great diversity of opinions which are entertained as to the effects which they produce on the body, frequently causing one drug to be given with the view of producing two opposite effects.

In a very learned and laborious work published by Dr. Pereira, one of the physicians to the London Hospital, and chemical professor at that institution, entitled, "Elements of Materia Medica,' occur the following passages on the subjects of opium and mercury, two drugs more universally in use than any other two in the whole list. "Several physicians," says Dr. Pereira, "as Dr. John Murray, and Dr. Anthony Todd Thomson, consider opium to be primarily stimulant; some, as Drs. Cullen and Barbier, regard it as sedative" (that is, just the contrary to stimulant); "one, viz., Dr. Mayer, as both—that is, a stimulant to the nerves and circulatory system, but a sedative to the muscles and digestive organs; another, viz., Orfila, regards it as neither; while others, as Muller call it alterative." Now here are five different men holding no fewer than five different opinions with regard to the effects produced on the body by this deadly drug, opium. When these five physicians give opium, it is clear that they give it with the view of producing five different and contradictory effects!

But Dr. Pereira proceeds thus with regard to mercury: "Again, mercury is, by several writers, as Drs. Cullen, Young, Chapman, and Eberle, placed in the class of sialogogues; by many, as Drs. A. T. Thomson, Edwards, Vavasseur, Trouseau, and Pidoux, among excitants; by some, as Conradi, Bertele, and Horn, it is considered to be sedative; by one, Dr. Wilson Philip, to be stimulant in small doses, and sedative in large ones; by some, as Dr. John Murray, it is placed among tonics; by another, viz., Vogt, among the resolventia alterantia; by one, viz., Sundelin, among the liquefacients; by the followers of Broussais, as Begin, among revulsives; by the Italians, as Giaccomini, among contra-stimulants, or hyposthenics; by others, as Barbier, among the incertæ sedis, or those drugs whose modus operandi is not understood.

After reading such a statement as this, one can hardly be surprised that the word physician should have been defined to signify, "a man who puts drugs, of which he knows nothing, into a stomach of which he knows less."

With regard to any danger likely to result from going into the cold bath when covered with perspiration, such danger is perfectly chimerical, and a mere popular fallacy—contrary to all the deductions of science—contrary to all daily and hourly experience ever since the creation of the world, and for which no shadow of a physiological reason can be given; while all physiological reasoning goes directly to prove that it is safer to go into cold water when the temperature of the skin has been raised, than when it has not been raised; and that if there be danger at all, it is going into cold water without first raising the temperature—and in this there certainly is some danger. And of course it is with the elevated temperature that we have to deal in this argument, and not with the mere presence of perspiration on the external surface. For it certainly can be a matter of no importance whether the skin be covered with a certain quantity of that peculiar grease called perspiration, or whether it be covered with an equal amount of hog's lard or white paint. And it is quite evident, and all modern writers agree that it is so, that reaction (the great object to be attained) will be most certainly produced, and internal visceral congestion (the great evil to be avoided) will be most certainly prevented, by going into the water when the surface of the body is warm. And I need hardly observe, that the body is not made hotter in proportion to the profuseness of the perspiration, but that, on the contrary, it is cooler than before that effect is produced, for perspiration is a cooling process. So that it will not do to say, "that although it may be good to go into water when the body is moderately warm, it is nevertheless bad to do so when it is extremely hot." For when perspiration is present, it is never extremely hot.

As to the sudden checking of perspiration, this too is a chimerical danger. For the oozing of perspiration always subsides *of itself*, almost at the moment that the means which produced it are withdrawn. And the perspiration which is still visible on the body, is merely that which has been *already produced*, and left upon the skin, by an action of the vessels which has now already ceased. The perspiration which is now seen upon the body has no more connection with the system than so much oil or other greasy matters.

I say, too, that supposition of danger is contrary to all daily and hourly experience. For are not our out-of-door laborers, our wagoners, our sailors, our hay-makers, and all our farm servants, constantly exposed, while bathed in perspiration, to the effects of a natural cold shower bath, in the shape of rain, and that too with perfect impunity? Is it not the constant practice of boys to bathe in rivers, without thinking for a moment, or caring a straw, whether they be in a perspiration or not? Does the North American Indian, when traversing his hunting grounds, and when he finds his path obstructed by a river, ever pause for an instant to consider whether he be in a perspiration or not, before he plunges into the flood? But the Indian is used to it. To be sure he is, and it is to that very use and want to which he owes his great strength, activity, and unimpregnable health. And why should not Englishmen use and accustom themselves to the same thing? What is to prevent it? Why should it not be? I cannot even conceive a reason.

If there were peculiar danger in being caught in a shower while perspiring, every showery day would crowd our hospitals with its victims, and April would be the most deadly month in all the year. Nature has not adapted the inhabitants of the earth to the circumstances of the earth's surface so bunglingly. On the contrary, the nature of every living thing has been beneficially fitted to the nature of those circumstances among which it was destined to dwell; and had a shower of rain possessed such deadly properties, our heads would have been furnished with a natural umbrella to defend it from the rain, as our eyes are accommodated with natural curtains to defend them from the dust.

In an exceedingly clever pamphlet lately published by Mr. Jackson, entitled, "The Spleen a Permanent Placenta, the Placenta a Temporary Spleen," it has been reasoned out with the most beautiful precision and great force, that the spleno-hepatic vein (one of the large veins within the abdomen) is the propelling organ which drives the blood through the portal system of veins, and circulates it through the liver; and that it is congestion in this vein which is frequently the cause of a great number of diseases (epilepsy among others). If these views be correct, they will account most satisfactorily for the good effects of cold water, externally applied, in relieving that large class of diseases depending on congestion of blood in the liver—or what is called a sluggish liver. The application of cold to the bowels would necessarily cause the spleno-hepatic vein to contract upon its contents, and so empty itself, and propel the blood onward through the liver, and thus remove all congestion there—just as cold applied to the back of the hand causes the veins there to contract upon their contents, thus emptying themselves, and shrinking to their proper size. Whatever causes vessels to contract, augments the velocity of the blood's circulation through them. And congestion of one sort or other, as we have just seen, is the proximate cause of all diseases whatever—and there is nothing which can so quickly and certainly produce this contraction of vessels, and removal of congestion, as the application of cold.

CHAPTER V.

PROPOSITIONS ON THE PRINCIPLES AND PRACTICE OF THE WATER-CURE.*

The Applications of the Water-Cure are in strict Accordance with the Facts and Phenomena of the living Organism.—A Knowledge of these of the greatest Importance to the Physician.—What constitutes Disease.—All Disease originally Acute.—Acute Disease a normal Effort of Nature.—In this Effort the Body may die from Exhaustion.—What constitutes a Chronic Disease.—Of accidental Injuries and skin Diseases.—How organic Disease occurs.—When a Disease is Curable and when Incurable.—There is necessarily an unnatural quantity of Blood in diseased Organs.—Preventing or removing this Condition necessary to be kept in view by the Physician.—The nervous System controls the Circulation of the Blood.—Curative Treatment to be made through this System.—It must not be too Violent.—How this Treatment is to be Applied.—Air, Diet, and Water.—These are the Agents used in the Cure of Disease.—Alcoholic and Medicinal Stimulants.—Their evil Effects.—The true Principle of the Water-Cure.

The following propositions will show that the applications of the water-cure are in strict accordance with the facts and phenomena of the living organism; and that without an intimate acquaintance with these last, it is utterly impossible to make the applications with safety to the patient, or with credit to the practice or the practitioner. Let the critical medical reader appeal, if he pleases, from our propositions to the doctrines of the schools as embodied in the works of the most celebrated modern writers on health and disease, and say whether we have not accepted those doctrines. In truth, the premises of health and disease, established by experiment and observation, stand untouched, as far as they go; far be it from us to contravene them. It is only in the conclusions of practice that we differ from the great body of our medical brethren. We assert the perfect right to do this so long as we can give scientific reasons for it. Such reasons are contained in these propositions. Time and experience are also daily accumulating facts of cure which come to the support of the justness of these reasons.

* From "Dangers of the Water-Cure Considered," by Drs. James Wilson and James M. Gully, England.

1. A series of unnatural symptoms constitutes a disease.

2. This disease is referable to a morbid condition of some of the textures of the body.

3. All disease is originally acute, that is to say, the symptoms are more or less rapid and pressing in their character, and more or less characterized by fever.

4. Acute disease is the effort of the morbid organ or organs to throw off their disorder upon some less important organ or organs. Thus, acute inflammation of the liver, stomach, or lungs, causes fever; that is, an effort to throw the mischief on the skin, the bowels, or the kidneys.

5. If, from the great extent of the mischief to be thrown off, and the feeble constitution, acquired or natural, of the individual, this effort is not successful, the body dies from exhaustion.

6. If this effort be only partially successful, more or less of the internal mischief remains, but gives rise to symptoms of a less rapid and pressing and more permanent character. These symptoms then constitute a chronic disease.

7. Except in the case of accidents to the limbs, we know of no disease which is not essentially internal. Skin diseases are invariably connected with disease of some internal organs, especially the stomach and bowels, and are regulated in their character and intensity thereby. This is so true, that where there is a skin disease, the crises effected by the water-cure invariably take place on the spot where it exists.

8. ACUTE DISEASE, then, is the violent effort of internal and vital organs to cast their mischief on external and less important organs.

9. CHRONIC DISEASE is the enfeebled effort of the same organs to the same end.

10. But as from the diminished power of the constitution this is always ineffectual, the morbid state of the organs tends constantly toward disorganization, or what is called organic disease. This is more certainly the case, if the original causes of the malady are at work.

11. Disease therefore is CURABLE when the power of the system is sufficiently strong to throw the morbid action from a more to a less important organ.

12. Disease is INCURABLE when the power in question is insufficient for the last-named purpose; and when it has become organic, that is, when a change of structure has taken place.

13. From these premises it follows that the aim of scientific treatment should be to aid the development of the power of the system and its efforts to rid its vital parts of mischief.

14. That mischief invariably consists in the retention of an unnatural quantity of blood in them, to the detriment of other parts of the organism—a retention commonly known by the terms acute inflammation, chronic inflammation, and congestion.

15. In endeavoring to develop the powers of the system, the dissipation of this inflammation or congestion must be constantly kept in view, as the end of which the constitutional efforts are the means.

16. But as the circulation of the blood every where is under the influence of the organic system of nerves, the power and efforts of these last are essentially to be strengthened in order to dissipate the inflammation or congestion referred to.

17. Curative treatment is therefore made through the instrumentality of the nervous system.

18. Violent and sudden stimulation of the nervous system of the internal organs, is invariably followed by exhaustion and increased inflammation and congestion. Hence the impropriety of alcoholic and medicinal stimulants.

19. But the gradual and judiciously regulated stimulation of the nervous system according to the organic powers, conduces to the development and maintenance of its strength.

20. This stimulation is the more steady and certain in its results the more universally it is applied to the entire nervous system.

21. To the external skin, therefore, and to the internal skin (as represented by all the lining membranes of the lungs and digestive organs), this stimulation should be applied, those parts containing the largest portion of the nervous system spread through them.

22. Pure air applied to the lungs, proper diet, and water applied to the digestive organs, and water applied to the external skin, fulfill this intention of stimulation and strengthening most effectually.

23. Further, as that portion of the nervous system (the brain and spinal cord) in which the will resides, requires the development of its powers, exercise of the limbs is requisite, the stimulation of the air, diet, and water aiding thereto.

24. Pure water, pure air, proper diet, and regulated exercise, are the great agents in effecting the cure of disease, by aiding the

natural efforts of the body, through the instrumentality of the nervous system.

25. In the due apportionment of these agents, according to the powers of the constitution and the phases of disease, as ascertained by minute medical examination, consists the scientific and the safe practice of the water-cure.

26. As strengthening of the system by the regulated stimulation of the nervous system, is the means, so the throwing off disease by more important or less important organs by that acquired strength, is the end of that practice.

27. During the efforts of the system thus aroused for so beneficial an end, if agents are employed which divert those efforts and tend to centre stimulus on the more important organs, augmented mischief is the certain result. Such agents are to be found in alcoholic and medicinal stimulants, applied to the internal skin and nerves; in hot and impure air applied to the external skin and nerves; and in exciting and factitious pleasures and anxious cares, applied to the great centre of the nerves, the brain.

28. These and the *mal-apportionment* of the stimulation included in water, air, diet, and exercise, give rise to the only "Dangers of the Water-Cure."

29. The proper apportionment of the stimulation in question originates and maintains a steady effort of the system to save its vital parts at the expense of parts which implicate life less immediately.

30. The result of this effort is shown in one of the following ways: 1. The re-establishment of obstructed and suppressed secretions; 2. In the elimination of diseased matters through the bowels, kidneys, or skin; 3. In the formation of a critical action of some sort on the skin.

31. Such result constitutes the CRISIS OF THE WATER-CURE.

32. The crisis, being the result of the extrinsic efforts of the vital organs, is to be viewed as the signal of their relief, not as the instrument of their relief.

33. Still as, during the crisis, the tendency from the internal to the external organs is most strong, it is more than ever necessary to avoid the causes which act in diverting this tendency and in re-concentrating the mischief on the internal parts.

34. At the same time, the tendency in point being then strongly established, it is not necessary to stimulate the system further in

that direction, and all treatment except that which allays irritation accordingly ceases.

35. A crisis being the evidence of cure of the internal disease, no recurrence of the latter is to be apprehended, unless the morbid causes are reapplied.

CHAPTER VI.

THE WATER-DRESSING FOR WOUNDS AND ULCERS.*

Definition of "Water-Dressing."—Mode of Application.—Water-Dressings used by some in place of Poultices.—Ill Effects that are sometimes caused by the Latter.—Water-Dressing a better Application.—Water as a Remedy for Wounds and Inflammation of ancient Date.—Doctrines of Hippocrates.—This simple Practice was set aside by Celsus and the Arabian Physicians.—Ambrose Paré.—Religious Superstitions concerning the Effects of Water. Gabriel Fallopius.—Pallazzo.—Laurent Joubert, Martel, and Denis. Van Helmont.—Lamorier.—Caldani and Danter.—A Miller of Alsace.—Baron Percy.- Baron Larrey.—Professor Kern.—Water not a Specific or Medicinal Remedy.—Necessity of paying Attention to the Temperature of the Water-Dressing.—Its Use in Lacerations, Punctured Wounds, Contusions, and Strains of Joints.—Gun-Shot Wounds.—The Division of Varicose Veins.—Boils.—Piles.—Gonorrhœa.—Chronic Affections of the Skin.—Corns and Callosities.—Water as a Preventive of Lock-Jaw.—Great Power of Water in preventing Pain. Cases.

The application of water in a liquid form can be used at all temperatures, from the heat of the living body down to the freezing point. This great range extends its efficacy to a variety of wounds and inflammation; but, except where cold is absolutely necessary, the remedy is usually employed at the heat of the body, or rather at that degree to which the application cools the part. The water is retained in some light and porous substances, charged or wetted throughout, and covered with some thin and impervious substance, to prevent evaporation. When water is applied in this manner, the impression it makes is permanent and equal; and as it bears some resemblance to other dressing for wounds and ulcers, in the form of its application, I have given it the name of *water-dressing*.

The substance that I have generally made the immediate object of application, is the finest and softest lint; and for the covering

* From a treatise on Inflammation. By James Macartney, M. D., F. R. S. etc., etc

material, either oiled silk, or a thin plate of Indian rubber. Simple as this mode of dressing may appear, it requires to be managed with care, and attention to many circumstances, which would appear trivial to persons unacquainted with the nature of the remedy. Two, three, or four layers of the lint should be first folded together, according to the size of the part to be covered, taking care also that the soft side of the lint is the outer one. In wetting the lint the first time, it is necessary to either float it in the water before folding it, or if it be first folded, it should be pressed between the fingers, to urge the fluid into the interstices of the lint, which receive fluid with difficulty, until all the air they contain be expelled. The lint, when applied, should just contain as much water as not to drop. The oiled silk, or Indian rubber, should project so much beyond the margin of the lint as may prevent evaporation, which will vary according to the shape of the part on which the dressing is laid, and the thickness of the folded lint.*

It is of great importance to use the wet lint without any bandage that can give to the part affected the least feeling of constraint. The figure of the parts sometimes renders this difficult to effect, without stitching the silk into a particular shape, which is much better than using any strict bandage.

The periods for changing the lint must vary according to the nature of the case; but as a general rule, three times during the day, and twice during the night (if convenient), will be sufficient. In cases where the inflammation is moderate, and the skin unbroken, the dressing will only require to be changed every twelve hours. At each time that the dressing is renewed, the lint and oiled silk should be carefully washed, and when it is applied to ulcers, fresh lint should replace that taken off, the utmost cleanliness being of the first importance.

French oiled silk is very much superior to the English; it does not adhere to the skin, and therefore does not fret it. Some other substance besides linseed oil, I am informed, enters into its composition.

The water-dressing becomes immediately the same degree of heat as that of the surface of the skin on which it is placed; but when it is desirable to combine it with cold, a bladder holding iced

* It should be remarked here, that Priessnitz objects to oil cloth and India rubber coverings over wet bandages, on the ground that they retain matter which should be allowed to pass off. Simple dry cloth is all he uses.—S.

water may be laid over the oiled silk; or where the comfort of warmth may be required, the dressing may be covered with flannel.

Some surgeons now profess to use water-dressing as a substitute for poultice, by which they show their ignorance of the nature and operation of the remedy. A poultice is made of materials, which, in a term far short of its renewal, become sour, and thereby render the poultice, after the first few hours, an irritating application. The greasy substances which are added to prevent the poultice adhering to the skin, do not always answer the end, and soon become rancid. A poultice favors the formation of pus, and causes a throbbing or pulsating pain, and a feeling of tenderness in the part, which are the natural attendants on the process of suppuration. It imbibes the pus it serves to create, and thereby becomes more irritating. A poultice, before it is many hours on, is a mixture of sour farinaceous substance, rancid oil, and pus, oppressing the part by its weight, and beginning to adhere round its edges to the skin, creating the sense of constriction.

In order to judge of the effects of poultices, it is only necessary to visit a hospital, where they are much employed, before the surgeon comes round, when the sufferings of the patients will be sufficiently obvious; and to contrast this state of feeling with that which arises after the poultices are taken off, and the wounds and ulcers bathed for some time with tepid water; the soothing and comforting effect of which is better known by the patients than the surgeon, and therefore they prolong it as much as they can.

Water-dressing has not only better, but very different effects from poultices; it either prevents or diminishes the secretion of pus: a wound may at first yield a little purulent fluid, but in a short time this will be furnished in so small a quantity, as hardly to stain the lint. The pus, even from an ulcer, rapidly diminishes under water-dressing. I remember a case of a very extensive ulcer of the leg, to which I applied it; the patient pulled off the dressing in the night, because, as he said, "it was stopping the discharge," he conceiving, like many surgeons, that no open surface could heal without suppurating. Granulations also, which are rendered exuberant by poultice, are either never formed, or exist in a very slight degree under water-dressing.

Instead of the throbbing pain produced by a poultice, being excited, all pain is removed by the use of this remedy. A man in a fight with another, had the nail of his thumb bitten through near the root. The water-dressing was applied. A day or two after I met him with a poultice on his thumb. On inquiring why he removed the first dressing, he said "there was no use in keeping it on any longer, as it took away all his anguish," he supposing a poultice the proper application for the cure. In a word, the tendency of water-dressing (if it be properly conducted) is to induce the cure of wounds and ulcers, not requiring excitement, by the approximating or modeling process already described.

The employment of water, as a remedy for wounds and inflammation, is no doubt of very ancient date. Hippocrates is said to have discovered, by the inscriptions in the temple of Æsculapius, that the priests had used water mixed with secret ingredients, in order probably to give the remedy more importance in the eyes of the people.

Hippocrates himself seemed to have understood more of the modes of application of water, and of its adaptation to particular circumstances, than we discover in the practice of many who have lived in later days. He used warm water in gangrene; sea water for chronic cutaneous diseases; cold water in fractures, erysipelas, and ulcers. His method of application was to bathe the parts with a sponge, afterward leave it on charged with the fluid, and wet the sponge as often as it became dry.

This simple practice was set aside by the Arabian physicians and Celsus having introduced a variety of absurd and complicated medicines into fashion, which held their ground until the fourteenth century, when the surgeons of that period fell as foolishly into the opposite extreme, as that of composing their medicines of a multitude of ingredients. They now endeavored to discover some one which would be universally applicable. This gave rise to the system of *secret dressing*, as it was called, each practitioner assuming that he possessed the panacea. Some of these secret remedies, when discovered, were found to be ridiculous; as for example, oil and cabbage, and an oil made of kittens, were much in use. At this period and for long after, water was employed, but accompanied with some absurd form of incantation, to which all its good effects were ascribed.

Ambrose Parè, who was a man of the greatest talent and experience of the age in which he lived, refused for some time to apply water to wounds, as the effects seemed to him to be so extraordinary, that they could only be produced by supernatural agency, which, from religious scruples, he did not consider it justifiable to employ. During the siege of Metz, in 1553, an ignorant quack, called Maitre Doublet, as Brantome relates, "performed strange cures with simple white linen, and clean water from the fountains or wells. But he was assisted by sorcery and charmed words, and every one went to him, as if he were Maitre Ambrose Parè himself, a man so celebrated and considered the first of his day."

Ambrose Parè, who equally detested fraud and folly, in writing his report of the proceedings of the medical department of the army, speaks thus: "I do not deny that water is a good remedy in wounds and recent injuries, having employed it myself with much advantage, but I object to the mysterious words, and the vain and unchristian ceremonies, that accompany this new and singular practice, which is so simple that it requires no aid."

The book on surgery by Gabriel Fallopius, published in 1560, strongly recommends the use of natural water as a "fruitful source of success."

Pallazzo published in 1570 a book on the true method of curing wounds by simple water, hemp, and flax. He recommends varying the temperature according to circumstances.

Laurent Joubert, in his work on popular errors, published in 1578, exposed the folly of using charmed water, and described common water as being most efficacious in procuring "a favorable termination and a good cicatrix."

Some time after this there was a sharp controversy between Martel, surgeon to Henry the Third, and one Denis, a surgeon of Vendome, and Danguaron, also surgeon to Henry the Third; the two latter contending for the use of charms. This dispute was terminated by the Chancellor of the University of Montpelier deciding in favor of simple water.

Soon after Van Helmont introduced his mode of curing by magnetic sympathy, and the water was only employed mixed with other ingredients, such as the powder of the Chevalier Digby.

In 1732, Lamorier published "on the Use of Common Water in Surgery." He asserted that there were few wounds which could not be healed by this treatment, more promptly and satisfactorily than by any other means.

Professor Caldani, of Padua, also recommended cold water as the best application in recent wounds. Danter published a learned essay at Gottingen, in which he recommended the use of water.

In 1785, a number of men were severely wounded in proving the cannon at Strasbourg; a miller of Alsace undertook their cure, by the leave of the Intendant of the province, with *blessed water:* these wounds were all cicatrized in six weeks. A second proving of the cannon wounded thirty-four men. They were dressed with common water by Lombard, the surgeon-in-chief, by which means they were all cured. The progress of the wounds was witnessed by Baron Percy, then a surgeon-major of cavalry. The success on this occasion produced a pamphlet from Lombard, in 1786, "on the Properties of simple Water as a topical application in the cure of Surgical Diseases."

Baron Percy always afterward employed warm or cold water, according to the season. He says they often had from six to eight thousand wounded in their hospitals. His experience, therefore, cannot be questioned, and so strong was his conviction of the utility of this treatment, that he said, "he would relinquish military surgery if he were prohibited from using water."

Baron Larrey is said to have treated, with great success, the most terrible wounds, with the water of the Nile, during the campaign in Egypt; probably from the want of other remedies being in his possession, as his predilection for complicated applications would have prevented him choosing so simple a one as water. In his writings he speaks of salt water being a proper remedy for wounds.

Professor Kern, of Vienna, was long known as the strenuous advocate of the employment of water in wounds and ulcers, and in the after treatment of surgical operations. He varied the temperature of the fluid, and consulted the feelings of the patient, by avoiding all useless bandages and medicated dressings for wounds, and his practice was, I have heard, proportionably successful. He claimed the credit of having invented water-dressing, an assumption that could only be made by a person ignorant of the history of continental surgery. Kern, I believe, however, carried out the principle of the treatment farther than those who preceded him.

The practice of most of the surgeons whose works I have mentioned, was to bathe the injured part with water in the first instance, and repeat the bathing frequently during the day. Only a few of those writers prevented evaporation by any impervious covering. Frequent ablution, either with warm or cold water, is, according to the nature of the case, an admirable remedy. It is a species of irrigation, but wants the convenience, and the unremitting operation of the wet lint and oiled silk. Within these few years, the practice of irrigation has been revived in France by Breschet, Berard, and Josse, with great improvements on the ancient system of temporary bathing; but, with these exceptions, the simple mode of treating wounds and inflammation cannot be said to exist in any of the civil hospitals of France or Italy. The dressing with dry charpie in the first instance, and after the wound is compelled to suppurate, with medicated ointments, and the use of complicated bandages, are as common throughout the South of Europe at the present day, as they were in the most barbarous ages of surgery.

It is quite manifest, from the history I have given of the employment of water in its liquid state, for the cure of wounds and inflammation, from the earliest periods to the present time, that I do not claim the discovery of the remedy; but that I have been the means of introducing it to the attention of the profession in these countries, is a matter of too much notoriety to admit of dispute. I have also connected the use of it with general views of the nature of inflammation, which (whether right or wrong) are peculiarly and distinctly my own; and I have demonstrated the possibility of open wounds healing without inflammation, and without the medium of either coagulable lymph, or granulations; a fact which, as far as my information extends, has not even been hinted at by any writer on surgery, either ancient or modern.

In all cases where it is not desirable to reduce the temperature of inflamed parts below the standard heat of the human body, I consider water, in the state of vapor, as superior to it in the liquid form; but in consequence of the application of steam being attended with some trouble and sacrifice of time, the water has been generally preferred, except in great and dangerous wounds, painful abscesses, and those internal inflammations, wherein common fomentation has hitherto been adopted. I do not attribute to water, under any form, a specific or medicinal power of controlling inflammatory actions; nor is such power necessary—for if the organic sense of injury and the feeling of pain be removed, by substituting an agreeable state of sensation, the motives to inflame cease to exist, and the natural actions of reparation proceed without impediment or delay. We have a very beautiful example of inflammation being not only excited, but maintained, by a slight irritation, and declining without any remedy, except the removal of the object which created the pain, in the common accident of a grain of sand or dust being lodged on the surface of the conjunctiva of the eye. I can conceive that water, either as vapor or fluid, might be capable of preventing, and perhaps of removing the impression of exposure, which most wounds more or less produce; and I am persuaded as much as I can be of any fact, not proved by experience, that if a serous cavity were to be opened in an atmosphere of steam of the proper heat, and detained in it, the cavity would not inflame, because it would not be sensible of any impression different from what it was accustomed to from its own vapor; for, as I have already mentioned, it is not the wound of the parietes of a close cavity, which spreads inflammation over it. When amputation is performed below the knee, inflammation of the joint does not occur; but if the head of the fibula be taken out at the time, and in doing this the slight capsule which divides its joint from that of the knee, be cut, inflammation is liable to come on the latter.

In the employment of water, those who have not been instructed respecting the nature of the application, do not pay sufficient attention to the influence of temperature. Some persons believe that they use in all cases cold water, which is impossible, beyond the moment of its application, if the dressing be covered with the oiled silk. It is only by perpetually adding the fluid, as in irrigation, or by covering the water-dressing with a bladder holding iced water, that a low temperature can be obtained. It is evident that warmth and confinement of the wound would be improper, when hemorrhage had either taken place, or was expected. In other circumstances, the temperature to be chosen is always that which is most easy and comforting to the patient.

Water-dressing may be employed in the common manner, after the pain of the injury is subdued by steam or fomentation, in all great lacerations, punctured wounds, contusions, and strains of joints. I have, in several instances of such injuries, prevented all suffering and inflammation by these means. Whereas in the common mode of treating these accidents, they would have been followed by extensive suppurations, much misery, protracted confinement, and in the end, perhaps, the patient left with a useless limb.

Water has been used with great success by many military surgeons in gunshot wounds, and in shattered limbs from explosions of gunpowder. I have seen a case in which this mode of treatment was carefully followed, and in which the patient never suffered any pain nor constitutional disturbance, except a little during one night, just before the piece of cloth was expelled. The edges of the wound did not slough, and the discharge was hardly enough to soil the lint. The gentleman walked out well the eighth day after he fought the duel; the ball remained imbedded in the ilium.

Mr. Bird, of Banagher, a very active and intelligent practitioner, has communicated to me some frightful injuries by gunshot wounds treated by water-dressing, with complete success; and one particularly severe case, in which amputation would have been formerly thought unavoidable. In consequence of a gun bursting in a man's hand, the carpus was torn open, the end of the radius broken, the metacarpal bone of the thumb was separated from the carpus, and the thumb thrown back on the hand. This man recovered the use of his hand, having only a stiff wrist-joint. Mr. Bird informs me, that since he commenced practice, he has treated twenty-two cases of gunshot wounds solely with water, and always with the same fortunate result.

I have seen under the care of the late Dr. M'Dowel, who practiced water-dressing extensively in the Richmond Hospital, cases of division of varicose veins, proceeding without the slightest appearance of inflammation.

Boils are completely under our control by this mode of treatment. If resorted to in the beginning, the boils will seldom exceed the size of peas, and produce no pain.

I have repeatedly cured inflamed and protruded piles by a wet sponge, covered with a plate of Indian rubber, which dressing conforms better to the shape of the parts than the lint and oiled silk. In these cases the complaint never returned.

I have never used water-dressing myself in gonorrhœa, not anticipating that it would succeed; but numerous accounts have been transmitted to me, of the disease being cured by the external application of water to the private part. The symptoms are described as being rendered very mild, and usually disappearing in from one to two weeks.

Water-dressing is particularly convenient and efficacious in many chronic affections of the skin, especially those that are dry and scaly. I have sometimes used the oiled silk, or the Indian rubber alone in psoriasis, which kept the parts moist by collecting and confining the insensible perspiration. On one occasion, where the disease had spread over the whole body, causing the greatest irritation, and a total want of sleep, I had the patient entirely enveloped in a dress of oiled silk with the best effects.

Water-dressing never fails to eradicate corns or any other callosities of the skin, provided it be persevered in for a considerable time.

If the effusions called ganglia, which form in the sheaths of tendons, be carefully dressed with water, or what is still better, the lead lotion, and be kept in a state of rest, the inflammation of the cyst will be removed, and the fluid which distended it absorbed. I have also reduced the size of the cartilaginous bodies found in similar situations by the same treatment, and I am disposed to think that it is possible to procure the entire absorption of the loose cartilages in the joints by these means.

I have never seen an instance of tetanus (lock-jaw) coming on, when wounds, however severe, and from their nature likely to produce the disease, where healed under water-dressing; and I know of but two cases in which it is said to have occurred, and possibly in these instances the remedy might not have been accurately employed. For I cannot conceive that tetanus could ensue, provided all pain and sense of injury were early removed, and that the wound healed by the approximating process without inflammation, or the medium of any new organized substance. In a letter from Dr. Bonyen, a very intelligent pupil of mine, now settled in Demerara, received the 23d of June, 1837, he states, that a medical man in extensive practice there, uses water-dressing after amputation and other operations; and that these wounds healed as well as the best-treated cases in cold climates, and that in fourteen amputations he had performed, he had not lost a single patient by tetanus.

The *immersion* of a wounded or inflamed part either in warm or cold water, according to circumstances, has perhaps more influence on the sensations than any other mode of applying the fluid. I have witnessed the greatest effect from it, when used either warm in place of fomentation to soothe pain, or cold to abate vascular action. It would be a most valuable remedy, if any means could be devised for its application, without the inconvenience of the inflamed part being placed in a depending position. A very striking case of the benefit of immersion was communicated to me by Dr.

Cardiff, then a military surgeon stationed at Kilkenny. A soldier received a thrust of a bayonet, which passed through his thumb, and between the metacarpal bones of his hand. After the bleeding had ceased, the hand was laid in tepid water, which speedily removed the pain. The immersion was continued for twelve hours, after which the hand was taken out and dressed in the usual manner (I presume with adhesive plaster), after which the pain returned with great severity and throbbing, so that it became necessary to remove the dressing and return the hand to the water. The immersion again removed all pain, and was now continued for twenty hours, and when removed, the common water-dressing was employed, no more pain was felt, and the cure of this frightful wound was accomplished without swelling, heat, suppuration, or any of the results of inflammation, and the cicatrix that remained was soft. The man went to duty on the eighth day after receiving the wound.

Baron Percy very truly says, "that if it were possible on the receipt of a gunshot, or other serious wound of the elbow, knee, foot, etc., to keep the part for the first ten or fifteen hours plunged in water, we should have fewer amputations to perform, and we should save the lives of a greater number of wounded."

A lady fractured her tibia close to the ankle joint; great swelling, tension, and pain immediately followed. At her own suggestion, the limb was placed in a bucket of warm water, which had the effect of removing the pain, and almost all the tumefaction, before I visited her for the purpose of adjusting the fracture.

CHAPTER VII.

PROCESSES OF WATER-CURE.

Water-Drinking.—Quantity recommended by Priessnitz.—Enormous Quantities sometimes drank.—Advantage of Water in Fevers.—Erroneous Notions concerning the Treatment of Fevers.—Rule to be Observed.—Water Drinking in Poisoning.—A Case.—Advantages of pure Water in New York.—Effect of Water taken at Meals.—Water Drinking for Indigestion.—Vomiting by Water.—Advantages of Drinking at Meals.—Living without Drink.—Water to prevent Vomiting and Hickup.—Some Laborers drink freely at Meals.—Water probably undergoes no chemical Change in the System.—Quality of Water.—That which is Pure and Soft the best.—Effects of Croton Water in New York.—How to obtain pure soft Water every where.—Injections or Clysters.—Their good Effects in various Diseases.—How they shall be Applied.—The Rubbing Wet Sheet.—Its Application and Uses.—The Leintuch or Wet Sheet.—Mode of Application.—Its Uses.—Compresses and Wet Bandages.—Their Object and Uses.—Warming or Stimulating Bandages.—Sweating Process.—How Sweating is Accomplished.—Rules for the Process.—It is little used by Priessnitz at the present day.

DRINKING WATER.

THE quantity usually directed by Priessnitz is from ten to twelve tumblers daily. His general advice is, "Do not oppress your stomach, although I wish you to drink as much as you can conveniently." Some have gone to great excess in drinking. At Graefenberg, enormous quantities are often taken without any apparent inconvenience. One gentleman, we are told, took by way of experiment thirteen and a half quarts in a day, little by little, taking a good share of exercise at the same time, and experienced only a slight headache in consequence.

Every one knows of cases in which a high burning fever has been broken up merely by drinking great quantities of cold water. How often have there been cases in which it was believed, both by friends and the physician, that the patient with burning fever could not live the night through, and the physician declaring that cold water, if taken, would be the sure death of the patient, and yet the friends, not always over particular to follow the directions laid down, have given water to the patient, or perhaps the patient in his delirium has broken through all restraint and satisfied himself to the full extent of thirst; and soon how changed! Sleep, which before could not be at all obtained, or if it could be, was only dreamy and disturbed, is now deep and refreshing; and in the place of a dry, parched, and burning skin, there is now most profuse perspiration. The friends now behold that the fever is "broken up:" the physician comes in the morning, and exclaims, "Astonishing! what the medicine has done!" But the medicine has been cast to the dogs.

If, in the whole range of human science, there is any error which shows pre-eminently how loosely mankind may reason, and into what great follies the human mind may be led, it is in the supposed effect of cold water in fevers. It seems, because it was well known to be dangerous for persons in great heat and perspiration arising from over-exertion—an artificial and most unnatural state—to drink largely of cold water, by parity of reasoning, it must always be dangerous *when there is great thirst.* But the cases are totally different. In the case of over-exertion, if the body is allowed to remain quiet, even in a warmer place, the flowing of perspiration—a cooling process—will soon cause the body to become cool; and indeed a cold will often be taken, unless great care is exercised to guard the body. Even in such cases, too, drinking very small quantities of water is safe and beneficial, especially if moderate exercise be kept up.

Drinking, then, in high fever, is highly salutary, and always perfectly safe, and should be reckoned as one of the most powerful means of reducing fever. Cases where it has proved injurious, cannot be found. To the utmost, the patient's thirst should be gratified.

In other cases than fever, we have seen most astonishing effects produced by drinking water. In a certain case, a woman of this city, as she believed, and it was no doubt true, had been poisoned by her husband: violent spasmodic action of the muscles of the extremities having come on, and a severe burning in the mouth, throat, and stomach, being present, and the woman nearly insensible, large draughts of iced Croton water were immediately given. The patient afterward said, that so parched and heated were the mouth, throat, and stomach, that the cold water produced no sensation whatever; but no sooner was the water taken, than most powerful vomiting ensued, and much to the woman's relief. Still the burning sensations to a considerable extent would soon return, and then copious drinking would again quickly cause the same good result. After a while, the water was taken tepid, and thus the patient drank and vomited many quarts. Other means were used, but drinking was the principal treatment. The next day, she was quite well. Cats and dogs that have been accidentally poisoned by arsenic set for rats, will take water greedily, and have thus apparently been kept from being destroyed.

It is said by those concerned, that in the hospitals of this city (New York) there have been no cases of *gravel* since the introduction of the pure soft Croton water, and that many cases have been cured spontaneously. The drinking this pure soft water, and its culinary use, are doubtless the causes of those favorable results.

There has been a great deal of prejudice concerning drinking water at meals. The common opinion is, that it dilutes the "gastric juice." But this opinion is founded in a wrong notion of digestion. The aqueous portion of the food taken is mostly absorbed before digestion proceeds to any considerable extent. This objection certainly is not made to the eating of fruits, and these are composed very much of water—by far the largest part; and so also the natural food of the infant—the mother's milk: the whey or watery part is absorbed, and the curd afterward digested. It is not true, therefore, that digestion is necessarily impaired by taking fluid into the stomach at the time of meals. Nor is it true that the gastric fluid is present in the stomach, as is by many supposed, before food is taken into the stomach, and that its action upon the coats of the stomach causes the sensation of hunger. The gastric secretion does not take place until the stomach is excited by the presence of food.

But whatever may be said concerning theories in this matter of drinking at meals, the real facts of experience furnish altogether the best guide. From very careful observation and experiment, we are certain that, in many cases, at least, of persons who suffer from indigestion, the complaint will be very sensibly mitigated, and in frequent instances be wholly removed, by free drinking pure soft water at the meals; and then again, if indigestion is really present, whether there has been drinking with the previous meal or not, full drinking of water is the best means that can be used to remove the distressing symptoms. There will generally, or at least often, be no thirst in these cases, so that the water is to be taken like medicine, "against the stomach." If there have been a debauch, sometimes vomiting will take place, but the vomiting that comes on from water drinking is comparatively easy, and causes great relief. At other times diarrhœa takes place, and still oftener neither vomiting nor diarrhœa, but a quick and certain subsidence of the symptoms. Here it may be said, that no violence should ever be done in drinking in the way of over-chilling the body. If we wish to cause vomiting, and in some other instances, water, warm or tepid, will be the most beneficial. Cold water can generally be borne, by a weak stomach, better with food than at other times; and why?—because the stomach is elevated in temperature soon after the taking of food. It is then better able to act against the coldness of the water.

What effect does cold water then have upon the stomach at meals? Do we not know that every person, day by day, through stimulants in the food taken, is literally being "drugged," and that the coats of the stomach are thus more or less inflamed and weakened? Suppose the face or hands are partially inflamed or feverish, does not every one know how strengthening and salutary to those parts is the application of cold water? Precisely in the same way does cold water, in suitable quantities, act upon the stomach, as every one can prove by trial.

There is another advantage in drinking with meals; it is this: less food is required to satisfy the appetite. It has been said, in objection to drinking at meals, that it over-distends the stomach. It is true that the stomach is almost always overtasked; but this distension will be much sooner removed, if a good share of it be from simple water. This is incomparably more easily removed by the action of the organ, than is too great a quantity of food.

Food is often taken that is of itself too dry, more so than is natural. Certain kinds, as dyspepsia or Graham crackers, dry bread, etc., are apt to swell in the stomach as a dried apple would do. If food is taken at all in this state, the greatest care should be exercised in mastication, but even then, drinking will be found salutary.

Some have lived weeks and months without drinking any liquid whatever. But in all such cases fluid must have been taken from some source. These have generally been vegetable and fruit eaters, and who have eaten largely of fruit; and these contain a large proportion of water. Dr. Alcott, a man well known for his physiological, hygienic, and other writings, lived without drink for more than one year, at the same time partaking freely of apples as a part of the regular meal. The moisture in the breath, perspiration, and other excretions of the body, which are constantly passing off, must be supplied from some source or other. Ordinary food, even, contains a much greater portion of moisture than would be at first supposed: baker's bread is said to contain about 35 per cent. The adult human body by weight is composed of about 80 per cent. water—the blood about 90 per cent., and the brain of nearly the same quantity. This supply of fluid must be kept up.

There is another good effect to be brought about by water drinking—to prevent vomiting. We have succeeded in arresting very obstinate vomiting, when the most effectual means of ordinary practice had failed, by giving water in small quantity frequently repeated. Hickup, according to our experience, can be more readily managed by water drinking, than by any other means.

Laborers who are much exposed to heat and fatigue, tell us they can get along with less drink, if they are careful to drink freely at their meals.

It has been supposed by some, that water undergoes a chemical change in the system; but there is not the least evidence that it is ever in any way appropriated to the formation of the animal solids of the body. It is true, however, that life can be sustained considerably longer in cases of starvation, if water is taken, than without it; but still the water undergoes no chemical change.

QUALITY OF WATER FOR DRINKING AND CULINARY USES.

It is agreed on all hands that for all the purposes of life, whether for culinary preparations, or for drink, *pure soft water* is the best. It was believed that the pure water of Graefenberg could not be the cause of the truly wonderful cures that were there performed. It was believed that Priessnitz had some remedial agent in the sponges used, and he was prosecuted accordingly: it was only as he from the first had stated—pure soft water, with attention to air, exercise, diet, and clothing. The water has been fully tested, and is found to be only pure and soft.

Since the Croton water has been introduced into the city of New York, there has been a manifest improvement in the health of the citizens. Still there are many who prefer the abominably filthy and hard water of the wells. Yet there is much of the Croton used, some preferring it, and others taking it more from convenience. During the past summer (of 1844), a season not particularly healthy, and very hot, it was stated in the public papers that the bills of mortality during some of the weeks of the hottest weather, were less than they had been for many years previously in the season corresponding—a significant fact to those who understand the effects of water, but a fact, the reasons for which were not at all commented upon in the public papers.

As in every thing in the present state of physiological knowledge, so in the matter of drinking water: people in general are guided by mere feeling. Any one who has been a time in the habit of drinking hard water, if he act merely according to taste, will prefer the hard water to which he is accustomed, to any soft water, however pure it may be. Horses will leave hard water, that is clear, for soft water that is even muddy.

Families can easily obtain soft water by depending upon the cistern and the clouds. Very cheap filters can be at any time constructed, so that cistern-water can be had very pure: for instance, a large common funnel, a keg with a hole in the bottom, or something of the kind, can be used, a sponge or fine rags being pressed closely in the opening, and thus the water can be made very clear: and if there is any fear of decayed animal matter being in the rain-water, a layer of clean sand and fine charcoal over the sponge or other substance, will serve to remove this. It is the charcoal that acts as a disinfectant, removing the animal matter. There is no way of filtering out the *hardness* of hard water. Some families in and about New York and Boston have double cisterns, so that rain-water, by pressure, passes from one to the other through a large filter box, and thus the water is made as pure and limpid as can be imagined: and yet, when such water is at hand, for drink, many prefer the hard water of the well.

INJECTIONS, OR CLYSTERS.

These constitute an important part of the treatment. They are highly valuable in various complaints. The bowels can at any time be easily kept free, and the evils and unpleasantness of constipation thus be at once removed. This application is also of great service in all bowel complaints. Severe diarrhœa, dysentery, cholera morbus, and colic, can often be speedily arrested by this application alone. In inflammation of the bowels it is of most signal benefit. The author has, in different instances, given immediate relief in this disease, when the bowels had been for days obstinately closed, resisting the action of the most powerful medicines.

This application should be made with an instrument by which no air will be introduced into the parts. Air may cause pain. It should always be carefully expelled by forcing water through the instrument a few times before it is inserted.

The quantity of water to be used will vary. As much as can be retained, be it more or less, can be taken. The temperature is to be made according to the feelings of comfort, never too warm or too cold. Many take cold water.

Some have a prejudice against this application, thinking that it will weaken the bowels like cathartic medicine or cathartic clysters, but this is not true. Pure water rightly used in this way strengthens.

ABREIBUNG, OR RUBBING WET SHEET.

A linen sheet of coarse quality, suitable for holding considerable water, and at the same time serving well for friction, is here used. It is better to press and not wring the sheet out of the water, and it may be allowed even dripping. The patient standing ready, it is to be thrown over the head or about the neck, so as to create a slight shock; active friction is made (*over*, not *with* the sheet) by the assistant behind, and the patient before, if able, or by another assistant. This should be continued from one to five minutes, when the skin will have become reddened and warm. This must be immediately followed briskly by a coarse dry sheet or dry cloths, until the surface is perfectly dry and in a complete glow. The patient is then immediately dressed for exercise, or for bed, as the case may be. The temperature of the water used should correspond with the strength of the patient. Those who are so feeble as to render it necessary for them to remain in bed, can be often much benefited by a judicious rubbing while in bed. This is a highly useful and convenient application, and, if judiciously made, will produce nearly, if not quite all, the good effects of a bath, and will often be found much more convenient of application.

WET SHEET, OR LEINTUCH.

The first reclining upon this sheet will be disagreeable. If it is to be used to reduce the temperature of the body, as in high fevers, it is well to have it of coarse quality, in order to hold more water. To apply it, the mattress of the bed or couch should be made bare, one or more large thick woolen blankets next, and the sheet last, upon which the patient is to lie. He is to be quickly and snugly enveloped, from the neck to the feet, first with the wet sheet, and then with the blanket. These adjusted with care, the packing is finished by covering over the whole a light feather bed, and a quilt, or a sufficiency of other bedding without the feather bed. After remaining twenty or thirty minutes, or long enough to become tolerably warm, some form of ablution suited to the patient's condition is administered.

In cases of acute rheumatism, or gout, where it would be troublesome for the patient to be moved, or in any case where it might be better for the patient to remain quiet for a longer time, two or three sheets can be used instead of one, to act as a refrigerant for a longer time. A long towel from the armpit down, upon each side, has been recommended, so that the whole body be exposed to the wet linen.

In cases of acute fever, the sheets must be changed according to the degree of heat, every quarter or half hour, until the dry hot skin becomes softer, and more prone to perspiration. This is usually the first process of the day, and is repeated or not, according to circumstances.

The wet sheet process is of great advantage in a variety of chronic as well as acute cases; such as are attended with an irritable and inactive skin, and in a multitude of skin diseases. A frequent change of the sheets in such cases would be unnecessary as a rule. Determination of blood to the head is to be removed or prevented by cold applications to it. Should the feet remain cold in the wet cloths, they should be extricated and wrapped in dry cloths only. At the close of the process the patient should be briskly rubbed until the surface is dry.

"The wet sheet produces two diametrically opposite effects, accordingly as it is used. If it be changed frequently, as fast as the patient becomes warm, as, for instance, in cases of fever, almost any amount of heat may be abstracted slowly and gradually from the body. But if the patient remain for half an hour, the most delicious sensation of warmth, and a gentle breathing perspiration are produced, while all pains and uneasiness are removed. It produces all the soothing influence upon the entire system which is produced by a warm poultice on an inflamed surface."*

* Dr. Edward Johnson.

For very delicate patients it has been suggested that the sheet be pressed out of tepid water, as introductory to the cold.

Respecting the application of cold water over the whole body: "Let us now suppose that heat is abstracted from the whole surface of the body; in this case the whole action of the oxygen will be directed to the skin, and in a short time the change of matter must increase throughout the body. Fat, and all such matters as are capable of combining with oxygen, which is brought to them in larger quantity than usual, will be expelled from the body in the form of oxydized compounds."*

"If therefore the body contain any morbific matters, these will be expelled in the form of such compounds."†

According to Liebig, the same results may sometimes be accomplished by a very scanty diet.

COMPRESSES AND WET BANDAGES.

Locally, water may be applied in various ways. Bandages are made to produce the same effect upon any part of the body, as the leintuch upon the whole body. As cooling or refrigerant applications, they should be applied of a size suited to the part inflamed, folded from three or four to eight times, dipped in very cold water, and are to be renewed from every three or four to ten minutes, according to the necessities of the case.

As to the effect of the various partial applications of cold water to the system, "they act by determining the force of oxygen from one part to another. They produce all the effects of both bleeding and blistering, except the pain."

"If," says Liebig, "we surround a part of the body with ice or snow, while the other parts are left in a natural state, there occurs more or less quickly, in consequence of the loss of heat, an accelerated change of matter in the cooled part.

"The resistance of the living tissues to the action of oxygen, is weaker at the cooled part than in the other parts; and this, in its effects, is equivalent to an increase of resistance in these other parts—the whole action of the inspired oxygen is exerted on the cooled part.

"In the cooled part of the body, the living tissues offer a less resistance to the chemical action of the inspired oxygen; the pow-

* Liebig. † Dr. E. Johnson.

er of the oxygen to unite with the elements of the tissues is, at this part, exalted.

"In the cooled part the change of matter, and with it the disengagement of heat, increases; while, in the other parts, the change of matter and liberation of heat decrease."

"And thus," says Dr. Johnson, "by the judicious use of cold water alone, all the good effects of blistering and bleeding are most readily and certainly produced, without any of the bad effects. The bad effects of repeated bleeding in certain diseases are well known to medical men. We know perfectly well, that it often happens that a patient is saved by bleeding, from dying of an inflammation, only that he may die of a dropsy; that a patient is often saved by bleeding from dying of hæmorrhage from the lungs, only that he may die the sooner of a consumption.

WARMING, OR STIMULATING BANDAGES.

These are applied by folding linen two or three times, and dipping them in cold water, or they may be made slightly tepid; they should be well pressed or wrung out, and are not to be changed until they begin to dry. They must be well adapted to the part, and also well secured from the action of the air by a dry bandage, which is better to be a non-conductor of heat, so that the part may be raised in temperature. The combined action of heat and moisture thus produced is highly beneficial in a great variety of indurations, swellings, tumors, etc. In the water-cure, they are also much used in derangements of the digestive organs, affections of the abdomen, diseases of the liver, etc.

For the abdomen, a convenient form is made by folding and sewing together two or three thicknesses of linen, of sufficient length to pass round the body two or more times, the width varying according to the size of the person; one end is wet and wrung out enough in length to cover the abdomen, or to pass round the body if desirable, and then applied as tightly as comfortable—and the dry folds over in the same manner; the whole secured by pins, or better by tapes attached for the purpose. There should always be enough of dry cloths of some kind to prevent a permanent chill.

SWEATING.

In this process, the patient, being naked, is closely enveloped in a large thick blanket, with the legs extended and the arms close to the body. The blanket must be tightly drawn and well tucked under, so that every part of the body, from the head down, is in immediate contact with it. Then over all there must be a sufficiency of clothing of some sort (cotton comfortables are good), all well tucked under, so as to retain all the animal heat. "Thus hermetically enveloped, the patient exactly resembles a mummy." This constrained position and the irritation of the blanket are at first disagreeable, particularly until perspiration commences, which takes place in from one half hour to two hours' time. Those that perspire with difficulty, should move the legs and rub the body with their hands all that the position will allow. It is however more desirable to obtain the end without the exertion, if it can be done. Sometimes the head, all but the face, is also covered. When sweating commences, the windows should be thrown open, so as to admit fresh air, and the patient be allowed to take small draughts of water, a wine-glass or more every ten or fifteen minutes. This will not only be refreshing, but will also promote the sweating. If there be headache, or a determination of blood to the head, cooling bandages should be applied, and changed as often as necessary. If, from the length of time of the envelopment, it be necessary, a urinal should be placed at the patient before the wrapping up. To allay the pain of swellings, tumors, etc., warming applications should be applied before the envelopment; otherwise the pain would be liable to an increase, before perspiration commences. Those who are very restless, should be confined by additional cloths and girths; otherwise the time would be too much prolonged. With the best that can be done, some will require four or five hours' encasement.

The best time for sweating in chronic cases, is early in the morning. As a rule, only once a day. The repetition would be the exception. In acute cases, the time of sweating will depend upon the fever, exacerbations, etc., and should be resorted to when necessary, without reference to the time of day.

When the process has continued long enough, the coverings (all but the thick blanket) are to be removed. The blanket must be loosened—about the legs in particular. An attendant should wet with a cloth the parts to be exposed to the air. The patient, if able, goes immediately to the bath, washes the head, face, neck, and chest very briskly, and then enters the bath immediately, and remains from one to six or eight minutes, keeping up constant motion and friction; and then immediately, on leaving the bath, the whole surface must be made thoroughly dry by rubbing with cloths, etc.

Those who are able should then take exercise in the open air, or in a well-aired room. Those not able should be well rubbed by attendants. No danger is to be dreaded from the sudden transition from heat to cold, in this kind of sweating, if every thing is properly done, as abundant experience proves.

This highly valuable part of the water-cure can very easily be made the means of much evil. It is an engine of great power, and therefore should be practiced with the utmost caution. In cold, phlegmatic habits, where the skin is inactive, the sensibility dull, and the circulation sluggish, it is productive of great benefit. But in the sanguine temperament, where the circulation is active and the sensibility acute, or if in any case it is carried too far, it is productive of great mischief. The *relationship*, or *equilibrium*, between the two great vital functions, circulation and respiration, would be destroyed. The velocity of the circulation would be increased, without a corresponding increase of respiration, thus destroying an equilibrium absolutely necessary to health, and which destruction, if maintained for a considerable time, must inevitably terminate with the most serious results.

"Profuse perspiration operates upon the body, first like the surgeon's lancet, in reducing the volume of the contained fluids. Secondly, it operates like the physician's blister, by determining from the centre to the circumference. It thus relieves congestion of the vital organs, and lightens the whole system. But it does vastly more than can be achieved either by bleeding or blistering; for it extricates from the body an increased amount of carbon and hydrogen, thus producing a *deficiency* of these elements *within it.* This deficiency of carbon and hydrogen is equivalent to a call for more food, in order to supply the place of the lost carbon and hydrogen. And thus it promotes appetite, which is more than can be said for either lancet or blister, by their warmest admirers."*

Priessnitz does not resort to sweating as much as he once did. We are told that where he formerly sweated fifty patients, he does not now sweat half a dozen.

* Dr. Edward Johnson.

CHAPTER VIII.

PROCESSES OF WATER-CURE—(CONTINUED)

Modes in which the Bath should be taken.—The Cold Bath not to be resorted to when the Body is Chilly.—Necessity of keeping in Motion while in the Bath.—Those who have weak Chests must be careful in their use of the Cold Bath.—Exercise beneficial after Bathing.—Full Baths should sometimes be discontinued for a period.—The Half Bath.—Its Uses and Effects.—Long-continued Hip or Sitz Baths.—Priessnitz's mode.—The Bath is sometimes taken after the Packing Sheet.—Means of reducing Feverishness.—Foot Bath.—Used to counteract Pains in the upper Part of the Body.—Headache and Toothache.—The Feet should be Warm before they are put into cold Water.—Exercise to be taken immediately after the Foot Bath.—This is much better than going to the Fire.—This Bath good in Fatigue.—To be used cautiously by the Gouty.—Head Bath.—Its use in Headache, Inflammations of the Eye, Deafness, and loss of Smell and Taste.—Rush of Blood to the Head.—Mode of taking the Head Bath.—Finger Bath.—Mode of treating Whitlow or Felon.—Eye Bath.—How and for what Used.—Leg Bath.—Its uses.—Sitz Bath.—Mode of administering it.—Its importance.—Douche Bath.—Its effects.—Douches at Graefenberg.—Mode of taking the Douche.—It should be used with great Caution.—Length of Time for taking this Bath.

DESCRIPTION OF THE GRAEFENBERG BATHS.

THE entire or public bath at Graefenberg is about thirty feet in circumference, and sufficiently deep for a man of the ordinary height to plunge into up to his neck. The water is constantly renewed by springs in the mountains, the waters of which are conveyed through pipes into the bath, and escape by an opening for that purpose, so that no impurities may remain; besides which, the bath is emptied and cleaned twice a day: but this remark applies to Graefenberg only, as at Freiwaldau, with but few exceptions, the houses are supplied with portable baths.

The immersion of the body covered with sweat, into cold water, is exempt from danger, provided the organs of perspiration are in a state of repose. The risk which is incurred of catching cold, if, on arriving at a river to bathe, we remain until the body is cold and dry, cannot possibly exist in this case: as we thereby abstract from the body the heat which it requires to produce reaction, and thus lose the good effect of bathing. Then if we walk fast, or a long distance to the bath, it is requisite to repose a little, in order to tranquilize the lungs, after which we must undress quickly, and

* From Captain Claridge's Hydropathy.

plunge head foremost into the water, having first wetted the head and chest, to prevent the blood mounting to those regions. This precaution is strongly enforced at Graefenberg. During the bath, the head ought to be immersed several times into the water. Great care is requisite in not exposing the body, between throwing aside the blanket after sweating and entering into the bath.

It is highly advantageous to keep in movement in the bath, and to rub with the hands any parts afflicted. The skin is thus stimulated and the sensation of cold abated. People whose chests are affected, must exercise moderation in the use of the bath, entering it only by degrees, and not staying in it too long. In general, the time for remaining in the bath is governed by the coldness of the water, and the vital heat of the bather; but no general rule can be adopted with respect to this. At Graefenberg, where the temperature of the water is from 43 to 50 degrees, no one stays longer in the bath than from six to eight minutes, many only two or three. Priessnitz advises his patients to avoid the second sensation of cold, which is a sort of fever, by leaving the bath before it is felt: by this means the patient will avoid a too powerful reaction, provoked by a great subtraction of heat. This precaution is indispensable at the epoch of the treatment, marked by fevers and eruptions. Then a reaction, produced by an immoderate use of the bath or douche, would compel the invalid to keep his bed for some days, without at all accelerating the cure.

On leaving the bath, which is found more refreshing than any one can imagine who has not experienced its effects, you are covered with a sheet, over that a cloak is thrown, and thus you go to your room, where the whole body is dried and rubbed; and then you must dress quickly, and walk to keep up the warmth. To effect this by the heat of stoves or beds, would be acting in direct opposition to the treatment. A glass or two of water immediately after the bath is agreeable, and should not be omitted while walking.

When irritation is highly excited during the cure, baths should be suspended, as they would augment it. A general washing of the body, and sitz baths, are then resorted to. Sweating is also replaced by the envelopment of the body in a damp sheet, the repeating of which operation, together with the sitz bath, will cause the irritation to cease.

THE HALF BATH.

The half bath is about the size of those generally used in our houses, and is only employed in cases in which the whole bath would be too much for the strength of the invalid, who may require to be bathed for a longer time, in order to excite the morbid humors. It is, in effect, less active than the entire bath, and being attended with less danger, is frequently administered to new-comers for about a week, preparatory to the large bath; the temperature of the small, or half bath, is never lower than sixty degrees.

The water in these half baths is only about three to six inches deep. When it is necessary that the invalid should have the advantage of an entire bath, water is poured upon him, or the attendant constantly wets the body and head with the water of the bath.

When these small baths are used, in order to be less exciting, the upper part of the body is sometimes covered, and the bath hermetically closed, so that the head only appears.

This is in cases where it is necessary that the invalid should remain in them for an hour or two. We have known Priessnitz order this for five or six hours at a time, and repeat it several days successively, in order to provoke irritation, and produce fever. Last year, a doctor afflicted with an atonic gout was subjected to this treatment, and was completely cured. It is, indeed, a common thing at Graefenberg to see invalids remain for hours thus enclosed in the small bath, and continue doing the same for days, until fever is produced; this brings the morbid matter to the skin, in the form of abscesses, which sometimes discharge themselves in sufficient quantity for the matter to fill several glasses. When this crisis takes place, the baths are suspended during the discharge of these humors, by which the system is much benefited.

The half bath is frequently taken by the patient immediately after he has been confined in the wet sheet. It is accompanied by a general sprinkling of the body with cold water and rubbing. While still sweating, the patient should hasten to the bath, throw off the covering, previously wetting the head and chest, and the attendant should pour a pailful of water upon the head, when the face and body must be well rubbed. This last part of the process is often continued for ten or fifteen minutes together, sometimes much longer. When the patient quits the bath he dries himself, dresses, and proceeds to take exercise in the open air immediately; but persons who have not the means of consulting a doctor acquainted with Priessnitz's mode of treatment, are not advised to attempt this.

In almost all cases of fever the patient is first wrapped up hermetically in a wet sheet, which is changed as soon as it becomes warm, and repeated until the fever has subsided. As each of these sheets will become hot from having extracted a certain quantity of the caloric from the body, it necessarily follows that a chill will succeed the subsiding of the fever; the patient is then placed in the bath and rubbed all over by two persons, with the bare hand, until all the symptoms are abated. The patient then joins in the promenade, or at the public tables. If at night feverish symptoms return, the same operation is performed, and repeated until a perfect cure is effected.

FOOT BATH.

The foot bath is employed almost exclusively as a counteracting agent against the pains of the upper part of the body. Priessnitz prescribes these baths for precisely the same purposes that the faculty order warm ones, yet every one knows that the feet, after a warm bath, become cold, and then the reaction is upward, while, on the contrary, after a cold bath the feet become warm and the reaction is downward. Headache and toothache, whatever may be their causes, particularly those that are of a violent nature, inflammation of the eyes, and effluxes of blood to the head, are almost always relieved by means of the foot bath. To this should be added the application of wet bandages, without dry ones over them. The tub, or basin, in which these foot baths are taken, ought only to contain warm water from two to three inches deep, or just enough to cover the toes; for the toothache, one inch is sufficient; and the bath may be applied for some fifteen minutes to half an hour. In cases of sprains, the feet must be put in water up to the ankles. The water, when it becomes lukewarm, should be changed. The feet, during the whole time, should be well rubbed by the hand, or against each other, in order to promote a strong reaction. Care must be taken that the feet are warm before they are put into water, and exercise should be taken immediately afterward, to bring back the heat to them. Rubbing them with a dry hand assists this very much. Cold foot baths are sure means of preventing tendency to cold in the feet; the application of hot water only weakens the skin, and renders the feet more susceptible to cold

When they are extremely cold, instead of exposing them to the fire to warm, it is much better to produce the effect required by exercise. If we want any proof of the reaction caused by the foot bath, and its powers of preservation from catching cold, we have but to feel our feet an hour or two hours after the bath, and we shall then find them extremely hot. If we cannot avoid being exposed for a long time to a piercing cold, it is well to take a cold foot bath two hours previous to going out. After great fatigue, a foot bath of this description, before going to bed, is most refreshing. Gouty subjects should not use these baths without advice; but to people in general, Priessnitz recommends their frequent use. He contends, that in the feet many of the most serious complaints commence.

Homer, when he stated Achilles to be invulnerable except in the heel, no doubt knew that the feet were the most important parts of the human frame. The poorer people, who wear neither shoes nor stockings, or whose feet are constantly exposed to a sort of foot bath, are seldom subject to those complaints which attack the upper region of the body.

An Irish gentleman, thinking to do his shepherd a service, who had lived in a low, marshy situation for many years, sent him to another estate, which was high and dry, and asking him how he liked it, he replied, "Not at all; he had never been well a day since he had been there, for there was not a drop of water to wet his feet."

HEAD BATH.

Head baths are used for rheumatic pains in the head, common headaches, rheumatic inflammations of the eye, deafness, loss of smell and taste. They tend to disturb the morbid humors, which nature generally evacuates in the form of abscesses in the ears. They are also used to prevent the flow of blood to the head, but in this case only for a few minutes, in order to avoid too great a reaction. These should be followed by exercise in the open air, in the shade. This bath is used as follows: a wash-hand basin should be placed at the end of a rug upon the floor. On this rug the patient should extend himself, so that his head may reach the basin, at the bottom of which may be placed a towel for the head to rest upon. Then the back of the head must be placed in the water; then one side; and lastly, the other side of the head.

All this is terminated by again placing the back part of the head in the water.

The duration of this bath depends upon the nature and extent of the disease. In chronic inflammation of the eye, each part of the head should remain in water for fifteen minutes; and as long for deafness, loss of smell and taste. All this will occupy an hour, during which time the water should be renewed twice.

If these baths and foot baths are continued with perseverance, success is certain. This success is generally announced by violent headaches, until the formation of an abscess takes place, which finishes by breaking.

For the common headache, the back of the head may be exposed to the water from ten to fifteen minutes, and each side from five to ten minutes; if it is obstinate, a foot bath and a sitz bath, both slightly chilled, should be used for half an hour each.

FINGER BATH.

For whitlows or felons, the finger is placed in a glass of water three times a day, fifteen minutes each time, the finger and hand bandaged; then the elbow must be placed in water twice a day, and a heating bandage placed on the arm above it; this will have the effect of drawing the inflammation from the hand.

EYE BATH.

Water is held to the eye, which for a minute is kept closed, and then opened for five minutes in a small glass, made for the purpose, in circumference about the size of the eye. The head bath is generally used with this bath, but the latter is repeated oftener, and in most cases where there is inflammation, a fomentation is applied to the back of the head on going to bed, and another at the back during the day. For weak eyes the forehead is bandaged on going to bed. Sitz and foot baths form part of this treatment.

LEG BATH.

The thighs and legs, when afflicted with ulcers, ring-worms, wounds, or fixed rheumatic pains, ought to be put into a bath so as to cover the parts afflicted. The object of these baths is for them to act as stimulants. They may be taken for an hour, and sometimes longer: they always determine abscesses, and where they already exist, they cause an abundant suppuration. They are also applicable to any other members afflicted in a like manner.

THE SITZ BATH.

For want of a better term, we adhere to that of the Germans, and instead of a sitting we call it a sitz bath.

This is a small flat tub, of about seventeen inches in diameter, with water seldom more than three or four inches deep; in this people sit as in a hip bath, with their feet resting on the ground, for different periods—a quarter of an hour, half an hour, an hour, or more, as may be deemed sufficient. This, in some cases, is repeated two or three times a day. The sitting bath is considered by Priessnitz to be of so much importance in his treatment, that those patients are considered quite as exceptions for whom it is not prescribed. It has the effect of strengthening the nerves, of drawing the humors from the head, chest, and abdomen, and relieving flatulency, and is of the utmost value to those who have led a sedentary life.

The object of using so little water in this bath, the half bath, and foot bath, is, that a reaction may the sooner be effected. If a greater body of water were used, it would remain cold during the whole time of its application, and cause congestions to the upper regions; whereas, in this case, it almost immediately attains the heat of the blood, and admits of an immediate reaction.

To prevent the former, the patient should apply a wet bandage to the head: and to succeed more effectually in the object for which the sitz bath is prescribed, he should rub the abdomen as much as possible with a wet hand.

DROP BATH.

"This term is applied to single drops of water falling from a height of several fathoms. For this form of bath a vessel is used filled with very cold water, and furnished with a very small aperture, through which water passes in the form of drops. The small aperture should be partially closed by a plug, to prevent the drops from following each other in rapid succession. By these means their operation is considerably increased, and it becomes yet more potent if we allow the drops to fall upon a particular part at certain periods, and rub the part during the intervals. The reaction about to commence will indeed be thus interrupted, but will afterward make its appearance in a more powerful, energetic form.

"The violent excitement and irritation of the nervous system produced by these baths, render it necessary to restrict the use of them to half an hour; nor are they, indeed, adapted for vital parts, or such as are abundantly supplied with nerves.

"They are often used with more effect in obstinate and chronic cases of paralysis, than the douche or affusion, with which they may alternate. Powerful and continued friction with a horse-hair glove is never in this case to be neglected after the baths."*

THE DOUCHE BATH.

The douche, of all the means employed, is the most powerful in moving the bad humors, and disturbing them from the position which they may have occupied for years: they are also used in the greater number of chronic diseases. The douche corrects the weakness which the skin may have contracted in the process of sweating, and also fortifies it. It hardens the body, and renders it capable of supporting all variations in the atmosphere. It exercises a powerful action upon the muscles and nervous system, by the reaction which it provokes. What is understood by a douche, at Graefenberg, is a spring of water running out of the mountain, conveyed by pipes into small huts, where it falls from the top in a stream about the thickness of one's wrist, which fall constitutes the difference between the douche and a shower bath; outside this hut is another for dressing, constructed like the first, in the rudest way imaginable.

There are six douches in the forest of Graefenberg: the fall of the first is fifteen feet; the second, ten feet; the third, twenty feet; the fourth, eighteen feet. The douches set apart for women have a fall of twelve feet each: the diameter of the fall is the same as in those of the men.

At the colony there is a douche which is available all the winter: this is not the case with the others. About half a mile out of the town of Friewaldau, there are four more douches, resorted to by both sexes. Nearly all the douches are at some distance from the places of residence of the patients, which occasions a walk to arrive at them, so that the body is in a glow, and better calculated to be benefited by the effect of the water, when submitted to the process.

Parts afflicted should, for the greater part of the time, be exposed to the action of the douche, though it must be received oc-

* Weiss's Hand-Book of Hydropathy.

casionally upon all parts of the body, except on the head and face, unless this is especially ordered by Priessnitz. Weak chests should also avoid it on that part and the abdomen, otherwise the fall of the water on the lower part of the stomach or belly is not injurious. The atony of this region will not, however, always resist these means. The relief afforded by the douche, sometimes in a few minutes, in arthritic cases and rheumatism, is almost miraculous.

The douche being intended to put the morbid humors in movement, ought to be discontinued when it produces feverish excitement, and be commenced again when that has ceased.

The time recommended for the douche by different authors, is from one half minute to fifteen minutes. This, as all other strong impressions on the body, as a rule, should never be made with a full stomach, and generally not more than once or twice daily.

"The most intense expression which can be made by the application of cold water is by the douche—and there must be in the system a very considerable amount of vital force to enable the patient to bear this mode of application. A misapplication may so far lower the vital resistance as to make the reaction exceedingly difficult, or even impossible. It may knock the patient so violently down as to make it difficult for him to get up again—thus giving rise to dropsical swellings of the legs and feet, venous congestion, piles, varicose veins, and other symptoms of deficient vital actions. It sometimes produces the most extraordinary effects, as weeping, laughing, trembling, etc. In its proper place, however, it exercises a most powerful influence over disease, and seems to exert an especial impression upon the absorbents. I have seen tumors of long standing most rapidly absorbed, and disappear, under the use of the douche."*

* Dr. Edward Johnson

CHAPTER IX.

PROCESSES OF WATER-CURE—(CONTINUED.)

Shower Bath, an excellent Mode of taking it.—Its great Value in a variety of Diseases.—A Bath for every One.—How often should we Bathe.—Daily Bathing advocated.—The Vapor Bath.—Alleged Objections to its Use answered.—The Vapor Bath in some cases a better Mode than the Wet Sheet.—The Tompsonians are often Successful.—Great disregard of the importance of making remedial Applications to the Skin.—A Case.—Practice of the ancient Romans, the Russians, and the American Indians.—Tepid, warm, and hot Applications of Water.—Many suppose, erroneously, that nothing but *cold* Water is used in the new System.—Cases in which warm or hot Water is useful.—A Case.—A Mode of Curing the Colic.—Caution in the Use of warm Water.—Temperature of Baths.—Curious Facts regarding the Sensations caused by Water.—Cautions in the Use of Water.—Important Rules.—Air and Exercise.—These are important Adjuncts in Water-Cure.—Clothing.—Diet.—Principles of Digestion.

SHOWER BATH.

THE shower is probably the best form of bath for daily use, provided an abundance of water can be had. There are many of these used in New York since the introduction of the Croton, and more particularly since the subject of water is of late receiving a greater share of attention. One advantage of the bath of this kind is, that it can be taken so quickly; and then also the constant shower of water is very cleansing and invigorating.

In this, as in every kind of bath, the head should be the part first to commence upon. If the hair is long it can be guarded by a close oil-cloth or India rubber cap, but always the face, temples, and neck, should first be wet. This prevents the blood from rushing to the head—an objection that has been made to the shower bath. If one is highly sensitive to the impression of cold, the shower will be more bearable, provided loud and continued exclamation be practiced while under the bath. The exertion seems to keep the blood outward. Brisk motion, as dancing and jumping, with friction, should be at the same time resorted to, and then the body should be quickly rubbed dry, and exercise be taken, or a weak person can go to a warm bed. The body should be made thoroughly comfortable.

We have known weak invalids who had scarcely ever taken a cold bath, to commence in midwinter with the shower, beginning in the morning immediately on coming from a warm bed, and in the course of a few weeks, such persons have gained an amount of health and strength which, for years, they had not known. Rheumatism, incipient gout, giddiness, indigestion, with its long train of symptoms, and the like, have often in a remarkably short time been removed; and individuals of a pale, sickly, and sallow look, have acquired the ruddiness and bloom of youth.

In a few instances, those who were weak and sensitive to cold, have been taken with a sudden neuralgiæ or rheumatic "twinge," but this is oftener than otherwise caused by the bath being continued too long, or the person not keeping up sufficient exercise and friction. This generally passes off at once, and has never, in our experience, been alarming. Still it should be avoided.

A BATH FOR EVERY ONE.

An intelligent correspondent writes us of an ingenious contrivance for bathing, as follows: "I purchased three yards of twilled cotton, cut it in two pieces, had them sewed together; then I got enough old rope (about the size of my finger) to go round it, and had my square piece of cotton cloth bordered all about its four sides with the rope. I then took it to the painter, and had it oiled over on one side with two coats, and dried. This made me a perfect bathing mat. I place a pail of water upon it, and with a sponge I wash all over. After I have done, I take it up by the four corners and pour out the water. It is wiped and folded up. When I travel, this always goes with me, upon my trunk." This individual knows well the power of water, for after having suffered for many years from a rheumatic complaint which had resisted the best of medical treatment, he was cured in a few months by water.

HOW OFTEN SHOULD A BATH BE TAKEN?

We know of no exception to the rule that a bath should be taken daily. Every sick person, in whatever condition, or however weak they may be, should have the whole body rubbed over with wet cloths, sponges, or the like, at least once every day. In some cases great caution will be needed that it may be done safely. Let those who have lain for days upon a sick bed without any ablution, as is generally the case in the common practice of medicine, try, when the body is warm, the rubbing it all over, little by little, following briskly with dry cloths, and then covering the parts warmly, according to the feelings of comfort, and they will find it a most powerful tonic, and an application productive of great comfort. Physicians have yet many simple lessons of this kind to learn.

We repeat, every individual, old and young, male and female, sick or well, should have a daily bath. And in case of indisposition, instead of less attention to bathing, bathing the more should be given. There is no condition in which Nature would say "stop;" but rather she asks at our hand assistance.

VAPOR BATHS.

Among those who advocate and practice water-cure, there seems to be a general opinion that vapor baths are injurious. The objection most commonly made is, that the vapor too much excites the circulation, causes a rushing of blood to the head, and by this undue excitation or stimulation the body becomes weakened. It is an easy matter to cause injury by vapor baths. If it is made too powerful, or is too long continued, severe headache, and even fainting, may be caused. But this is the abuse. If a patient is wrapped in a dry blanket or a wet sheet to perspire, precisely the same injurious effects can easily be caused. With a good apparatus, there is no difficulty in regulating the vapor bath so that it will be as mild as one pleases—as mild in temperature, even, as the wet sheet in the way ordinarily used to cause mild perspiration.

It has been objected, that in vapor baths the heat is from a foreign substance, and that therefore it must be debilitating and weakening. But the same objection may be made respecting the sweating blanket, or the wet sheet causing perspiration. The natural heat of the body being 98 degrees Fah., there is constantly passing off in every direction a considerable amount of heat, unless it is some way obstructed; but if this heat is obstructed, as by the non-conducting blankets, as used in the wet sheet or sweating envelopment, and is retained at the surface of the body, or is thrown back upon the surface, the effect is not different from what it would be if the same amount of heat from any other source were applied in a similar way.

In many cases, we are confident, from experience, that a vapor bath suitably arranged, with a cool or cold bath after it, is better than to lay for hours in an envelopment. The time thus gained by the vapor bath is very valuable for exercise in the open air, and is often better than for the patient to be laying in a room perhaps not over well ventilated, as is generally the case.

To prevent too much blood at the head, a cold wet cloth, or a frequent washing the head and temples in cold water, is very useful. A headache or faintness are the first symptoms denoting that the bath is too powerful. The vapor bath should never be used in such a way as to cause headache or faintness. Such effects are never needed, and are always more or less pernicious.

The Thomsonians, or "steam doctors," as they are sometimes called, have been unmercifully and ignorantly vilified by many whose ignorance in certain cases superseded that of the ignorant ones among the "steamers," in proportion as it was more "scientific." Who does not know that the Thomsonian has often relieved patients in a most remarkable manner, when the "scientific" practitioner was compelled to "give up." A good vapor bath, and a thorough cleansing of the skin, will often cause such speedy relief, that it is reckoned an accident rather than otherwise that relief is obtained. The remedy appears too simple to cause any marked result.

Physicians generally seem to think it a thing of little consequence to pay any regard to the skin. Day after day, week after week, and month after month, patients are allowed to lay suffering for want of a cleansing of the skin; and in cases, too, where such a cleansing of the skin would cause more sudden relief than any thing else that can be done. We knew a physician of very extensive practice, who had under treatment a person with obstinate fever. After having done his utmost without any good success, he thought he would try vapor to "get up an action," as it was called; and to do this, some common barrel hoops were cut in two, and the half hoops were placed over the patient in bed to elevate the clothes; and then by hot stones or bricks wound in wet cloths, placed under the bedding thus elevated, a genial, pleasant vapor was caused all about the body, and thus by this simple means the patient was at once greatly benefited. It was just the thing needed. The patient rapidly recovered.

We lately had a patient who had been treated many months, and who, on leaving home, was given by his physician written directions, and to "wind up," it was recommended that, by all means, he should take vapor baths, should he be where they could be obtained—as if a vapor bath could not be had any where. He had been treated all this time without any. It is easy to give a bath of this kind in the following way: A number of bricks or stones are heated red hot. The patient is to sit upon a cane bottom or open-work chair (the clothing being removed), with a couple of woolen or other blankets pinned about the neck. A vessel of water—a common tin pan is as good as any thing—is placed under the chair, and into this water the hot bricks or stones are to be dipped, little by little, so that the vapor rises from the surface of the water. The body can thus be easily brought into perspiration.

The ancient Romans frequently used the vapor bath, and the cold one immediately following. The Russians go from vapor baths even at 150 degrees Fahrenheit, and plunge in very cold water, or roll in the snow. William Penn saw the vapor bath and the cold immersion used with remarkable success among the Indians of our own country; and at the present day, among the red men of the forest, the vapor is an important agent in the treatment of a variety of diseases.

TEPID, WARM, AND HOT APPLICATIONS OF WATER.

One great objection to the new system, is the supposed *chilling* effect of the treatment. It is supposed by many that the new mode consists wholly of horrible applications of *cold* water. Physicians themselves are not always over-particular in avoiding exaggeration on this point. It is found to be quite a good "bug-bear," with which to frighten people, by basely stating that weak infants, children, and old persons, are all to be subjected to the one horrible thing—*cold water.*

In many cases, no cold water at all is used, unless it be a little in the way of drink. It may be laid down as a rule, that whenever warm or hot applications are more agreeable to the feelings of the patient in subduing severe pain, as in severe colics, certain inflammations of the bowels, cramps in the stomach and bowels, pain in the back, pleurisy, or pain within the ribs or chest, etc., etc., the best rule we know of, is to consult the feelings of the patient. If there is high, burning inflammation, cold applications will be the most agreeable, and the best; but when there is pain without high, burning inflammation, the warm or hot applications are to be used. Let the following case illustrate:

An individual had eaten too heartily at dinner, and of food, in his case, indigestible. Very improperly, a full supper was taken upon this indigestible dinner, which soon caused, in the stomach and bowels, an excruciating colicky pain. In similar cases, the man had removed the difficulty by clysters and vomiting, caused by lukewarm water. At this time, however, these means failed, giving only partial relief. The author being called, he directed that the patient have warm bricks to his feet, and at once large towels folded over, to be slightly wrung out of water as hot as could be borne, and applied all over the abdomen and a part of the chest. These were changed unremittingly, as hot and as often as the patient desired, and very soon brought relief—sooner than could have been done by any drug opiate whatever. The bowels were also again freely purged, and the acid and indigestible substances removed from the stomach by much drinking of tepid water. After all pain was removed, and the stomach and bowels were well cleansed with pure clean water, it would have been well to have applied the tepid wet sheet to sleep in. This not being convenient, and not being very essential, it was omitted. A good night's rest was obtained. The individual lived nearly fasting the next day, drinking, however, a large quantity of water, mostly with the chill off, and then returned gradually and cautiously to a more full diet, and thus avoided all pain. In inflammation of the stomach and bowels, in almost every case where those frightful relapses take place, impropriety in food is the cause. In this case, had not relief been soon given, there would inevitably have resulted a very violent inflammation—in the stomach and bowels, always a most formidable disease.

A medical friend whom we highly esteem—a man who is never afraid to break away from old usages, provided he can see a better way—lately informed the writer, that in a case of most excruciating colic which fell under his treatment, when ordinary means had failed to bring relief, he caused the man quickly to be wrapped in a blanket wet in hot water, and this simple application caused immediate relief. It is astonishing to witness what can be often done by so simple a means to relieve pain. The same principle was used by the ancients to some extent, and has been more or less through all periods of time. The relief caused by applying the warm skin of an animal just slain, or by putting the patient into the warm carcass of an animal, an ancient mode, is upon the principle of warmth and moisture to soothe.

To propose a warm or tepid sheet, would perhaps only excite the ridicule of some who advocate water-cure. But it is certain that these are sometimes the best. We sometimes prescribe warm wet sheets, for there are cases in which it would not be safe to apply the cold one. It is not productive of any sort of good for a weak person to lay shivering in a cold wet sheet an hour or more, hoping afterward to get warm. Injury has been done by such means. It may be laid down as a rule, that when the body is cold, it should not be made colder, but instead it should be made warmer; and if this cannot be done by natural means, as by exercise, then artificial means should be used. Still the direct effort of heat is always weakening. The question, then, in warm or hot applications, is, whether they are not on the whole of evils the least.

Warm and hot foot baths are often very useful. But in such uses of water, a cold application following should be used to counteract the weakening and relaxing effect of heat.

TEMPERATURE OF BATHS.

Sensations from water alter very considerably, according to the temperature of the atmosphere, state of health, etc., etc. Hot baths are from 98 degrees Fah., the temperature of the blood, upward. Warm baths are generally reckoned from 92 degrees to 98 degrees; tepid, below 92 degrees. A tepid bath to one, may appear cold to another. As a rule, the colder the bath, if well borne, the better. The direct effect of warm baths is to weaken. Whenever they are taken, the time should be very short, and they should be immediately followed by a cold plunge, dash, shower, or at least rubbing with a cold wet cloth. It is well known by some housekeepers, that "washing day" can be borne with much less fatigue, if most of the water used be cool or cold.

As to different sensations, here is a curious fact. Atmosphere 55 degrees F.; body comfortable. Took three basins of water at 60 degrees, 70 degrees, and 80 degrees. Placed one hand in the water at 60 degrees, the other in the water at 80 degrees. Let them remain thirty seconds, and then placed both hands in the water at 70 degrees; to one it was cold, to the other warm.

It is said that in a road over the Andes, at about half-way between the foot and summit, there is a cottage, in which the ascending and descending travelers meet; the former, who have just quitted the sultry valleys at the base, are so relaxed that the sudden diminution of temperature produces in them a feeling of intense cold; while the latter, who left the frozen summits of the mountain, are overcome by distressing sensations of extreme heat.

CAUTIONS IN THE USE OF WATER.

Every one knows water may be made the means of great mischief. According to the celebrated Dr. Currie, of Liverpool, water may be safely used at any time when there is no sense of chilliness present, when the heat of the surface is steadily above what is natural, and when there is no general or profuse perspiration. For a full bath, general affusion, and drinking, these rules were by Dr. C. deemed fully sufficient for safety; and yet we are often told, that such men as Dr. C. and Priessnitz can manage water safely, and with it do wonders, but that practitioners in general would not be able to make those nice distinctions, and would consequently do much mischief. Better by far had it been if drugs were no more dangerous than water.

To the above may be added, as a rule, no strong impression should be made with water, externally or internally, within about three hours after a meal. A bath upon a full stomach may be very injurious. But if there is indigestion, colic, or inflammation, water should be used at once, in a way suited to the case.

Perspiration caused by the envelopment, or by vapor baths, does not come within Dr. Currie's rules. It is well known that a cool or cold bath rightly taken is not dangerous immediately after sweating, if this is not caused by over-exertion.

AIR AND EXERCISE.

It will be observed that these important adjuncts to any kind of treatment, share largely in the water-cure. Priessnitz insists that all who are able shall take an abundance of out-door exercise regularly. The value of such exercise is inestimable. Every one who observes at all respecting it, knows the invigorating effect it has upon the system. The cases given by different authors in this work, will furnish sufficient directions in reference to these adjuncts:

"Priessnitz's first endeavor is to alleviate pain, so that the patients may avail themselves of air and exercise. How far this object is attained may be judged of, from the circumstances that out of five hundred or six hundred, the usual average number of patients under his charge, there are seldom a dozen of persons in bed at one time. If their complaint be fever, he is so completely master of the case, that no one ever keeps his bed, and seldom his room, for more than two or three days, excepting in cases of typhus, a malady which generally takes twelve or fourteen days to eradicate, but hardly ever longer. The same remark will apply to rheumatism. If the sufferer can only reach Graefenberg, he may be sure of immediate relief, such as elsewhere would be called a cure, and which is repeated many times a year; but the cure can only be regarded then as just commenced, it being Priessnitz's object to eradicate the cause of malady from the system. What is understood by a cure at Graefenberg, is a perfect cleansing of the body of all impurities, a radical cure of that which has been the source of disease. Cases of no very long standing succumb to the treatment, sometimes in two or three months; others resist for one or two years. Supposing, for example, a young man to be attacked by gout, let him apply to Priessnitz, and he will be cured immediately; but another, who has inherited it from his family, and who has been a bon-vivant himself for a number of years, cannot expect to be made a new man, but with the exercise of patience; yet he will have this satisfaction, that during the cure he will find himself, in other respects, in perfect health, never be confined to his room, and be able to take plenty of exercise."*

CLOTHING.

Priessnitz requires of his patients that they lay aside their flannel and cotton. He holds "that they weaken the skin, render people delicate, and less able to contend against atmospheric changes." When objections are made, he says, "Wear it, then, over your shirt; but when you are accustomed to cold water, you will not miss it. After the bath which you have now taken, run or walk until you provoke perspiration. You need then have no fear of catching cold."

DIET.

Some who advocate the water-cure, as practiced by Priessnitz, have made objections to the diet. It is not pretended but that it is improvable. When it is said of his patients that "they eat too much," it is only saying what is true of civilized man the world over. When Professor Mott, of this city (New York), in one of

* Captain Claridge.

his lectures, said there was as much need of temperate eating societies as there was of temperate drinking societies, he by no means meant to be understood as placing a low estimate upon popular temperance societies; he was fully aware of the undeniable fact, that excessive alimentation is a most fruitful source of disease. Admitting that the diet at Graefenberg is not in all respects what it should be, as it is not, to obtain the best results in treating disease, it only goes the more strongly to prove the power and value of the water-cure. In some important particulars, Priessnitz has shown his good sense and judgment, all must admit, who are well informed on the subject of diet. "He deprecates all exciting things, such as tea, coffee, wines, and spirits, and recommends cold aliments rather than hot. A rule for dieting (in disease, second in importance to no other), is that which relates to *quantity*. In the process of starvation, it is a well-known principle, that the substances or parts of the body least essential to life are the first to be wasted, and on this same principle, in cases of shipwreck and other accidents, tumors have been known to disappear rapidly, and old ulcers to heal in a very short time, with those who have been thus subjected. This rule, of course, will not apply in *all* cases of disease.

"I know a gentleman," says Dr. Johnson, "who was entirely cured of an obstinate permanent stricture, by adopting a very severe course of abstinence, as it regards both food and drink, for two or three weeks. I am also acquainted with several other very severe cases of disease, entirely cured by the rigorous adoption of a severe diet—but *always in connection with a very mild course of the water treatment.*"

DIET AND DIGESTION.

The following rules are drawn from Dr. Beaumont's well-known Observations and Experiments, perseveringly made upon a healthy young man, whose stomach was exposed by a wound which healed, leaving an external opening. The rules are valuable for all, whether sick or well.

1. Bulk is nearly as necessary to the articles of diet as the nutrient principle. They should be so managed that one will be in proportion to the other. Too highly nutritive diet is probably as fatal to life and health as that which is insufficient in nourishment

2. The more plain and simple the preparation of food, and the less of seasonings of any kind, the better for the health. Stimulating condiments (salt, pepper, vinegar, mustard, etc.), instead of being used with impunity, are actually prejudicial to the healthy stomach. Though they may assist the action of a debilitated stomach for a time, their continued use never fails to produce an indirect debility of that organ. They affect it like alcohol, or other stimulants. The present relief afforded is at the expense of future suffering.

3. Thorough mastication and slow swallowing are of great importance.

4. A due *quantity* of food is of the utmost importance. There is no subject of dietetic economy, says Dr. B., about which people are so much in error, as that which relates to *quantity*. Dyspepsia is oftener the effect of over-eating and over-drinking, than any other cause.

5. Solid food, if properly masticated, is more easy of digestion than soups and broths.

6. Butter, fat meat, and all oily substances, being always hard of digestion, tending to derangement of the stomach, are better omitted.

7. Alcoholic liquors of every form, the various stimulating condiments, as mustard, pepper, spice, etc., tea, coffee, and narcotics of every kind, all tend to debility, derangement, and disease of the stomach, and through it, of the whole system.

8. Simple pure water is the only fluid necessary for drink, or for the wants of the system. The artificial drinks are all more or less injurious. "*Tea* and *coffee*," says Dr. B., "the common beverage of all classes of people, have a tendency to debilitate the digestive organs. Let any one who is in the habit of drinking either of these articles in a weak decoction, take two or three cups, made very strong, and he will soon be aware of their injurious tendency; and this is only an *addition* to the strength of the narcotic which he is in the constant habit of using."

9. Violent exercise very soon after a full meal is injurious, but gentle exercise promotes digestion. Sleep soon after a meal is better avoided.

10. Strong mental exercise and emotions of the mind, as grief, anger, fear, etc., particularly with a full stomach, tend to impair digestion.

CHAPTER X.

THE CRISIS OF WATER-CURE.

The Crisis a remarkable Feature of the Water Treatment.—This is sought much at Graefenberg.—Symptoms preceding the Crisis.—Meaning of the Term.—In some Cases of Cure there is no perceptible Crisis of any kind.—Priessnitz's Doctrines concerning Crisis.—It often happens on the part originally Diseased.—Sir Charles Scudamore's explanation of the Crisis.—Boils do not occur in healthy Subjects.—Crisis, Boils, and Rashes act as Counter-Irritants, as well as by purifying the Blood.—A Water Patient must often be Worse before he can be Better.—Too active Treatment should not be Practiced with a view of causing a Crisis.—A case of Injury by too severe Treatment.—Priessnitz's Skill and Prudence should not be lightly called into Question.—Does Water cause Dropsy?—The real Cause of this Affection.

One most remarkable feature in the water-cure is the Crisis, as it is termed. It is said that at Graefenberg it is really amusing to observe with what anxiety it is looked for by the patients. In most cases it proves the certain harbinger of a good cure. "The patients themselves are constant witnesses of this fact, and it is no wonder, therefore, that they should look forward with pleasure and hope to its advent in their own persons. A patient is no sooner missed from the table, than the question goes round, 'Has so-and-so got a crisis?' And if the reply be in the affirmative, the report spreads like the news of a fresh victory, and his friends assemble around him—not with long faces to condole him—but with merry smiles, and laughing jests, to congratulate him on his happy fortune." "The following allegorical lines from Southey," says Capt. Claridge, "might with great justice be literally applied, by the individual who has passed through the crisis, and been restored to health:"

"Most blessed water! Neither tongue can tell
The blessedness thereof, nor heart can think,
Save only those to whom it hath been given
To taste of that divinest gift of heaven.
I stopped and drank of that divinest well,
Fresh from the rock of ages where it ran;

It had a heavenly quality to quell
All pain. I rose a renovated man;
And would not now, when that relief was known,
For worlds the needful suffering have foregone."

"The crisis is generally ushered in by a sense of uneasiness, a loss of sleep and appetite, an alternate change from heat and cold, and lastly by all the symptoms of fever, which is sometimes violent, but always of short duration, if properly attended to. At its termination, the alvine and other evacuations are more plentiful, and accompanied by a more copious separation of extraneous matter than ordinarily; sometimes by several of the excretory passages at the same time. This increased secretion is generally accompanied by a variety of eruptions of the skin, by boils, abscesses, ulcers, etc."

"The term crisis applies to any very marked disturbance of the system, or cutaneous change; as the crisis fever, odorous perspiration, odorous urine, vomitings, diarrhœa, hæmorrhoidal discharge of blood, and various kinds of eruption on the skin."

In very many cases of cure, there is said to be no perceptible crisis of any kind. There appears to be no very general rule respecting it. In some old and obstinate cases of gout, mercurialism, etc., it may take place as many as from three to five times, before the cessation of the disease, and the re-establishment of perfect health.

"The very important matter of *crisis* is always sought for with much solicitude both by Priessnitz and the patient. He believes that it could not be produced in a healthy man; and that its occurrence is a sure proof that nature is successfully exerting herself to throw off the disease, by the exit of bad humor from the mass of blood. It is a sort of wholesale theory, and equally serves for all persons, and for every known disorder; and assuredly is the most convenient for one ignorant of medical science. I conceive that Priessnitz must have been gradually led to this idea of mordid blood by the observations which his experience enabled him to make; for, as before explained, he entered into the water-cure practice* by accident, and not from tuition. His principles have arisen out of practice as an empiric art, and were not as a precursor first implanted in his mind. He has, in innumerable instances, so

* I employ this term in its just signification, meaning experience, not charlatanism, from which I believe Priessnitz to be entirely free.

that the contrary forms the exception to the rule, witnessed the formation of crisis in the progress of the water-cure, among which boils take the lead in pre-eminence and importance of character. But the term also applies to any very marked disturbance of the system, or cutaneous change; as the crisis fever, odorous perspiration, odorous urine, vomitings, diarrhœa, hæmorrhoidal discharge of blood and various kinds of eruptions on the skin. It was a fact of ordinary occurrence, presenting itself to the mind of Priessnitz, that the great crisis of boils, in proportion to their free suppuration, proved in the highest degree remedial, removing chronic pains and internal sufferings of long standing; and that no marked amendment did take place until the event of some crisis. Also the additional fact must be mentioned, that very frequently indeed the boil crisis would appear in the immediate vicinity of the disease, sometimes on the very spot. It is no longer surprising therefore that the idea of humor in the blood should be strongly confirmed in the mind of Priessnitz, and have grown with him into a rule of practice. The patient very naturally cares not for the absence of scientific explanations, but renders his faith to fact, and to the long list of very extraordinary cures which have been performed, after the failure of regular medical art. But it will not be uninteresting to examine more closely this doctrine of the bad blood, with reference to crisis and treatment.

"In the case of morbid poisons, as, for example, small-pox, measles, and scarlatina, nature evidently makes a vigorous effort to free the blood from the virus, by producing in the skin a characteristic eruption, attended by a symptomatic fever. After a certain period, health returns, and no reminiscence of the poison occurs. I adopt this illustration to show that the blood can in this manner, by the medium of the skin, clear itself of the offending cause, however difficult the explanation may be. In the very familiar examples of cutaneous disease, as erysipelas, the shingles, nettle-rash, etc., we commonly refer to the blood as the source of disorder, although we can only generalize our notions; or, by other theory, we may regard these disorders as the offspring of some internal vitiated secretion, as acrid acid in the stomach, or bad bile, affecting the skin by supposed sympathy—which is equally figurative language, if we are driven to close and searching analysis.*

* A breaking out, as it is called, on the lips and chin, would probably be

"Boils and carbuncles do not occur in healthy subjects; and, when they happen naturally, are always looked upon as indicating a bad habit of body. The surgeon may choose other description, and call it weak and unhealthy inflammation, affecting the outward texture of the body differently from phlegmon or true inflammation. I will not, therefore, for the sake of language, attempt to dispute the plain notion, so familiarly adopted, of the nature of crisis in the water-cure treatment; but I do think it of great importance that it should have its sober limits, and not be made an ignis fatuus to the practitioner or the patient. The benefit arising from crisis must not be referred merely to the depuratory or cleansing process for the blood. Boils and rashes act as counter-irritants, in the ordinary and most accepted view, and in this way also prove useful; on the same principle that we see advantage derived from blisters, and artificial eruptions produced by external applications, tartar emetic, croton oil, etc.; and even the use of setons and issues is connected with this principle of counter-irritation equally with the idea of discharging the offending humor from the blood. It is very evidently the formation of an artificial disease, with the hope that it may be a substitute for the real one, and cause its removal.

"It certainly happens in this way that much inconvenience must often be sustained by the patient in the progress of his cure; and he must submit to be worse, before he can be better.

"The occurrence of boils is not, however, invariably necessary to the cure. Nature determines this, and may give another kind of crisis; and even none that is notable may be the pleasing fate of some, who still receive every benefit and recover.

"From all that I have seen, and my opportunity has been extensive, I am deeply impressed with the conviction that the employment of a very large amount of treatment, at one and the same time, in order to urge the circulation to produce crisis, demands most prudent consideration, and especially in irritable constitutions. I am free to admit that, in chronic cases of long standing, superficial measures would be of little or no avail, and that there must be efficient treatment. If too active measures be pursued in these exceptionable instances to which I allude, a sudden and too severe crisis might be produced, creating high suffering and possible danger. Instead of the favorably suppurating boils, such as are of un-

produced in any one, by eating for a continuance rich sauces, especially if made with bad butter.

toward character might arise. I am sure that these unfavorable consequences may always be avoided by ordinary care, and do not belong to the water-cure treatment, as of right, more than any accidental untoward result belongs to the regular practice of physic.

"Whenever a threatening appears of too strong a crisis, the treatment is to be immediately reduced; and, being nicely adapted also to the particular circumstances of the case, all anxious embarrassment will be removed.

"In conclusion of this subject, I advert with regret to reflections which I have seen in print on the skill of Priessnitz, on account of a particular case which occurred at Graefenberg, unfavorable in respect to the constitution of the patient, and having a fatal termination. In its treatment at the latter period, there had been on the part of the individual much improper deviation from the directions laid down, owing to an impatient desire of urging crisis for the sake of a more speedy cure. From this cause, fever crisis set in suddenly and with destructive violence. Continued high irritation and fatal exhaustion ensued.

"A lamented event of this kind, happily most rare, should serve as occasion for such reflections as I have already suggested. No remedy that is powerful for good, can be so weak an instrument as not to be also capable of evil. Neither the skill nor the prudence of Priessnitz should be lightly called in question by any one. I am convinced that, with regular superintendence of a case, he would never provoke a crisis beyond his power of convenient control. The very large number of patients in his list, varying from two to five hundred, could not allow of watch being kept over every case, and he must be sought for rather than seek. He is most attentive on every important occasion; and it must be the fault of the patient if he do not report progress; and more especially if he do not seek prompt aid in the event of the least unfavorable occurrence.

"Another and very important consideration presents itself on the subject of crisis: for how long a time is its occurrence to be viewed as an indication for the continuance of treatment? Evidently it requires judgment to know what may be referred to the influence of the constitution not yet delivered from its errors; and what to simple morbid action of the vessels of the skin, existing as a secondary and a local disease. I know an instance of the occasional formation of boils on the legs, causing much inconvenience, although the general health is quite restored: the full water-cure treatment, which was carried on nearly two years, having been laid aside for one, with the exception that the patient applies water-dressings to the skin when it inflames, or to a boil, and uses a cold bath daily."*

DOES WATER CAUSE DROPSY?

"Many object to the drinking of cold water, on the ground that animals only drink to quench thirst. This is true, but they do not live in our artificial state, nor are they subject to the influence of the mind. It cannot be denied that the nearer people approximate to nature, the less they need adhere to any prescribed rules; but man resorts to water to establish his health, therefore the quantity must be increased, not only for the purpose of allaying his thirst, but to dilute, purify, and restore, in quantities which must depend upon the inconvenience or pain experienced. By this simple means, serious indispositions are often prevented. Another argument made use of against drinking cold water is, that it produces dropsy. In the first place, it is evident, that if this were true, such a complaint ought not to exist among us, for whoever heard of an Englishman drinking too much water? But we affirm, on the contrary, that this disease is caused by the injudicious administration of drugs; the use of too large a quantity of them; by omitting to drink cold water, and by neglecting to wash or bathe the body daily in that element.

"If the skin is so much relaxed that it no longer throws out those matters which daily reach it from the interior of the body, fluids are collected underneath the skin which ought to be evaporated, and which cause inflation, paleness, and cold. This is what is called dropsy.

"The more the human body is injured by drugs, the more it is in need of strong perspiration, because it endeavors, by the aid of this physical agent, to relieve itself of all diseased matter. From this it may be inferred, that no persons are more in need of the cold water-cure than those who have taken too much physic. Further, strong poisons, of whatsoever nature they may be, whether mercury, blue pill, calomel, bark, or spirituous liquors to excess, frequently cause death by dropsy; sometimes this disease is caused

* Sir Charles Scudamore's Medical Visit to Graefenberg.

by catching cold, but only those are liable to it who have produced a disposition to the complaint by relaxing the skin. The only remedy formerly known was to draw off the water by tapping, which operation, often repeated, gives a respite to life for a short time. This illness, in its infancy, may always be speedily cured by hydropathy, and, in its most advanced stages, if there be any strength left in the constitution, this disease will be eradicated by the water-cure; it being the property of this treatment to revive the activity of the skin, and enable the latter to indulge freely in the necessary ejection of perspiration.

"From the returns of the year 1841, within the city of London, and bills of mortality, among a people altogether opposed to the use of water, we find that from dropsy alone the deaths amounted to no less a number than 584. Any one who never takes physic nor intoxicating liquors, and keeps to a water diet, may be perfectly sure of never being attacked with dropsy."*

CHAPTER XI.

DISEASES TO WHICH THE WATER-CURE IS MORE ESPECIALLY ADAPTED.†

Water a Remedy applicable in all Diseases.—The true Nature of this Means.—The great benefit of Water in acute Diseases.—Neuralgic, or painful Disorders.—Indigestion.—Its Nature, and the proper Principle of treating it.—Leucorrhœa, or Fluor Albus.—Nature of this Affection.—Gout and Rheumatism.—These are often Cured at Graefenberg.—Epileptic Fits.—Spinal Irritation.—Difficult Menstruation.—Influenza.—Concluding Remarks.

I SHALL now proceed to enumerate a few of those diseased conditions of the body to which the water-cure is most especially adapted. But I would here premise that this mode of treatment, when properly modified, and carefully adapted to the peculiarities of individual constitutions, and to the nature of the disorder, can seldom fail of conferring more or less benefit, let the diseased condition be what it may. This is true from the very nature of the

* Captain Claridge.

† From Dr. Edward Johnson's "Hydropathy, or the Water-Cure."

remedy, the effect of which is to *strengthen the general system.* And undoubtedly a certain amount of strength may, by it, be accumulated in the body, although the actual disease itself may not be eradicated. In cases where it is impossible that the disease should be cured, the general health and strength may be so much improved as to render it far more easily endured.

I must also premise, that besides those diseases which I am about to mention, as well as many others concerning which want of room must necessarily keep me silent, there are a multitude of anomalous and undenominated disorders, so entirely varied in form, character, and symptoms, that any attempt to enumerate them here is perfectly out of question—and yet many of these are unquestionably such as can be entirely removed by hydrotherapeutic treatment, upon the principles herein laid down as the foundation of that mode of cure.

ACUTE DISEASES.

The diseases over which the water-cure is said to possess the most rapid and striking influence, are *acute diseases.* Fevers, febrile diseases, inflammations, etc., etc.—such of them, of course, as are curable by *any* means—are said to be removed with a certainty and rapidity which is little less than magical. A fever which, under ordinary treatment, would confine the patient to his bed for six weeks or two months, is frequently overcome in *two or three days,* and the patient is thus restored to health before there has been time for the approach of that extreme weakness and emaciation so constantly the result of a long illness, even after the disease itself has been vanquished.

In all curable acute diseases, therefore, the water-cure is peculiarly and especially available.

NEURALGIC, OR PAINFUL DISEASES.

In all painful disorders also—disorders the chief character of which is *severe and acute pain*—this treatment possesses the most extraordinary, and even unaccountable powers of relief. Severe pain is a sensation almost entirely *unknown* at Graefenberg.

INDIGESTION.

There is a most extensive class of symptoms, manifesting themselves in various groups, in different persons, attacking almost every individual more or less severely, and more or less frequently, throughout the whole range of the upper and middle classes; sparing neither age, sex, nor condition; undoubtedly the cause of more human suffering than any other disorder, and which class of symptoms has received the general appellation. These distressing sensations are exceedingly various, and indeed only agree among themselves in being universally accompanied by evidences of a disordered stomach. The term indigestion is an exceedingly absurd one—inasmuch as it implies that the faulty action of the stomach is always the *cause*—whereas the faulty action of the stomach is much more frequently the *effect* of disorder in some other organ. Ignorance of this fact (well known to medical men, however) has led persons to do themselves infinite mischief, and actually to bring on disorder in a previously healthy stomach, by a misapplication of remedies. For instance, a man gets a headache and a disordered condition of the stomach, at one and the same time. He never hesitates a moment as to what he should do, but forthwith sets about physicking his unfortunate and most innocent stomach—taking it for granted that it is the disordered stomach which has produced the disordered brain; whereas it much more frequently happens that it is the disordered brain which has produced the disordered stomach. He addresses his remedies to the wrong organ, thus doing no good to the *one*, and infinite mischief to the *other*.

I believe that indigestion hardly ever (now-a-days) commences in the stomach. But the healthy functions of the stomach are continually disturbed by a distressed, irritated, fagged, worn-out condition of the brain and nervous system—from which system alone the stomach, like every other organ, must derive all its vigor. But how can the stomach derive *vigor* from the brain and nervous system, if the brain and nervous system have *no vigor themselves?* Indigestion is almost peculiar to the upper and middle classes, and among these is nearly a *universal* disease. There must, therefore, be a universal cause for it, which cause must be *peculiar* to these classes. But *excess*, either in eating or drinking, is not *now*, by any means, a *universal fault* in, nor is it peculiar to, these classes.

But there *is* a morbid cause, which *is* almost *peculiar* to the upper and middle classes, and which *is*, also, almost *universal* among these classes.

This cause is a morbid, undue, and excessive *excitement* of the *brain and nervous system.* And the morbid sensibility which necessarily results from this constant excess of nervous excitement, I take to be by far the most frequent source of indigestion. For it must be remembered that the stomach derives its digestive powers from the eighth pair of nerves, along which nerves the nervous influence is transmitted to the stomach like electricity along the conducting wire, or steam through a tube. If this nerve be divided in a healthy dog, while digesting his meal, digestion instantly stops and becomes impossible.

Among the upper and wealthy classes, this excessive excitement is derived from artificial, and unnaturally refined sources of pleasure. The theatre, the ball-room, music, dancing, gaming, political ambition daily disappointed, fashionable emulation perpetually on the strain—petty contentions of all sorts—late hours and luxurious habits—these, in the upper ranks, are the causes of excessive excitement—morbid sensibility—anxiety—indigestion.

In the middle classes, the *same* morbid results are obtained, by the *same* means, from sources somewhat different. And the cares of business, the anxieties of speculation, solicitude for the welfare of a numerous family, pride hourly contending with poverty, debts, doubts, dangers, and difficulties—these do for men of the middle rank, what the causes above enumerated do for those of the upper.

Some of the more prominent features of this many-headed monster I will here enumerate. They are nausea, pain about the region of the stomach and sides, headache, heart-burn, a sense of fullness, distension, or weight in the stomach, a feeling as if a ball were lodged in the throat, acid or offensive eructations, flatulence, vomiting, especially of a clear liquor (like pure water), sometimes of an acid quality, and often in large quantity, a sensation of *sinking or fluttering* at the pit of the stomach, and loss of appetite; costiveness or irregularity of the bowels, with a morbid appearance of the evacuations; pain of the back, and turbid urine; a disagreeable taste in the mouth, especially on waking; a feeling of stinging, or heat, as of cayenne pepper, in the mouth; toothache, palpitation, pulsation in the region of the stomach, irregularity of pulse; short, dry cough, and occasional difficulty of breathing; giddiness, languor, lassitude, depression of spirits, with fear of death, or of impending evil.

Whenever this long train of distressing symptoms has arisen from excessive irritation of the nervous system—from morbid sensibility, without organic lesion—as it does in nineteen cases out of twenty—it can be cured, beyond question, by the hydropathic treatment—by exalting and accelerating the change of matter.

LEUCORRHŒA, OR FLUOR ALBUS.

This most distressing, enfeebling, and exceedingly common disease—a disease which resists almost every other mode of treatment—depending, as it does, upon chronic inflammation of the uterus, is well calculated to be effectually removed by the invigorating method adopted at Graefenberg, and other hydropathic establishments.

Attempts have lately been made to show that leucorrhœa depends upon an ulcerated condition of the os uteri. It is extremely probable that the os uteri may be frequently found in an ulcerated condition in females laboring under leucorrhœa, but the more probable inference is, that the ulceration is the *effect*, and not the cause, of the morbid discharge—whose acrimonious nature is often fully sufficient to account for the ulcerated condition of the os uteri. Besides, supposing the ulcerated condition to be the cause of the discharge, that condition could not have come on without previous inflammation. But, whichever of these two conditions, inflammation or ulceration, be the true cause, the cold water remedy is equally well adapted to remove it—seeing that *both causes* are themselves *caused* by a *weakened condition* of the organs concerned.

GOUT AND RHEUMATISM.

The cases of rheumatism and gout which have been cured at Graefenberg, are almost without number. And when it is considered that these diseases depend upon inflammation of particular structures of the body, and that this inflammation again, in *its* turn, depends upon a *weakened* condition of the nervous system, it is sufficiently easy to account for the fact.

EPILEPTIC FITS.

Whenever this disease depends, as it very frequently does, upon a clot of blood pressing on the brain, it is curable by the hydropathic treatment, united to that of a *severe diet*. Besides the cases given in the list of cases in this work, I have been witness to another very remarkable one. The patient was the subject of epilepsy for four years, and the fits recurred regularly every ten days. He has not now had a fit for three months, and is about to return home perfectly cured.

SPINAL IRRITATION.

Spinal irritation, resulting from subacute or chronic inflammation of the vertebral theca, and giving rise to a long train of the most distressing symptoms, is perfectly curable by cold water treatment.

DIFFICULT MENSTRUATION.

Painful, excessive, suppressed, or *insufficient* menstruation, is another distressing affection over which the hydropathic remedy possesses the most absolute control.

INFLUENZA.

Of late years a vast number of persons have suffered greatly from protracted influenza; and occasionally this disease is so obstinate as to resist all ordinary remedies. It yields most readily, however, to the Graefenberg method of cure.

Constipation, hysteria, rheumatic gout, catarrh, rheumatism of the head or of the heart, bilious headache, sciatica, lumbago, mercurial diseases, secondary symptoms, inflammation of the kidneys, impotence, neuralgic or painful affections of the nerves—all these are completely under the control of the cold water treatment.

But my limits will not allow me to devote more space to the particular mention of individual diseases. More will be found in the list of cases.

Besides these, however, there is a whole host of anomalous, undenominated diseases, which cannot be referred to any particular class, which come within the scope of the cold water-cure. And there is probably *no disease* which cannot be benefited, more or less, by the exaltation of the living energies, and the improvement of the general health and strength.

In fine, all those diseases depending upon functional weakness—all those depending upon nervous debility, and morbid sensibility—all those depending upon inflammation, acute, subacute, or chronic, *uncomplicated with permanent organic lesion*—all those depending upon morbid matters in the blood or other humors—these constitute that long list of diseases which are peculiarly calculated, from their nature and causes, to be removed by the hydrotherapeutic remedy.

It is not, however, to be inferred that this remedy is unable to cure *any cases* of organic lesion. On the contrary, whenever these cases are, from their nature, capable of cure *at all*, without the aid of surgical operations, the cold water treatment undoubtedly offers a better and more rational chance of success than any other—as some of the cases herein related *prove*—as, for instance, the cases of fistula, epilepsy, and paralysis.

CHAPTER XII.

GRAEFENBERG CASES OF WATER-CURE.*

Acute Rheumatic Fever.—Inflammation and Swelling of the Breasts, with general Fever.—Paralysis.—Sciatica.—Constipation.—Dyspepsia.—Dyspepsia and Rheumatism.—Gout and Rheumatism, complicated with Venereal taint.—Gout in the Hands and Knees.—Rheumatism, with Psoriasis.—Case of Psoriasis communicated by George Anthony, Esq., an English surgeon, now at Graefenberg.—Skin Disease.—Psoriasis.—Skin Disease following Gonorrhœa.—Fistula in Ano.—Urinary Fistula.—Gonorrhœa.—Consumption.—Cough, Weakness of the Chest, and Injury of the Back.—Deafness.—Hip Disease.—Scarlet Fever.—Symptomatic Fever (related by the Mother).—Cartarrh, or Cold.—Baldness.—Headache, with Giddiness.—Secondary Syphilitic Symptoms.—Another Case of Secondary Syphilis.—Third Case of Secondary Syphilis.—Fourth Case of Secondary Syphilis.—Impuissance, complicated with Gout.—Contracted Joints.—Hernia.—Hæmaturia, or Voiding of Blood from the Urinary Organs.—Cerebro-Spinal Disease.—Suppressed Measles.—Deafness.—Epilepsy.—Hypochondriasis, Psoriasis, Sciatica.

Most of the following cases fell under my own immediate notice, and were examined by me *personally*, and their previous history and progress narrated to me by the *patients themselves*. There are two or three, however, for the history of which I am indebted to George Anthony, Esq., an English surgeon who had been residing at Priessnitz's establishment for a considerable time, and who took notes of such cases as fell under his notice. This gentleman had quitted his profession for a very lucrative appointment in the East, to which he proceeds in the latter part of the summer (1843)—that he went to Graefenberg merely as a matter of curiosity, and to fill up his time previously to his quitting Europe, and that the

* From Dr. Edward Johnson's "Hydropathy, or the Water-Cure."

cases noted by him cannot, therefore, be supposed to be *colored favorably* by any interested bias toward hydropathy; against which, indeed, he evidently entertained at first a very natural and professional prejudice.

For two other cases I am indebted to Col. Bowen, late of the Coldstream Guards; but the greatest bulk of them fell under my own immediate notice and personal examination.

Before I proceed to the detail of cases treated at Graefenberg, I will mention two remarkable ones which I treated myself by cold water alone, more than twenty years ago—that is, before its efficacy as a remedial agent was known *even to Priessnitz himself.* I mention these merely to show how early in life I had been led, by observation and general reasoning, to form a high opinion of cold, in the treatment of disease.

ACUTE RHEUMATIC FEVER.

Somewhat more than twenty years ago I became the subject of a very uncommonly severe attack of acute rheumatic fever. I was attended by Dr. Birkbeck and Dr. Thomas Davies, who afterward became physician to the London Hospital. I was also daily visited by some other medical gentlemen living in my neighborhood. They were exceedingly kind and attentive to me, for which I shall never cease to feel most grateful—and I am quite certain that my case was treated in the most scientific manner, that is, according to the accepted medical science of that day.

I was three times bled in the arm, and took frequently repeated doses of calchicum, which produced excessive and continued vomiting. These powerful means, however, failed to remove the pain, but reduced me to so slow a degree of exhaustion, that the fever began to assume the typhoid or nervous character. My wife was now told not to calculate upon my recovery, and ordered to give me brandy, repeatedly, and at short intervals, during the course of the night. At this time my skin was excessively hot and the bedclothes oppressive. I begged and prayed for cold water to drink, and to have myself washed all over in cold water. Every thing that was delicious and desirable in the universe seemed to be represented by these two words—cold water. My wife at last yielded to my entreaties—and the more so, inasmuch as she had often heard me enlarge upon the efficacy of cold ablution in fevers and many other diseases, and lament that popular prejudice would not suffer me to employ it so frequently as I desired. She had, moreover, herself, on one occasion, been plucked from agony and sudden danger by the use of snow.

The cold ablution, and large draughts of cold water, were immediately exhibited, and industriously and frequently repeated night and day.

In a week, with the exception of the debility consequent on the loss of so much blood, *I was quite well.*

INFLAMMATION AND SWELLING OF THE BREASTS, WITH GENERAL FEVER.

The second case occurred in the person of my wife about a year previously to that which I have just mentioned. On the evening of the third day after her first accouchement, I came home from Guy's Hospital, where I had been detained since morning, and found her groaning and weeping with intense pain, the breasts red, and enormously enlarged, which the frightened nurse was vehemently rubbing with brandy and oil. The skin was excessively hot and dry, and the pulse was leaping along at the rate of 120. It was in the month of January—so I walked into the street with a pail, which I filled with snow, and bringing it into the sick room, I piled a heap of it over both breasts, continually adding fresh snow as it melted. In a very few minutes the milk span out in streams, to the distance of more than a foot, and the tears of torture were at once changed for those of pleasure, accompanied by that hysterical sobbing, which is the common result of a sudden transition from intense suffering to perfect ease. The mere absence of pain in these cases takes all the characters of the most delicious and positive pleasurable sensations. In half an hour the inflammation had subsided, the breasts had become *comparatively* flaccid, the fever had entirely subsided, and not only all danger, but all inconvenience, had utterly vanished. But for this timely succor, suppuration must have supervened in both breasts, and large abscesses would have been the *inevitable consequence.*

PARALYSIS.

Herr Von Wulffen, an officer in the Prussian army, was seized in 1842 with a paralytic stroke. Of this he recovered. But the disease continued to recur at short intervals, until he had almost entirely lost the use of one side of the body—so that he could only walk very imperfectly and with great difficulty. In addition to this, he was extremely rheumatic, and the glands of the neck were swollen. After resorting to an infinite variety of curative means, which left him exactly where they found him, he came to Graefenberg.

After his arrival at Graefenberg and commencement of the treatment, this gentleman did not experience a single attack for two months, although before his arrival he would frequently be attacked two or three times in a month. The swelling of the glands of the neck subsided, his rheumatism was entirely removed, and his health completely re-established.

At the expiration of two months, however, he one day took an extremely long walk among the mountains, and came home very much fatigued, cold, and with wet feet. And now, instead of going to bed, he went into the hot and crowded billiard room, where he continued to play for some time. After this he suddenly lost the power of distinct utterance, could with difficulty articulate his words, and began to talk, all at once, quite incoherently. Priessnitz was sent for, who threw cold water over his face and chest, and then ordered him a foot bath, with three men to rub his feet for half an hour. This recovered him. He was then told to walk, but after having walked for ten minutes, he became so weak that he was obliged to go to bed. His friends now left him, in order to go to dinner. When they returned, they found him quite in his senses, but perfectly speechless, and unable to write. In fact, his tongue, and right hand, and foot were palsied. Priessnitz now ordered him a wet sheet (merely damp) for ten minutes—then another, a little wetter, for ten minutes more—and then a third, very wet indeed, for ten minutes more again. Feverish symptoms now followed, with violent headache, and great prostration of strength. For these symptoms he was put into the tepid bath for half an hour, and well rubbed by three men the whole time. Vomiting now took place, and in the evening he was up in the saloon at supper, as well and as sensible as any one there, and laughingly assuring his friends that he was now not only in full possession of his tongue, but of his teeth too. Since this time, which is now some months ago, he has had no return, has the perfect use of all his limbs, and is otherwise in good health.

Herr Regenhard, of Vienna, had suffered for many years from

nervous disease and severe dyspepsia. Three years since he had a paralytic seizure of the right half of the body—not severe—and from which he recovered. Six months afterward he had a second attack—more severe—from which, however, he partially recovered. Four months later he had a third attack, and afterward a fourth and fifth, the intervals between the fits becoming shorter and shorter, until they returned every fortnight. His right leg and arm now became nearly useless. He was advised to try the baths at Toeplitz, which he did, but without any good result. He returned to Vienna; he took the best advice which that capital could afford, but entirely without benefit. One of his physicians at last, with a candor and honesty which done him honor, confessed that he believed his case to be beyond the reach of any ordinary medical treatment, and recommended him to try the water-cure. He came to Graefenberg in company with my friend Mr. Niemann, who was also going to Graefenberg on his own account. He arrived there in May, and was then in his sixtieth year. He was immediately put under a very mild treatment (merely an abreibung, rubbing the head with a wet cloth, and a coph bath). In six weeks he had crises, but (which is very remarkable) only on the side affected. Not a single pimple appeared on the sound side. When the crises appeared, he took leintuchs with abgeschrecktes bath. No cold bath, no douche, no sitz bath. He continued to have crises till October (five months). He then left perfectly recovered, never having had a single attack after he commenced the treatment. His friends at Graefenberg have since received two letters from him, perfectly well written by that same right hand which was paralyzed and useless when he first came to Graefenberg, and which had been to him nearly a profitless member for the three previous years.

In gratitude for his recovery, he has made several ornamental presents to the grounds about Graefenberg, which still remain, and will remain there, monuments of the curative power of cold water. Indeed, Graefenberg abounds with such monuments, both in iron and stone, erected by Gratitude in commemoration of recovered health, and of a size and durability which gives them a fair chance of endurance for hundreds of years.

Captain Wardle, of the Fiquelmont dragoons, the nephew of Colonel Wardle, celebrated for certain charges which he preferred against the Duke of York, became suddenly deprived of the use of one entire side. He was blind of one eye, deaf of one ear, and the leg and one arm of one side were paralyzed. He was twenty-two years of age. Under the water-cure he entirely recovered. The sight of the eye was perfectly restored, his hearing entirely regained, and the full use of his limbs returned. After his recovery, Colonel Bowen saw him on guard at the theatre of Prague, the picture of youthful health and manly strength. He is still on military duty at Prague.

SCIATICA.

Mr. Wrangler, merchant, had been affected with sciatica for eighteen months. He was living at Milan, and the physicians there recommended him to have the actual cautery* applied to the part. This, however, he refused. He then went to a water establishment in the Tyrol, superintended by a physician, but one who was grossly ignorant of the principles on which the water-cure proceeds. This gentleman succeeded at last in persuading him to submit to the actual cautery, for his sufferings were so great that he would have submitted to almost any thing, in the hope of relief. He showed me the deep scar left by the hot iron, and which was as large as my extended hand. From the actual cautery, however, he received no benefit, and, in consequence of injudicious treatment, he became exceedingly ill, and then proceeded to Vienna, where he placed himself under the most celebrated medical practitioners, and underwent every conceivable mode of treatment. While submitting to treatment at Vienna, his bowels suddenly became constipated, and would never relieve themselves without the aid of medicine; and his thigh dwindled away until it was but little larger than his wrist, and he could not walk a single step.

He was now brought to Graefenberg, where he has resided for the last nine months. He gave me the history of his case himself, and was good enough to let me examine the affected parts. He is now perfectly well, entirely free from pain, full of flesh and animal spirits, and the withered thigh has entirely recovered its original very fleshy dimensions. He is not in the slightest degree lame, and can climb the mountains with the best of them, and in any weather. He is covered with the usual critical eruption, as soon as which subsides, he will return to his family at Milan. He

* The actual cautery is a hot iron.

is forty-eight years of age. His treatment consisted of the leintuch, succeeded by the tepid bath, the sitz bath, and douche.

SCIATICA WITH LUMBAGO.

Monsieur Varnod was afflicted with sciatica for *three years* so severely that it was with great difficulty he could walk even with the aid of a stick. Every ordinary means of cure had been resorted to without effect. He was at last prevailed upon to visit a water establishment at Innspruck. With great pain and difficulty he was got down to the side of the cold bath; and here it required a great exertion of courage in a lame man, and one who could not on any sudden emergency move his limbs without excruciating pain—I quite agree with him, that it required great courage in one so situated to allow himself to be tumbled heels over head into the water. With fear and trembling, however, he submitted, and to his utter astonishment found that while in the water he could move his limb without the slightest pain or inconvenience. The pain had entirely vanished, and from that moment to this it has never returned, nor does he exhibit the slightest indication of lameness or weakness in either of his legs. He is now at Graefenberg for another disease—a disease of the skin.

CONSTIPATION.

Herr Fricks, the father of the young man whose case I am about to relate, put himself under treatment also, for an obstinate constipation which had annoyed him, and interfered greatly with his health, for 17 years. So obstinate and torpid had the bowels become, that it would frequently require four or five lavements before their contents could be emptied.

This gentleman was treated by leintuchs and sitz baths—four of the former daily (two in the morning, and two in the evening, each couple of leintuch's being succeeded by the tepid bath), and two of the latter also daily.

In a fortnight this gentleman's bowels began to empty themselves without assistance, daily and plenteously, and have continued to do so up to the time when I left Graefenberg.

Mr. Niemann, a gentleman about 35 years of age, was affected by obstinate constipation. During five entire years he never once was able to pass a motion, without the aid of either medicine or an injection. He is now at Graefenberg, and for the last four months has had a regular and healthy evacuation every day, without the use either of injection, or of a single grain of medicine of any kind whatever. Had not this gentleman's constipated condition of bowels been thus fortunately removed, I feel quite sure that every unprejudiced medical man will allow that, sooner or later, severe disease, in some shape or other, must have been perfectly inevitable. This gentleman had no crisis.

DYSPEPSIA.

Mr. ——, 48 years ot age, had been accustomed for many years to indulge in a very free mode of living. His daily regular allowance of wine was one full bottle, in addition to sundry glasses of ale, and a couple of glasses of brandy and water in the evening. This was his regular daily quantity. Under this excitement his health soon began to suffer, and it grew gradually worse, until, about twelve months since, he was in so shattered a condition, that he found it necessary to adopt some rigorous and continued means to repair the mischief his constitution had sustained. The symptoms of which he complained were, excessive languor, physical weakness, drowsiness, and depression of spirits, foul tongue, relaxed throat (to such an extent that he was obliged to have his uvula removed by the surgeon's knife), capricious appetite, and all that long train of the most distressing symptoms which characterize a severe case of dyspepsia, accompanied by hypochondriasis. He had been affected, too, for many years, with large furunculi, or boils, of such severe and irritable character, that when one appeared on the chin, it would cause the whole of one side of the face to swell so violently as to entirely close the eye on that side. For these furunculi he consulted a London physician, who ordered him to take a pill every day before dinner, consisting of aloes, rhubarb, and an extract of chamomile. These pills stopped the appearance of the furunculi, and from that moment all his distressing symptoms became aggravated.

After very many fruitless attempts to regain his health, he repaired to Graefenberg. At this time he was so weak that he could not walk the length of a single street. At Dresden, which is a small city, in attempting to walk from one exhibition to another, he found himself unable to do so, and obliged to dispatch his servant for a coach while he waited for its arrival. His breath, moreover, was so short that he could not maintain a conversation for more than five minutes together. In six weeks after his arrival at Graefenberg he could sing; and his strength is now so great, that he walks up and down the snow-clad mountains, often as early as six o'clock in the morning, without any difficulty, in all kinds of weather, and he declared to me that he believed himself able to run continuously, at a moderate pace, for a distance of three or four miles without stopping. Every day I see him climbing the hill-side in large jack-boots, breasting the acclivity with the firm and vigorous step of perfect health and strength. This gentleman bathes, and douches, and takes one or two wet sheets every day, wears umschlags round the body, and drinks nothing but pure cold water. Yet this gentleman had been all his life accustomed to luxurious living, and the daily use of wine and spirits. He declares that when he came to Graefenberg he did not know even the taste of water—for when he cleaned his teeth in the morning, he always took great care to expel every drop of water with the tip of his tongue, fancying that if he suffered it to enter the cavity of his mouth, it could not fail of producing some deadly mischief; and he would as soon have thought of swallowing poison as of drinking a cup of cold water. And this gentleman did not leave off the use of stimulants gradually—he left them off entirely at once—and so far from experiencing any evil consequences, he immediately became sensible of relief.

I will just mention that this gentleman had for a great many years (perhaps 20) a large fatty tumor on his back—so large as to be quite visible through all his clothes, and giving to him an appearance of deformity. When I examined this tumor a few days ago it had almost entirely disappeared.

DYSPEPSIA AND RHEUMATISM.

Herr Baumann, a builder, from Saxe Weimar, 45 years of age, suffering under rheumatism, dyspepsia, nervous debility, and with a constitution, to all appearance, quite broken. The first crisis made its appearance in the form of the usual eruption, and he felt himself relieved. Some time after this, however, he had another crisis, consisting of what are called furunculi, or boils. He now began to mend rapidly. His dyspeptic symptoms left him, his rheumatic pains ceased, his nervous debility gradually vanished, and his health is now firm, strong, and good.

Mr. J. B. S——, a gentleman of Manchester, came to Graefenberg in June last. I had the history of the case from his own mouth. His case was one of confirmed and obstinate dyspepsia of four years' standing. Being a man of property he took the advice of the most eminent physician, who, having failed in relieving him, finally recommended him to travel in a warmer climate. In obedience to his advice he went to Rome. Here he improved a little for a short time, and then became again as ill as he was when he sat out.

While traveling on the continent, he accidentally made the acquaintance of a Captain Fuminelli, of Venice, to whom he related his case, and the object of his travel—a search after health. The captain, now the strongest man in Venice, and who had himself been raised from a sickly condition to one of high health, by the sole use of cold water, at once strongly recommended him to repair to Graefenberg, and he came accordingly. When he arrived his symptoms were these—first, great general physical debility, so that he could not walk even a small distance without great fatigue and exhaustion. He was the subject of constant heart-burn—his tongue exceedingly foul—his appetite capricious—and his stools invariably presented the appearance of little, hard, stony balls. He was perpetually annoyed by *sighing and gaping,* which he could not resist even when engaged in conversation—proofs of great vital debility. In addition to all this he had a constant and severe pain in his left side.

This was his condition for four years. These were the symptoms which had obstinately resisted the most judicious medical treatment under the ablest medical advice in England. The first sensible effects of the treatment were manifested in the changed appearance of the alvine evacuations. These became large, hard, dry, and solid, and their expulsion exceedingly painful. For this he was ordered a wet bandage round the body, covering the whole abdomen and stomach. In two days his motions assumed a perfectly natural and healthy appearance. He now made rapid progress. His tongue became cleaner, the pain in the side greatly relieved, the heart-burn left him, his appetite became steady and good, his strength greatly increased, and he felt so well that he made up his mind to discontinue the treatment and go home. He was not, however, yet quite well, for as soon as he left off the treatment his health flagged, and he describes his feelings as resembling those of one who suddenly loses some long-continued cause of excitement. He felt low, depressed, and was obliged to resume the treatment. After having undergone the treatment for some weeks longer, however, he entirely recovered both his health and strength, and could spend a whole day in climbing the mountains without suffering more fatigue than would necessarily be felt by a strong and healthy man. He has now been in perfect health for four months, during the whole of which time he has entirely dicontinued the treatment, with the exception of an ordinary cold bath every morning. He only remains at Graefenberg on his wife's account, who has also been undergoing the treatment, and whose case he has likewise kindly permitted me to publish.

Mr. J. B. S——'s crisis occurred about the eighth week after he commenced the treatment, in the form of a thick rash, which entirely covered his legs, thighs, and arms. Immediately after the appearance of this eruption, the pain in the side began to decrease, and with it the eruption also disappeared. He declares to me that he cannot remember the time when he felt himself in such good health and strength as he is at this moment.

GOUT AND RHEUMATISM, COMPLICATED WITH VENEREAL TAINT.

For thirteen years, Captain Vogt had been the subject of severe pains in his wrists, ankles, knees, and the long bones of his legs and thighs. While suffering thus, he contracted the venereal disease, of which he was not properly cured. From this time his rheumatic pains were aggravated tenfold, so much so that he was at intervals confined to his bed for several weeks at a time.

In this forlorn condition he arrived at Graefenberg, and was immediately put under treatment. The first crisis which manifested itself was a return of the chancre, which he had contracted six years before. This, however, got perfectly well in a fortnight. He has been here eight months, and when I examined him a few weeks since he was completely recovered, free from all pain, active with his limbs, and able to take any reasonable amount of exercise on foot or on horseback. He is covered with a critical eruption all over his limbs and body, and he only waits for the subsidence of this to return home. He was on full treatment the whole time, with the exception of the sweating blanket. He wore umschlags night and day, which, during the day, were renewed five times.

GOUT IN THE HANDS AND KNEES.

Mr.——, 45 years of age, had gout in his hands and feet for

twelve years. He began the treatment in July, 1842. At six in the morning, leintuch for half an hour—tepid bath for five minutes. At eleven and at five the same treatment repeated. He wore umschlags. On the second day he sweated for two hours—took a tepid bath for two minutes—after which a cold bath for one minute—then another tepid for two minutes. At eleven o'clock he took a foot bath for twenty minutes. At five o'clock he took a leintuch, for half an hour, with tepid, etc., etc., as in the morning. This treatment was pursued for ten days. After the tenth day, immediately after the sweating, a cold bath for a minute. In the third week he douched in addition to the other treatment, and wore wet bandages on the knees. He got well rapidly.

RHEUMATISM WITH PSORIASIS.

Mr. G——, an officer in the army, aged 59 years, about twenty years since began to be affected in the muscular part of the legs and thighs with very severe pains. At last they became so exceedingly sensible of cold and damp that, in frosty weather, while sitting within doors, he was always compelled to have the lower half of his body enveloped in a cloak, and no barometer could indicate a coming change in the weather with greater exactitude than this gentleman's legs. This state of things lasted, with little variation, for twenty years, not confining him to the house, but imbittering his life, interfering with his prospects, and poisoning all the springs of enjoyment. During these twenty years he was three times sent home under a medical board as unfit for duty—once from the West Indies, once from the Mauritius, and once from New South Wales. His legs, I forgot to mention, had also become, very early in the disorder, covered with that obstinate itching disease, called psoriasis; and for several years any attempt to lean forward in the act of writing gave him acute pain in the region of the stomach. After having taken the advice of a multitude of physicians to no purpose, he was recommended to travel. He visited Wild Bad, in the Black Forest, Wild Bad Gastein, on the Norrishe Alys, Buxton, Bath, Ramsgate, and spent one whole winter in Italy; but all in vain. At last he heard of the water-cure and determined to visit Graefenberg, where he still remains, the very merriest man of the whole two hundred, who are now, in the very depth of winter, and with the snow a foot thick, daily undergoing the water treatment at that place.

He has had crises, both in the form of rash and of furunculi. He has also had diarrhœa, which confined him to his bed for three days. During these three days he wore umschlags night and day, changed every hour—with sitz baths. When the feet became very cold he had them rubbed with cloths dipped in cold water, and wrung out. In the evening he became feverish, for which he was put into a shallow bath for five minutes. This immediately removed the fever. When he was first attacked with diarrhœa his appetite went, and he could only take a little rusk in cold water. It soon, however, returned and became better than ever. He is now in excellent health, his pains and the eruption rapidly leaving him, and he is looking forward with the utmost confidence to a perfect cure.

CASE OF PSORIASIS. COMMUNICATED BY GEORGE ANTHONY, ESQ., AN ENGLISH SURGEON, NOW AT GRAEFENBERG.

Mr. Burch, a farmer from Somersetshire, aged 50 years, a stout, strong man, came to Graefenberg in the middle of October last (1842). He was examined, and the progress of his case watched, with great interest by Mr. Anthony, and many others, resident at Graefenberg.

His whole body and limbs were literally covered with that most obstinate, and, generally speaking, hitherto incurable disease, called psoriasis. Deep fissures had formed in many parts, and an enormous quantity of scurf and scales were swept out of his bed every morning, while the itching with which he was annoyed was almost intolerable. It was that form of psoriasis which is sometimes called, though I think erroneously, lepra figurata. He had been afflicted with this abominable scourge for *many years;* and had consulted many physicians of acknowledged eminence without the slightest benefit. Every mode of treatment which he had adopted had utterly failed of making the slightest impression on the disease.

When he consulted Priessnitz, he was told that he would certainly get well, but that it was by far the worst case he had ever seen, although he had seen great numbers, and that it might take two or three years to effect a perfect cure. On hearing this he became disheartened, since circumstances would not allow him to sacrifice so much time. He was determined, however, not to return without making a trial. He went down the hill on which Graefenberg stands, into the town of Friewaldau, in which many of Priessnitz's patients, who cannot find room in Graefenberg, take lodgings. He here commenced the treatment, drinking large quantities of cold water, and confining his diet to bread alone. He continued this plan for about six weeks, when, to his joyful astonishment, as well as that of Priessnitz himself, the eruption almost entirely disappeared. In this case, the crisis showed itself in the shape of diarrhœa.

In order to produce perspiration he slept under a German feather bed, close to a German stove, which gave him a profuse perspiration every night—an effect which his medical man had often labored to produce in vain, and which he had never experienced for many years.

Having now remained as long as circumstances would possibly permit, he left Friewaldau to all appearance perfectly well, with the exception of a few isolated spots. On his way home he was accompanied as far as Prague by Mr. Ellis, a gentleman who is still at Graefenberg undergoing the water-cure. Here he all at once returned to a very free diet. From a very scanty diet, and one consisting solely of bread, milk, and water, he leaped at once to the full diet of the fashionable continental hotels, with wine, etc. The consequence of this was a fit of the gout and a relapse. But from the very marked and powerful impression which was made by the treatment upon the disease in the short space of six weeks, no rational doubt can exist, and no doubt was entertained by any of the gentlemen who saw the progress of the case, some of whom were medical men, that the disease would have been entirely removed could the patient have submitted a little longer to the treatment, and confined himself for a longer period to a more rigorous diet. It should be remembered that this gentleman was 50 years of age—that his disease had existed not merely for many months, but for many years—and that the various modes of treatment which he had adopted under the ablest advice had not only been unable to cure it, but even to make the slightest impression upon it.

SKIN DISEASE—PSORIASIS.

Mr. Spangenberg, a gentleman of Hamburg, a young man of very high attainments, and the son of the late very eminent Dr. Spangenberg, (about 24 years of age), had been afflicted with a scaly eruption over his face, and entire body and limbs, for twelve years. The disease first made its appearance in the form of red, itching patches. These became covered with small scurfy laminæ, or scales, which were easily rubbed of, leaving the patches red and shining as before. In a very short time, however, the scales were reproduced, and fell off as before. The itching was excessive, and this distressing condition continued for twelve years, in spite of the most varied and persevering efforts, under the most able medical advice, to remove it.

In this pitiable state he came to Graefenberg, covered from head to foot, face and all, with a disease at once loathsome, and, in an uncommon degree, distressing. His complexion was exceedingly fair, his eyes blue, and his hair flaxen—his temperament irritable. And it required a good deal of tact to accommodate the intensity of the treatment to the excessive sensibility of his skin, which made it frequently necessary to change it; for whenever it was urged too far, the disease was aggravated. By constantly varying the treatment, however, his skin became gradually accustomed to the impressions of the various baths, and when I arrived at Graefenberg, his treatment consisted of two leintuchs every morning, one immediately after the other (the former for half an hour, the latter for three quarters), immediately succeeded by the cold bath. At twelve o'clock he took a wet sheet and sitz bath. At five he took another leintuch, for an hour and a half, succeeded by another cold bath. All night he wore wet linen pantaloons, from his ancles up to his arm-pits. He also wore wet bandages round his arms. All day he wore wet bandages round the entire body and arms, which were renewed five times *daily*. In the summer months he took the blanket and douched; but these it was found necessary to discontinue.

This gentleman's crisis assumed the form of diarrhœa, immediately after the occurrence of which, his disease began to disappear. I saw him almost every day, and examined him repeatedly. When I left Graefenberg, he was so nearly well that a few isolated, dark-colored spots, indicating the parts where the disease had been most virulent, were all that were left.

SKIN DISEASE FOLLOWING GONORRHŒA.

The following case I detail for an especial purpose—for the purpose of showing in what manner the most obstinate diseases, especially of the skin, and painful rheumatic affections (so called), are constantly produced.

Herr Von Nehemet, a Hungarian gentleman, three years ago contracted gonorrhœa. After having vainly endeavored to rid himself of his malady for nine months, it *suddenly disappeared* on taking a large *dose of cubebs.*

Soon after this sudden disappearance, an *eruption* showed itself on his face and nose, for which he took Pulnau water, which seemed to remove it. He was now, *to all appearance,* well; but the suddenness with which both the original disorder and the eruption had ceased, made him distrust the soundness and permanence of the apparent cure. Distressed with this feeling of insecurity, and his family being at Graefenberg, he determined to go thither too, and submit himself to the Graefenberg treatment. He was soon satisfied that his fears were but too well founded. For, shortly after he began to adopt the remedy, a crop of small ulcers made their appearance round the fundament. Similar ones soon showed themselves on his legs, and presently his hands and fingers became covered with pustules.

By slow degrees, however, the whole of these symptoms vanished, and his health was perfectly restored. He left Graefenberg while I was still there.

Now, I think it cannot be doubted that when this gentleman's original disease so suddenly disappeared, his system *still retained the poison* with which he had been first inoculated. Nor can it be doubted, that if that poison had not been thrown to the surface by the treatment adopted, he must have become, at some future time, the subject of severe disease, of some kind or other.

I am persuaded that multitudes of anomalous disorders, whose causes seemed buried in obscurity, are occasioned by *suppressed poison*—and often by a poison of the kind here alluded to.

FISTULA IN ANO.

The young Count Thun, a youth sixteen years of age, became sensible of uneasiness in the neighborhood of the rectum while passing his motions. This uneasiness gradually increased until it became so severe as to prevent him from riding on horseback. The parts were now examined by a surgeon, and found to be thickened, enlarged, and hardened. In a short time the pain became excessively severe, and other advice was taken, both at Vienna and Prague. It was determined to puncture the part. This was done, and a discharge of matter mixed with blood ensued. The disease was now pronounced to be fistula. Attempts were made to effect a cure, by means of injections thrown into the sinuses through the puncture; and that the case was one of perfect or complete fistula is proved by the fact that a portion of the injected matter always escaped through the sphincter, proving beyond question that the sinus opened into the bowel. A great variety of injections having been used with no benefit whatever, the case was pronounced to be incurable without an operation. To this measure the young count could not be persuaded to submit. He had now been under medical and surgical treatment for twelve months. He had five fistulous openings around the anus, and his system had been so much reduced that it was with the utmost difficulty he could walk, even when assisted by the arm of his father.

When I saw him he had been at Graefenberg eight months. For the first three months he took daily three wet sheets of an hour each—each being immediately followed by the cold bath. He wore umschlags round the body and under the crotch night and day. At the expiration of three months, he began to douche every day; and he has only now just begun to undergo the sweating process. He takes all his food, both meat and drink, perfectly cold. He has never taken a sitz bath; nor has he had any crisis.

After hearing the detail of the case from the father, whose memory was assisted by the son himself, I requested that I might be allowed to examine the parts. This request was immediately complied with. The scars left by the healing of the sinuses were distinctly visible. But the thickening has disappeared, as well as the pain, which I ascertained by making firm pressure entirely round the anus, and especially upon the scarred parts. Four out of the five openings were perfectly and soundly healed, but there yet remained one, formerly as large as the tip of the little finger, but now not larger than a pin's head, to be healed.

Prepared as I already was by à priori reasoning from the nature of animal life up to the nature of animal disease, and from the nature of disease up to the true nature of remedies, to award great efficacy to the cold water-cure, yet I must confess that if I had not witnessed this case, and also the one which follows, with my own eyes, I should have had great difficulty in believing the truth of the statement.

URINARY FISTULA.

Baron Lauengen, of Lauengen, captain of cavalry, struck himself a severe blow against the pommel of his saddle. Inflamma tion and much tumefaction ensued. After a time the swelling of the part was enormous, and fluctuation was distinctly felt. An opening was made into it, very low down, from which there immediately escaped a very large quantity of urine. This puncture never healed, but the urine continued constantly to flow through it. He suffered from this state of things for two years, which two years were spent in fruitless endeavors, under the advice of the very best continental surgeons, to heal this fistulous sore. He then came to Graefenberg, where he has been, if I remember right, only eight months. He was kind enough to suffer me to examine the part, which I found to be perfectly healed and sound, the scar where the opening had been still remaining distinctly visible near the raphe.

GONORRHŒA.

A gentleman of Transylvania, a healthy man, twenty-eight years of age, contracted gonorrhœa. In spite of all the means which could be devised by his medical advisers, the disease continued for fifteen months. Four months after he had got well he contracted the disease a second time. The treatment he had gone through on the former occasion had been so painful as well as unsuccessful, that he could not make up his mind to submit to it again, but resolved to go to Graefenberg. He was three weeks on the journey, and he had had the disease three weeks before he started. The disorder was of a virulent kind. The treatment which was adopted in this case was as follows: At half past six in the morning he took a wet sheet. After the wet sheet he took a tepid shallow bath, at twelve degrees of Reaumur. After this (immediately) the cold bath, and directly after this the shallow bath again. At ten o'clock he took a tepid sitz bath, at twelve degrees, for half an hour. At five o'clock the wet sheet and all the treatment of the morning over again. He drank thirteen glasses of cold water daily, and wore umschlags round the abdomen day and night. This treatment continued for a week, but on the fourth day the disease had entirely disappeared. It was thought desirable, however, to continue the treatment a little longer. In the second week he took the two wet sheets as at the beginning, but went immediately after each into the cold bath, without the intervention of the tepid shallow bath. At ten o'clock in the morning he douched for five minutes, but not on the seat of the disease, nor on the stomach, nor on the head. At twelve o'clock he took a sitz bath *cold* for one hour and a quarter. At the end of the second week he left perfectly cured.

CONSUMPTION.

Extracts (translated from the Italian) from a letter received by J. B. S ——, Esq., at Graefenberg, from Captain A. F——, of the Marine Artillery, Venice.

VENICE, 10th February, 1843.

* * * * "Mr. and Mrs. H. are much obliged by your kindness, and have heard with great pleasure the good effects of the cure, on which they sincerely congratulate you, and return their kind compliments to you and your lady. The reading of your letter has determined H—— to visit Graefenberg next summer. He will profit by your advice, with respect to the method which you recommend him to adopt while there. Colonel S—— is very well; he says that he feels himself ten years younger (since his visit to Graefenberg, 1842), and sends his compliments to you both.

"With regard to my own case, it is given in few words. From my twenty-fifth to my thirty first year, I was subject to frequent affections of the chest, for which my physicians ordered me to lose blood, and gave me palliatives, which treatment left me constantly liable to relapses. They said I was of a plethoric habit, and that I must have the mass of my blood diminished. These diseases were produced by weakness brought on by a too sedentary life, too much application to study, and too free indulgence in wine and spirit. My constitution was extremely delicate, and the least draught of air caused inflammation of the lungs.

"These affections of the chest returned three or four times a year, until the last time, 1827, the lungs were so much weakened that I could scarcely breathe. At this same period (I was then thirty-one years of age) I was at Zara, in Dalmatia, and had a severe attack, which lasted several months, and of which I could not recover. I was confined entirely to my room. The physician said that it would be death to me if I exposed myself to the open air. I had a consultation of physicians, at which Dr. Pinelli, the principal physician in Dalmatia, attended, and I was declared consumptive. I was studying at that time the German language, and while reading the '*Conversations Lexicon*,' I was struck with the article 'Huffeland.' In this article great praise was given to his (Huffeland's) work on Macrobiotics (or the art of prolonging life). I obtained this work, and it seemed to me that I recognized my own case in it. As I was already quite given up by the faculty, I thought that in my position as an officer it would be best for me to attempt an *heroic* cure, and to put an end to my disorders, either by death or recovery. I bade adieu to all my physicians, *in a half-dying state,* and began to wash myself in my room with fresh water, by means of a sponge—repeating this operation several times a day—and limiting my diet to vegetables, fruit, and water.

"I began to feel benefit in a few days, and soon acquired courage to go out. In the course of the forty days I was strong enough to begin sea-bathing. It was the month of August, 1827.

"The sea-bathing, which I took every morning, *in all weathers,* joined with exercise immediately after the bath, continually strengthened me more and more, and in the space of five months I found myself the strongest and the healthiest of any of my companions. From that time to the present day I have had no illness of any kind. I drink no wine, because I do not like it. But I *could* drink it without any evil result.

"I prefer vegetable diet; but, for several years that I was at sea, I took animal food, without the least inconvenience. I expose myself to all weathers—and go without a cloak, even in winter, in order to put my health to the proof. I go from a hot atmosphere into a cold one, *et vice versa,* without any precaution. I wear no flannel, and lead a very irregular life.

"In 1835, when I was on board ship, I was attacked, in the Port of the Pirœus, with an epidemic fever, which raged there on account of the marshes, and which attacked three fourths of our crew. On the *second* and *third* attack of fever, I took, each time, a bath in the sea, and recovered, while my companions were ill for *several months.*

"The only precaution which I observe is to bathe every day in the sea, in all weathers, and in all seasons, when I have the opportunity; and to take a douche bath* for one minute, and wash myself all over with cold water, as soon as I get out of bed. I drink a great deal of cold water—from twenty to twenty-five beakers every day—chiefly in the morning before breakfast. But when-

* Three buckets of water poured over him.

ever I have been so situated that I could do *none of these things,* I have still felt myself perfectly well.

"In short, at the age of forty-seven, I feel myself stronger than I was at twenty-five, before I was attacked by disease in my chest. This is the method which I followed before I had any knowledge of the method of Priessnitz, with which I only became acquainted five years ago when I returned from the Levant, and which has determined me to continue it, and to recommend it to all my friends.

"If Dr. Johnson wishes to make use of this information, I have no objection whatever. I only request him to put merely the *initials* of my name.

"I request you to write to me before you leave Graefenberg, and to believe that I am, and shall always be, with the most perfect esteem, etc., etc., A. F.,

"Captain of the Marine Artillery"

COUGH, WEAKNESS OF THE CHEST, AND INJURY OF THE BACK.

Mrs. J. B. S——'s case related in her own words.

"From a child, I never recollect to have had strong health. I was constantly suffering from the illness incident to children, besides much cough, with tendency to weakness of the chest, for which at an early period I was ordered to wear a flannel dress next the skin. When at school, and while playing, I fell backward over a garden roller, to which I paid no attention, although finding it difficult either to walk fast or to run for a few days. From this circumstance I think may be dated the weakness in my back, which was first evinced in a difficulty to rise from the ground, if I had been stooping or kneeling while at work in my garden; the feeling being a total prostration of strength, from the lower region of my back (precisely the part hurt) to the knees. Still I struggled against the weakness, until I found myself incapable of walking up a slight hill with ease. Application was then made to the physician, by whom I was ordered to rub the part well with a liniment principally composed of essential oils, and which produced a discharge equal to that of a perpetual blister, and for a time restored strength to my back; but the disease invariably returned.

"This state of debility continued until 1841, when I think it increased; if I walked up a long staircase, my strength was exhausted; the same indeed after any slight exertion. In 1842 I came to Graefenberg. I was ordered *to leave off flannel,* a leintuch for one hour, to be succeeded by the abgeschrecktes bath, in which I was well rubbed for a few minutes; an abreibung and sitz bath at eleven o'clock, and the same at four o'clock in the afternoon. In a fortnight I was ordered to plunge *once* in the cold bath, returning thence to the abgeschrecktes to assist the circulation of the blood. At the expiration of five weeks from my first arrival at Graefenberg, I was suddenly seized with an utter prostration of strength; so much so, that my legs dragged, and I feared paralysis. This was succeeded by ague, shiverings, and burnings, pains from head to foot, but principally across the loins. A profuse natural perspiration relieved me of much uneasiness; and, when Herr Priessnitz came, he ordered an immediate abreibung with umschlags around the waist, to be repeated frequently so long as the pain continued violent in the loins. If I were better in the morning, the bathing was to be continued as usual. This was done. When I attempted to walk after being dressed, I found myself incapable of the exertion, being weak almost as an infant. During two days I ate only a little bread, and drank water, the food that my appetite asked for. In four days my strength had considerably returned, and in a week I was as well as usual. After this fever, I was ordered to douche, which in a very short period produced considerable swelling in my left foot; then I was ordered a foot bath, Priessnitz saying, 'it was probable a crisis was approaching;' which took place in a few days, and which discharged as an issue for seven weeks. Another succeeded, which lasted for five, and another afterward for three weeks, more violent than the preceding, with a multitude of little ones; and after each one I felt stronger and stronger, and now have to rejoice that all pain in the back, with that prostration of strength, and every other symptom of debility, headache, etc., etc., have apparently bid me farewell."

DEAFNESS.

While I was staying at Graefenberg, during the first week in January of the present year (1843), Herr Fricks, a young Prussian, aged twenty-seven years, arrived from Stettin.

He had been totally deaf for ten years, his deafness having been produced by a severe attack of typhus fever. During the course, however, of the whole ten years his hearing returned three times, but only remained *a day or two,* when he became again as deaf as ever. Having undergone treatment *for twelve days,* a large quantity of matter issued from his nose. He immediately regained his perfect hearing, and remained quite well up to the time when I *left Graefenberg*—a period of about six weeks.

I will here relate an accident which befel this young man, in order to show that the water treatment is an edged tool which cannot with impunity be trifled with—and that, like every other remedy which is not mere chip in porridge, it is only safe in the hands of those who know how to adapt its use to the peculiarities and powers of individual constitutions.

He had been packed in the blanket; but, after having lain there for three hours, did not perspire. He was ordered therefore to be taken out and put into the tepid bath. The bath-servant, however, either to save trouble, or from misunderstanding, put him in the *cold* bath. The moment he came out he fell down, and remained perfectly senseless for more than an hour. Constant friction, however, with the wet hands, at length restored him.

General Baron Esch, commanding the cavalry at Prague, a gentleman well known in the military world, and who made his first campaign with the Duke of York, at Dunkirk, in 1799, was afflicted with a confirmed deafness of several years' standing, for which the most celebrated physicians in Austria had all been repeatedly consulted without relief. At last he was induced to go to Graefenberg and consult Priessnitz, who told him he thought he could cure him, but would not say what length of time it might require. He was immediately put under treatment, and at the expiration of six weeks he had perfectly recovered his hearing. This case was related to me by Colonel Bowen, late of the Coldstream Guards, who is now undergoing the treatment for chronic inflammation of the eyes, and who was a personal friend of General Esch, and had the statement from his own lips. The general also related to Colonel Bowen the case of a young dragoon officer under his command.

HIP DISEASE.

One of the first cases which attracted my attention, after my arrival at Graefenberg, was a case of hip disease, in Elizabeth St——, a child eight years of age, and the daughter of highly respectable parents at Hamburg. On inquiry of the child's governess, she stated that the hips had become enlarged rather more than two years ago—that the tumefaction gradually increased—that the child constantly complained of pain in the knee—that the leg and thigh became gradually wasted—that the knee-joint became firmly contracted, and bent nearly at right angles, so that she could only walk with two crutches, the other limb being weak, and the general habit of the child *delicate*, and, in fact, scrofulous. Every medical man, if any such be present, will immediately recognize in this account, a very common form of scrofulous disease of the hip joint. When I saw the child, however, all these symptoms had disappeared, excepting some remaining enlargement of the hip, and a little limping in the gait, arising from a trifling shortening of the limb. But the account thus given of the child's condition when she first went to be submitted to the treatment, was fully confirmed by the testimony of more than a dozen persons, who saw the child when she was first brought to Graefenberg, and who had watched her progress with great interest. But besides this, the shortening of the limb, the appearances of the hip, with the general constitutional aspect of the little patient, were precisely such as would have led any surgeon to foretell, without information, that the patient had suffered, or was about to suffer, the peculiar train of symptoms which the governess mentioned.

When I left Graefenberg, I saw this child galloping about in the snow, by the side of her governess, without any thing to distinguish her from a perfectly healthy child, excepting a little limp in her gait.

SCARLET FEVER.

In the month of May, 1842, Mrs. Klauke (aged about 25), was seized with pains in the head, and back, and calves of the legs. Her face, neck, arms, and legs, and subsequently the whole body, became brightly scarlet, and she complained of a soreness in the throat. The pulse was rapid, and skin dry. She was packed in the leintuch for half an hour; then rubbed all over in a tepid bath for twenty minutes with the wet hand. She was now ordered to wear an umschlag round her stomach night and day. When she felt cold, she was rubbed down with the wet sheet—when hot, packed in the leintuch, and so on all through.

The tepid bath was suspended, until by the application of a succession of sheets the fever was reduced. Then the tepid bath was repeated. Every morning she was packed up in a blanket, in which she was allowed to perspire for an hour; then she was put into the tepid bath. This treatment was continued for a fortnight. At the close of the sixth day all fever was extinguished, and at the close of the whole treatment her strength was undiminished.

In addition to the above, a lavement of cold water was administered every night. During the whole time she ate and drank as usual, and one evening went to a ball (in the saloon of Priessnitz's establishment), and danced for hours, while her whole body was crimsoned with scarlatina. On returning home from the dance, she was rubbed down with a wet sheet, went to bed, and slept soundly.

SYMPTOMATIC FEVER. (RELATED BY THE MOTHER.)

Alexander Klauke, aged three years, was a fine lively child, but with a disposition to inflammatory affections of the stomach and bowels. A month previous to the present disease, he had an attack of inflammation of the stomach, accompanied with strong fever, and determination to the head. In the evening the child was put into a bath not quite cold, in which he remained about twenty minutes, additional cold water being added as the temperature arose by the heat from the child. During this time, cold water was poured from a tumbler glass on the head, repeated at intervals of a minute, and, as is usual, his whole body was rubbed cautiously by the maid. He was then taken out of the bath and placed on the sofa, covered over with a sheet and blanket, with the back part of his head in cold water, for ten minutes. By this time reaction had taken place, when wet compresses were applied to the head and back part of the neck, and the body, from the arm-pits to the hips, wrapped in a similar way. He slept quietly till three o'clock in the morning, when the same process was repeated, the previous symptoms having returned. The child was again placed in bed, where he slept till morning, and was then found to be quite well, and went out as usual.

A month after this attack he was taken ill in a similar way, but with symptoms much more severe. The fever running high, and accompanied by delirium. The treatment was commenced by placing him successively in nine wet sheets, from which the water was but slightly wrung out. In each of these he remained about five minutes. Toward the last, the heat being diminished, he was allowed to remain ten minutes. To the head and breast, a thick wet compress was applied in addition, these being the parts where the heat was greatest. The feet were cold, and as long as they remained so, the wet sheet was only applied down to the knees; in the meantime, the feet and legs were rubbed strongly with the hands. While the extreme heat continued, the wet sheet was covered by a thick dry one instead of a blanket, as is usual, the feet only being covered with the blanket. After the last wet sheet, he was placed at once in a tepid bath, where he remained an hour, the same process of rubbing and pouring water over the head being practiced. The first day the same process was repeated four times, the duration of the last being not so long, when the fever was not so high. During the night the wet cloth was changed every half hour. On the morning of the second day the child refused to go into the water, calling out himself at intervals for additional wet sheets. Orders were given that the inclination of the child should be obeyed. In the course of the morning the child desired himself that he might be put into the bath, where he remained until the heat in the arm-pits and on the back of the neck was the same as on the rest of the body; this being the general guide for the duration of a bath.

The same treatment slightly varied was continued four days, when the child was well, and was sent out to play with the other children. In eight days after this a pustule appeared on the foot, which discharged matter freely.

CATARRH, OR COLD.

Mrs. ——, an English lady now at Graefenberg, on her husband's account, was subject, in England, to very severe attacks of catarrh, which usually lasted her a month before she could get entirely rid of it. Soon after her arrival at Graefenberg she had a very severe attack. She was treated by the wet sheet and tepid bath alternately for *two days*, which entirely removed every trace of the catarrh.

BALDNESS.

Assessor Willert came under the hydrotherapeutic treatment for a very old rheumatic affection. When he arrived at Graefenberg his entire head was perfectly bald and smooth. I had an opportunity of examining his head soon after I myself reached Graefenberg; which I did with the more care, having heard that it was expected, during his treatment, that his hair would probably return. Shortly before I left Graefenberg I was requested to go and examine Assessor Willert's head once more. I did so, and found it every where covered with a fine new hair, nearly half an inch in length. There can be no doubt whatever that this gentleman's head will shortly be covered with hair as luxuriant as at any former period of his life. His age, judging from his appearance (for I did not inquire), is about seven or eight and thirty.

HEADACHE, WITH GIDDINESS.

To Herr Slatinsky, a gentleman (about forty years of age) whose case I am now about to relate, I was introduced by Mr. Niemann. On going to his room I found his body literally covered all over with large dark brown spots, some about the size of a farthing, some as large as a half-penny, and others somewhat larger, and many of them running one into another, giving to his skin a dark marbled appearance. He had also had crises in another form about his legs and arms, very much resembling what, in England, are commonly called boils. They seemed to me to partake of the nature of what are denominated, in medical phraseology, furunculi—not malignant, but in a very mild form—discharging a ropy matter from one small pinhole in the centre. All these, excepting one on the breast, were perfectly healed.

The eruption on the body, however, had but just made its appearance, and the patient was in high glee, and exhibited his mottled skin with all the pride and satisfaction with which a man exhibits to his friends some long-desired object—a horse, for instance, or some precious antique—which he has just succeeded in obtaining after much labor and difficulty. The whole time he was undressing a smile of exultation was playing round his mouth, which plainly said, "What a happy fellow am I! and how much I am sure you will envy me when you see the treasure I am about to show you—the blessed blotches wherewith I am blessed!" And this is the feeling which is common to all the patients at Graefenberg on the appearance of the crisis—for it is invariably hailed as a certain harbinger of a speedy and perfect restoration to health. As the crisis disappears the health returns—and I have never either seen or heard of a single case in which these eruptions did not entirely vanish again, leaving the skin perfectly healthy and clear as before.

For the three years previously to his coming to Graefenberg, this gentleman had been grievously afflicted with violent pains in the head, accompanied by dizziness. He was unable to attend to any kind of business. He could neither read nor write for more than two or three minutes together. He felt as though two nails, one on either side of the forehead, were being violently thrust into his brain. And he could never stoop nor turn round without imminent danger of falling. This was his condition for three years, from which all the ordinary medical treatment had failed to relieve him.

I forgot to mention that, in addition to his other sufferings, he was afflicted with piles.

On the appearance of the first crisis all his symptoms were relieved, but not removed. Since the appearance of the second, however, his headache, his giddiness, his piles, have entirely left him, and he now only waits till the critical eruption shall also leave him, when he will return to his country, his family, his friends, and his home, freed from a load of misery and disease which could not but render life rather a curse than a blessing.

SECONDARY SYPHILITIC SYMPTOMS.

Count Pyatcshavich, a Polish count, contracted syphilis. Under a course of mercury all his sores healed except a large one in the groin, which resisted all medical treatment. His health at last began to flag. He lost both his flesh and his strength, and became reduced in substance even to emaciation. This state of things continued for one entire year, when, hopeless of relief by ordinary means, he yielded to entreaty, and, in spite of strong prejudice against the treatment, came to Graefenberg. In six weeks he was perfectly well, and I myself saw him depart, the picture of health and strength—a fine young man standing six feet without his shoes, and as strong as a giant.

ANOTHER CASE OF SECONDARY SYPHILIS.

—— Robertson, Esq., a Scottish gentleman, contracted chancre in Sicily, 1838, which was healed by external mercurial applications. He took mercury internally also, but it failed in producing ptyalism. The chancre returned in a short time, and continued to heal and return at intervals, during the space of six months. During these six months he took *four pounds by weight of Lafecteur's rob* (a concentrated preparation of sarza and other drugs), and sixteen pounds by weight of Dupuytren's rob. He was then ordered to rub in mercury for what were called secondary ulcers; and these ulcers never healed until all these medicines and all mercurial applications were discontinued. But under the use of simple purgatives, washing the sores with nothing but goulard water, they healed in eight days. But by this time his system had become so broken up that pressing fears were entertained for his life. He had become quite emaciated—the slightest exertion, or a sudden noise, would cause him to faint—his spirits were depressed even to frequent weeping—the inside of his mouth, his tongue, cheeks, and throat, were covered with excoriations and sores—*the skin of his face and forehead were covered with blotches*—and his stomach and bowels in so irritable a condition that when he took a plate of hot soup he was obliged to sit upon a commode while eating it. For this excessive irritability he was obliged to take large quantities of opium, which he did under the advice of his physician.

At this time the joint of his knee was larger than the thickest part of his thigh. He was now removed to Naples, and placed under the care of another physician, who gave him iodide of potassium. From this he derived great benefit, the sores healing and the blotches disappearing. He was desired to travel, but never to return to a hot climate. His health now became considerably better, but the disease was still in him, for it was not long before the blotches returned, and he was obliged to have recourse again to the iodide of potassium. And indeed he soon found that, in order to keep the disease under, it was necessary to take the iodide of potassium constantly. He now took warm sea bathing at Peterhead, which brought out several ulcers in the part first affected. After this he took sulphur baths, and also some iodine administered by Mr. Callaway, one of the surgeons to Guy's Hospital in the Borough.

He now came to Graefenberg, and submitted himself to a full course of the water-cure. When he came there, the skin of his face was so excessively irritable that he could never go out without an umbrella to protect his face from the wind.

He had not been under the treatment long before the disease, which had been hitherto only suppressed, was driven by the water to the surface of the body. He became covered with venereal eruptions, and no fewer than twenty-one ulcers reappeared on the part originally infected. As soon as these appeared, his general health began to mend, and in a few months he was perfectly well, and offered for a wager of any amount to walk eighty miles in two days—forty miles each day. He has just left Graefenberg for Vienna, and related his case to me only a few days before he went. This gentleman was so popular at Graefenberg, and (having the command of several languages) so kind in interpreting for foreigners when they first arrived, that a dinner was given to him at Friewaldau, at which I had the honor to be present.

This gentleman also mentioned to me a case of gleet which came immediately under his own notice. It had existed for seven years, and obstinately withstood every mode of treatment which could be devised. Under the influence of the water treatment he got perfectly well in a few weeks.

THIRD CASE OF SECONDARY SYPHILIS.

Mr. Kindermann, a government reporter at Frankfurt-on-the-Oder, was affected with secondary symptoms. He had a venereal fungous growth on the verge of the anus. There were also deep ulcerations on his thighs. Having failed to obtain any relief, and his health having been to all appearance utterly ruined, it was proposed to convey him to La Charité, the great hospital at Berlin, as a last resource. His physician, however, declared that such a step would be perfectly useless, and nothing could save his life. Soon after this he was strongly urged to visit Graefenberg, whither he was conveyed in the latter end of March last year. In the beginning of July of the same year, he left Graefenberg in perfect health and strength, and is now again residing at Frankfurt-on-the-Oder.

This gentleman is about twenty-six years of age.

He sweated every morning, with cold bath—two leintuchs in the afternoon with cold bath again—once a day he took a sitz bath—and he wore umschlags night and day. He was covered with crises, observed a strict diet, and almost lived in the open air.

FOURTH CASE OF SECONDARY SYPHILIS.

About seven years ago Herr Von Goltzsch contracted chancre, which was cured by mercury. From that time his general health began to decline. Every now and then he had sore throat, and was scarcely ever free from what he at that time believed to be rheumatic pains. For six years this state of things continued, during the whole of which time he was so weak that a strong child running against him was sufficient to push him down. At last his shin bones became attacked with the most excruciating pains the moment he became warm in bed, which made it impossible for him to sleep. Shortly after this, nodosities made their appearance along the whole course of the bones. He was now strongly urged to come to Graefenberg, where I had the pleasure of seeing him, and of examining his legs. He has been under treatment for eight months, during which time his throat has not once been sore. He has entirely lost all his pains, and, on questioning him as to the state of his physical strength, his emphatic reply was, "When I came here I was as weak as a child; but now I would not turn my back upon ten devils."

IMPUISSANCE, COMPLICATED WITH GOUT.

The uncle of the reigning Duke of Nassau, between sixty and seventy years of age, had been afflicted with gout so severely, that when he arrived at Graefenberg, he was almost bent double. In addition to this he had become impuissant.

He remained at Graefenberg for two years, married while there, and in due time became the father of two children; and was, moreover, perfectly cured of the gout.

There are probably no two affections over which the hydropathic remedy exercises a more marked and beneficial influence than it does over the two just mentioned.

CONTRACTED JOINTS.

A Hungarian girl was brought here with the knee joint so much contracted, that she was obliged constantly to walk with two crutches. In six weeks she left Graefenberg, walking exceedingly well without any crutch at all.

HERNIA.

A young man affected with inguinal hernia, consulted a surgeon at Milan, who undertook to cure him.

The surgeon applied a plug of wood to the rupture, supported by a strong band of iron, which produced ulceration to a great and painful extent. At the end of six months the hernia was no better, and he suffered severely from the ulcerations.

He then repaired to Graefenberg, where he has been prosecuting the hydropathic treatment for six months. The ulcerations are quite healed, and his rupture so much better that he has already left off his truss, and Priessnitz assures him that there is no doubt of his perfect recovery.

HÆMATURIA, OR VOIDING OF BLOOD FROM THE URINARY ORGANS.

Herr Zelowski had bleeding from the urinary organs almost daily for six months before his arrival at Graefenberg. On one occasion he voided a large tumbler full of pure blood. He was also the subject of piles. After ten weeks of treatment, he was entirely free from both disorders. He gave me the history of his case himself, on the evening before he left Graefenberg.

CEREBRO-SPINAL DISEASE.

Monsieur de Gallette, an officer in the Imperial Guard of Russia, aged thirty-five years, was affected about two years since with severe giddiness in the head. He could not look vertically upward without falling either on his knees or on his side. Any sudden motion of the head deprived him in a moment of the use of his lower extremities, which immediately yielded to the weight of his body, and let him down.

He lost also the perfect command of his tongue, so that he could not articulate the words which he desired to utter. His memory too quite failed him, and all his faculties were so disordered, that he became quite foolish and unfit for society. One day, in a room full of company, he took up a decanter of water and emptied it completely upon his own head, not knowing what he was about, and wondering where the water came from which was running down his clothes. This gentleman has been four months under the water-cure. His giddiness has left him, he can articulate every word with the greatest facility, he has quite recovered his memory, and all his mental faculties are as perfect as ever they were. He complains now of nothing but physical weakness, from which, however, he is daily recovering. But the most remarkable part of this case still remains to be told. This gentleman has been quite bald for *fifteen years* over the entire roof of his head, and down on either side to within an inch of the tips of his ears, for which he has always worn a wig. When he had related his case, he requested me and some other gentlemen to raise the candle and examine the bald part of his head. We did so, and then perceived that a fine downy hair is beginning to grow all over the bald part, which promises in a month or two entirely to cover it, and supersede the necessity of a wig. The hair is already a full quarter of an inch in length, but exceedingly fine. A hundred persons can vouch for the truth of this statement, among others Colonel Bowen, Mr. Hoppner, and Mr. Anthony, an English surgeon, who examined the case with me.

SUPPRESSED MEASLES.

In June, 1812, Major Heise, in the Hanoverian service, while on active duty, had measles, during which disease he received orders to march to Valladolid, in Spain, and perform the route from Madrid to Valladolid on horseback. On the march he was exposed day and night to the open air. The measles suddenly disappeared. Six months after this his body and limbs became covered over with a dry scaly eruption, exhibiting a yellowish brown patchy appearance, when the scales fell off, accompanied by intolerable itching. Every expedient was tried in order to get rid of this eruption. He visited the baths of Germany, Switzerland, and Italy. He took Russian vapor baths for twenty years. But all perfectly in vain. Six years ago he was attacked with diarrhœa and prolapsus ani, occasioning from ten to twelve motions daily, with constant desire to return to the water-closet. With these symptoms he came to Graefenberg. Added to this, he had nervous twitchings of two years' standing. Two weeks after he had been under treatment he had fever, with delirium, with loss of sleep and appetite, for which he took leintuchs and tepid bath. This lasted a week, and was succeeded by good appetite and returning strength. Crises, consisting of furuncles, now set in, which lasted nine weeks. At the end of three months, he was ordered to go to Vienna and to adopt the following more moderate treatment, viz., three abreibungs daily. Five days after his arrival, diarrhœa and frequent desire for stool left him. At first his treatment consisted of leintuchs, cold baths, sitz baths. On returning from Vienna, he took six leintuchs of half an hour each, and each being immediately succeeded by a cold bath daily—douche for five minutes daily. Umschlags were worn night and day on his body, legs, and head. He was here six months, at the end of which time he went away entirely free from pain, in fresh and strong health, and in all respects perfectly well. Just before I left Graefenberg, Priessnitz received a letter from Major Heise, in which he expressed his great gratitude for his recovered health.

AGUE.

A general officer in the British army, well known at the Horse Guards, still staying at Bœmischdorf, and whose permission I have to give his name to any private applicant, was attacked with ague. After enduring two or three fits, in the hope that it would leave him, he sent for Priessnitz. When Priessnitz arrived, he was in the third or sweating stage. He was immediately placed in a bath at 16 degrees of Reaumur, or 68 of Fahrenheit. Here he was kept for twenty minutes, being well rubbed all the time by two men. After this he walked about the apartment for half an hour, and then went to bed. The ague left him, and never returned.

DEAFNESS.

Colonel Bowen, late of the Guards, has been residing at Graefenberg seven months, without the slightest benefit in his own case. He cannot, therefore, be reasonably supposed to be blinded by any violent prejudices in favor of hydropathy. But he related to me the following circumstances concerning an intimate friend of his own—and it was afterward confirmed by many others who were themselves under treatment at the same time with the colonel's friend. General Baron Esch, lately dead, but at that time commanding the cavalry at Prague, a gentleman extensively known in the military world, and who made his first campaign with the Duke of York, at Dunkirk, in 1799, was afflicted with deafness, of several years' standing, and which had resisted the most judicious treatment. He was at last prevailed on to submit himself to the water remedy—and in six weeks he had *perfectly* recovered his hearing, in the fullest sense of the word. Witnessing, with his own senses, the singular effect which had thus been wrought on his friend's ears, it was *this* which determined Colonel Bowen to try the *same* remedy on his own eyes—but hitherto without effect.

EPILEPSY.

The next case which I shall mention, is one of epilepsy. On

being introduced to this patient, a young Hungarian of about 27, he told me that he had been the subject of epilepsy for four years, having a recurrence of the fits about every ten days. He had been under treatment for four months, and was kept on a very scanty diet the whole of that time. He is now perfectly recovered, having had only one fit since he commenced the treatment, and that occurred *shortly* after his *first arrival* at the establishment. He was very pale, and considerably wasted, but was then gradually returning to a full diet, with a view to his returning home.

I suppose this case to be one of epilepsy, depending on irritation, set up in the brain, by the presence of some foreign body, probably a clot of blood; and that this clot, under the deprivation of food, had entered into combination with oxygen, in order that it might assist in protecting the vital organs from the destructive action of that element, and had quitted the system in the form of oxydized products. The cases of palsy probably depended on similar causes, which are removed by similar means.

This gentleman has made copious notes, both of his case and his treatment, which he intends to publish as soon as he returns to Pesth.

HYPOCHONDRIASIS, PSORIASIS, AND SCIATICA.

The gentleman (an Englishman), about 60 years of age, who was the subject of these three severe afflictions, belonged formerly to the civil service in India. I made his acquaintance at Graefenberg immediately on my arrival, and am indebted to him for introductions to several valuable cases besides his own. He had labored under these affections for eight years. Shortly after he had become the subject of sciatica and psoriasis (which latter disease his French medical advisers denominated dartre farineuse), his mind became excessively excited by some family occurrences, with the particulars of which he did not, of course, think it necessary to acquaint me. In a short time, what with this excitement, the torture arising from his sciatica (inflammation of the sheath of the great sciatic nerve where it passes through the structure of the hip), and the intolerable *itching* produced by the skin disease, the equilibrium of his mind became so much disturbed that he was not considered in a fit condition to be left by himself. Always in a state of high excitement, there were times when he was perfectly insane.

For eight years the sufferings of this poor gentleman, bodily and mental, were indeed awful. When I asked him to give me a detailed account of his sufferings, he sat thoughtful for a moment, and then, going to a table, he took up a small pocket-book, and opening it at a particular page, and placing his fore-finger between the leaves, he reseated himself. "Some time ago," he said, "I was perusing the book of Deuteronomy, and in the course of my reading, the passages which I have copied into this pocket-book riveted my attention. They were so exactly characteristic of my sufferings, that I almost fancied myself the particular object of the divine wrath, and that I was even then realizing the fearful denunciations which those passages of Scripture contained. No language of mine can so truthfully or so forcibly convey to you the horrors under which I was laboring both in body and mind. Read them," continued he, "and judge whether I have not great reason to be thankful that I am *now* such as you see me." He handed me the book, and I read as follows: "The Lord will smite thee with the botch of Egypt and with the emerods, and with the scab, and with the itch, whereof thou canst not be healed. The Lord shall smite thee with madness, and blindness, and astonishment of heart. The Lord shall smite thee in the knees, and in the legs, with a sore botch that cannot be healed, from the sole of thy foot to the top of thy head: and thy life shall hang in doubt before thee; and thou shalt fear day and night, and shalt have none assurance of thy life. In the morning thou shalt say, 'Would God it were even;' and at even thou shalt say, 'Would God it were morning!'"

"At the time," continued he, when I had done reading, "that I was perusing these passages, those terrible denunciations were most of them actually realized in my person. I trembled as I read—for at that moment I was covered, '*from the sole of my foot to the top of my head*' with an intolerable itching botch. I was even then '*smitten in the knees and in the legs with a sore botch,*' and was covered with *scabs*. Madness, and blindness of the understanding, and astonishment of heart, were also mine. I had indeed '*no assurance of my life,*' for I was often sorely tempted to destroy it; and every morning I wished it were night, and at night I longed for the morning—and every effort I had made to get '*healed*' had been utterly in vain."

This gentleman had then been under the water-cure about three months. His sciatica had entirely left him—the eruption was nearly gone—the itching had wholly ceased—while the state of his mind was calm, cheerful, rational, and full of thankfulness.

So fully satisfied was he that he should get entirely well, that he left Graefenberg about a week before myself, in order to bring the whole of his family back with him—partly that he might have the comfort of their society for the rest of the time that it would be necessary for him to remain under the cure, and partly in order to submit his daughter, who had ill health, to the same remedy which had proved so signal a blessing to himself.

CHAPTER XIII.

GRAEFENBERG CASES OF WATER-CURE—(CONTINUED.)*

Nervous Headache.—Deafness and Constipation.—Indigestion, severe Headache, etc.—Indigestion, Nervous Debility, and Hypochondriasis.—Nervous Debility from excessive Study.—Indigestion and Pain in the Side.—Great suffering from Nervous Weakness.—General Fever.—Indigestion and sore Throat.—Inflammation of the Stomach and Bowels.—Nervous Debility, with frequent Cramps.—Nervous Debility and Sleeplessness.—Indigestion, Distress, and Depression of Spirits.—Gout and Rheumatism.—Syphilitic Eruption, Hernia, Sciatica, Biliousness, Indigestion, etc.—Indigestion, Rheumatism, and spitting of Blood —Gout.—Gout and Rheumatism.—Hereditary Gout.—Cutaneous Eruptions and universal Pains.—Great Nervousness.—Urinary Fistula, or Opening.—Hemiplegia, or Paralysis of one Side.—Catalepsy, or Trance, general Debility, and Indigestion.—Seminal Weakness, with great Nervous Debility.—Debility, Nervousness, and Baldness, following the use of Mercury.—Does Water bring Mercury from the System? —Defective Hearing and Smelling, with general Debility.—High Fever, with Delirium.—Dyspepsia, Sleeplessness, and Nervousness.—Rheumatic Neuralgia.—Gout.—Menorrhogia, or excessive and debilitating Menstruation.—Great Debility and depression of Spirits, following Nervous Fever.—Insensibility following an improper Bath.—Insensibility following Over-drinking.—Secondary Syphilis.—(A Horrible Case).—Inflammation of the Brain, with Delirium.—Dyspepsia, Headache, and Fullness at the Head. —Debility, Sleeplessness, Depression of Spirits, etc., from excessive mental Application. —Scrofulous Disease of the Knee Joint.—Scrofulous enlargement of the Knee Joint.—Skin Diseases.—Leprosy, Tetanus, and Hydrophobia.

NERVOUS HEADACHE, DEAFNESS, AND CONSTIPATION.

THAT I may present to the reader a familiar picture of the nature of the different processes of water-cure, I will give some account of my own treatment, adopting the maxim of Seneca:

"Longum iter per præcepta, breve et efficax per exempla."

I have for many years experienced inconvenience from rheumatic and nervous headache, with noises and deafness in the left ear; always dependent on medicine for the function of the bowels, yet very seldom requiring active treatment.

I waited a few days, to recover from the fatigue of traveling, before I began the treatment. At 6 A. M., Tuesday, April 18, I was visited by Priessnitz and the bath attender, who rubbed me down with the wet sheet for two or three minutes; following it

* From Sir Charles Scudamore's Medical Visit to Graefenberg.

with an equally diligent application of the dry one. The cold application being accompanied with such immediate friction, no severe shock was experienced. It was merely disagreeable, and that only in the first impression. The reaction was quickly established, and a safer mode of bathing cannot, I think, be imagined. The best results must follow from this effective cleansing process for the skin, tending to maintain it in health and to remove its diseased conditions. By the recommendation of Priessnitz, I put my flannel waistcoat over my linen.

The wet bandage was applied round my body, the dry part being closely rolled over it. The cold sensation was unpleasant at first, but quickly removed by exercise. I next used hard-rubbing for my head most freely with cold water in a basin, and was careful, by Priessnitz's desire, to chill the nape of the neck. I next took a long walk, and drank three half-pints of water at suitable intervals.

At 11 A. M. sheet process repeated, and, in addition, a sitz bath, with water at 65 degrees Fah., to reach to the navel. I continually rubbed the abdomen and loins with the water, and remained a quarter of an hour. The unpleasant first impression does not last more than a minute, and it is not disagreeable to remain for any length of time, unless the water should be changed. At 5 P. M. this treatment was repeated. I came in from a walk, much heated by exercise in the sun, waited a few minutes till the pulse became quiet, and then had the wet sheet applied with a most refreshing and satisfactory effect.

19th.—Placed in the wet sheet; the first lying down on it and investment with it were very disagreeable; but, immediately after the packing up with the blanket, etc., sufficiently comfortable; and in a few minutes more, so much so that the effect was quite soothing and tending to sleep. At the end of three quarters of an hour, warmth came which would have produced perspiration, and, this not being desired, I was taken out, and immediately entered the shallow bath, at 62 degrees, and was well rubbed with the water for about two minutes. The immersion being so slight, the impression of the cold water was very bearable, and the warmth of surface was afterward quickly restored. Rubbing wet sheet at 11 A. M. and at 5 P. M., this and the sitz bath at 62 degrees. Each time rubbed the head.

20th.—Same treatment. Examined my animal heat before

being rubbed with the wet sheet; it was 97·5, and the sheet 50 degrees; no alteration produced—showing the mildness of this refrigerant process.

After the leintuch this morning, went first into the shallow bath at 62 degrees, and then into the plunging bath, which was 44 degrees, and cutting cold; returned quickly to the shallow bath, which now seemed pleasantly tepid. I found the animal heat reduced one degree by the plunging bath, although the sensible reaction was excellent; and, after the dry rubbing and dressing, I was comfortably warm.

23d.—Same treatment. In using the sitz bath found the temperature of the water raised by the warmth of the body 2 degrees in 5 minutes, 4 in 10, and 6 in 15. Hence the necessity of a change of the water, if a continued cold sitting be desired.

Being, in the common language, bilious from the change of diet, and such a free use of milk mornings and evenings, the bilious secretion suspended with loss of appetite, took blue pill and colocynth at night, and next morning the improved Cheltenham salts. It was my object to save time; and I was confident that I should have this error more quickly corrected than by leaving it to the sole influence of the water-cure treatment.

25th.—I used the lying sheet and shallow tepid bath yesterday, but no other treatment. Every success and benefit from the medicine.

26th.—To-day resumed the plunging bath, and went on with the same treatment to the end of the month, but changed the midday process for the use of the regular head bath and foot bath; having recourse to the latter also, from being much subject to coldness of feet. I received the head bath for a quarter of an hour, allotting five minutes to the back, and the same to each side of the head.* I lay on the floor, and had a good proof of the superior conducting power of air over water for sound, in the strong perception of any contiguous accidental noises. From this application of cold water I always felt sensible invigoration of the nerves of the head.

The foot bath was also sensibly useful, tending to comfortable warmth of the feet; and the further rubbing of the ankles and muscles of the leg much relieved the consequences of fatigue.

* I find a shallow wooden vessel, with a rounded groove to receive the neck, answer the purpose for this process very well.

May 1st.—In using the leintuch this morning, applied a long towel, wetted, from the arm-pit down the side, and found its effects agreeable ; the sensations, from the complete contact of wet linen, more pleasant on that side than the other. Indeed, the effect of this process is very soothing ; and it becomes a punishment to be unpacked. Every one would willingly go to sleep in the wet sheet. If, in any particular case, the feet fail to become warm with the rest of the body, socks may be worn.

May 5th.—To-day used the douche, the temperature of which was 44 degrees, for two minutes : it immediately reduced the animal heat one degree ; but I had a comfortable reaction. I felt very sensibly how much the most active this is of all the processes, when the douche is strong and the water cold. I used it afterward occasionally during my stay, but not regularly, as I did not require full treatment.

I proceeded regularly till the 16th, when I tried the experiment of lying on three wet sheets instead of one. The first impression on lying down was that of greater coldness; but, when packed up, this subsided into a sense of pleasant coolness that was refreshing. This remained, so that at the end of an hour and a quarter I was not warmer than I had been in ten minutes with the one sheet. It was particularly agreeable that the back remained cool so long. In an hour and a half, I had the same general warmth as with half an hour of the one sheet. In another quarter of an hour, I was becoming so warm that the animal heat had risen half a degree. Had I remained longer, I should, doubtless, have perspired freely. I was much satisfied with the experiment, as showing the long-continued refrigerant power of the three sheets, in comparison with the one.

Two days after, I made the experiment of using the sweating blanket. On awaking at 5 A. M., I had some headache : pulse rather full, at 56 degrees ; animal heat 98 degrees. In the course of ten minutes after being packed up, I was comfortably warm ; least so in the feet, where I desired more weight. At the end of an hour and ten minutes, when the warmth of the whole body was much increased without sensible perspiration, the pulse was increased to 66 degrees, full and soft ; the animal heat 99 degrees. At the end of two hours, the perspiration was universal, but not copious, pulse 68, animal heat 100 degrees. In another half hour, perspiration in a greater degree, but not streaming, pulse 68, animal heat 101 degrees. At the end of two hours and three quarters, I quitted the bed, for the full bath, into which I plunged instantly, while hot and perspiring, made two immersions, and came out exceedingly refreshed.* On being dressed, the pulse was as in the beginning, and the animal heat 97·5.

On the following day, returning from a long mountain walk, the sun shining, my pulse was excited and my animal heat 101 degrees.

I waited a few minutes only for a quiet circulation; I wiped off the flowing perspiration, and then, while yet hot and perspiring, was freely rubbed down with the wet sheet, holding more water than usual. I was highly refreshed and agreeably cooled: my pulse became natural, and the animal heat, examined during dressing, was 98 degrees.† Hence another proof of the perfect safety of applying sudden cold to the heated body with perspiring surface, when the animal heat is raised beyond the natural standard.

I proceeded with regular treatment to the 20th, and then desisted. After this period, in consequence of a severe cold from remaining in wet clothes, when I had no opportunity of changing them, I was attacked with slight general fever, rheumatic pains, and severe throbbing headache. I immediately had recourse to a leintuch, followed by the shallow tepid bath, and two affusions with cold water. The relief was immediate: the animal heat, which had been increased to 100 degrees, was immediately reduced to 97·5. One repetition of this treatment was so successful, that in twenty-four hours I found myself quite well.

The final result of the whole proceedings has been a most satisfactory improvement of my health, in all the failings which I mentioned; and I have not found the least occasion for medicine during the last two months. On my journey homeward, which was most extremely fatiguing, I took every opportunity in my power to use, on first rising, the rubbing wet sheet, hip bath, head and foot bath, and always with the greatest comfort and advantage: a plan which, together with early rising, drinking cold water freely,

* It is to be considered that with the elevation of the animal heat, the nervous energy also is simultaneously increased, or more diffused.

† In a paper on heat, which I had the honor of reading at the evening meeting of the College of Physicians, March 5th, 1838, I quoted the experiment of Sir Joseph Banks, Dr. Fordyce, and others, showing the impunity of passing immediately from an apartment heated to 260 degrees Fah. into a very cold atmosphere; the effect indeed being agreeable, refreshing, and useful.

and an active walk, I follow up with the highest advantage and sensible comfort and benefit.

In relating the following cases, I avoid all mention of names; knowing that the violation of this proper delicacy has given great offence at Graefenberg, and disturbed the feelings of many persons.

INDIGESTION, SEVERE HEADACHE, ETC.

A. B., aged 44, for the last seven years during a residence in India, liable to severe headaches; complaining frequently of heat on the top of the head, and a weight at the back. After a time, these headaches became much worse periodically, accompanied with sickness approaching to faintness, and a momentary loss of recollection. These periodical returns at length becoming so frequent as every twenty-five days, and the illness much more severe, accompanied with pain in the lower part of the spine, he was advised to try change of air, from the sultry climate of India, to the Neilgherry hills, where, during a residence of two years, he became much better, the periodical returns being forty-five and forty-six days apart. As his general tone of health improved, the illness also became slighter. His health not being however established, he was directed to return to his native climate, and proceeded to Europe by the overland route, via Malta, where he changed his route and proceeded to Graefenberg, via Naples, Leghorn, Florence, Trieste, Vienna. During this journey, his complaint returned every twenty-sixth, thirtieth, or thirty-sixth day, and the illnesses were not so slight as they had been during the latter period of his residence on the Neilgherries. He complained a good deal of cold feet and frequent headaches. The latter might perhaps be attributed to improper diet at the hotels, and the fatigue and irregularity incident to traveling. It was the opinion of his medical friends in India, that there was no organic disease, and that his complaint was to be attributed to indigestion and the exposure to the climate of India. He had a return of illness on the 29th of March, in the carriage between Olmutz and Graefenberg. Priessnitz saw him on the 30th, and commenced treatment on the 31st, with abreibung and head bath, the back and sides being immersed for a quarter of an hour. On the 1st of April, he had leintuch at 5 A. M., followed by a tepid bath. Leintuch again at 12, followed by an abreibung and head bath; at 5 P. M. an abreibung. This treatment continued until the 20th of April, when he had a return of illness in the night. Priessnitz being sent for, he directed his head to be wetted before using the leintuch, and an abreibung after it, instead of the tepid bath; the abreibung to be repeated at 9 A. M., 12 noon, 3 P. M., 6 P. M., and 9 o'clock P. M.; in addition to which he was to have an abreibung every fifteen minutes for one hour after the faintness. This treatment of six abreibungs a day, and leintuch at 4 in the morning, head bath at 9 A. M. and 12 noon, continued several days; was then reduced to five abreibungs in a day, then to four; and lastly, he went back to the former treatment, which continued until the first of May, when he had another return of illness. Priessnitz was then of opinion that the present treatment proved too severe for him, and must be modified; that the tepid baths were to be left off; but that he must continue the leintuch once in the day, head bath once, four or five abreibungs in the course of the day, and a foot bath twice in the day; and that as soon as the present illness had passed off, the head bath was to be discontinued, and the head to be simply rubbed with water. He directed an abreibung every fifteen minutes, to be repeated four times after any faintness; also one foot bath after a paroxysm. On being told that the patient was fatigued with the exertion of dressing and undressing every fifteen minutes while ill, he directed that he should go into bed between each abreibung, be kept quiet, and that if he fell asleep he was not to be disturbed.

During the first three weeks of the time that this gentleman was under treatment, he was *remarkably* well; had no headache whatever, and never complained of indigestion since the 20th of April (it is now 12th of May); he has occasionally complained of headache, but is nevertheless better than he was before he arrived; his general tone of health is improved; the pain in his back quite gone, so that he can run *down* a hill without uneasiness, whereas even walking fast *down* a hill formerly used to shake and jar his system. His feet are always warm; he no longer starts in his sleep as he used to do, and can sleep on his back as well as on his side, which he could never do before, since he resided in India; and he no longer complains of indigestion after dinner. Before adopting the treatment, he was always dependent on the aid of medicine for the bowels; since, he has not had the least occasion for any. It must also be mentioned, that although the two last attacks of illness occurred within very short intervals of time, the headaches were slight, and the illness only a mild one. His chest appears to me to have become wider. I saw this gentleman almost daily, and left him in a fair way of recovery.

INDIGESTION, NERVOUS DEBILITY, AND HYPOCHONDRIASIS.

A gentleman, aged 25, had brought himself into a state of great nervous debility from excess of study. He was at length incapable of any mental application, had great nervous depression, and was hypochondrical. The sight so much weakened that he could neither read nor write, and even blindness was apprehended. Often had severe headache. Greatly lost both flesh and strength; the digestive functions torpid. He related to me that he first came to Graefenberg three years ago, in the state of indisposition above described. His treatment then as follows: The plunging bath in the morning on first quitting the bed. After breakfast, the douche from five to ten minutes, even in the coldest weather. In the afternoon, a sitz bath for half an hour; drank water in the usual quantity. For five months there was no change in the treatment. He observes, "I had no crisis, not even the water-rash; my health improved gradually. After this, I returned home, where I used a cold bath every morning, and avoided all sorts of spices and fermented liquors. My health improved more and more; my eyes grew stronger again; I could read and write; and, of my former complaint, there remained merely a pressure on the chest; inability for strong mental exertion, accompanied with some dislike for society. Three months ago I returned to Graefenberg, when Priessnitz ordered me to be packed up in a wet sheet morning and afternoon, followed by the plunging bath; to douche for two minutes; to take two head baths; and a sitz bath for a quarter of an hour. He recommended me to make a practice of walking in the air with my head uncovered, however cold the weather." I saw much of this very interesting person, who quitted Graefenberg during my stay. He was quite well. The digestive functions became regular very soon after the commencement of the treatment. This is an example of no sensible crisis occurring, although the treatment was very active.

ASTHMA AND HERNIA, FOLLOWING BRONCHITIS.

A female servant, aged 35, has suffered from difficulty of breathing during the last five or six years, in consequence of an acute attack of bronchitis, which she underwent in India; was unable to ascend a hill or to make any extraordinary continued exertion without much distress. Has also, during the last few years, while residing in India, suffered from severe affections of the bowels. One of these, the last, occurred in August, 1842, and was very severe, and attended with symptoms of much inflammation, for which she was leeched and blistered. She recovered but slowly from this attack, and it was shortly followed by psoas abscess, which pointed below Poupart's ligament (in the groin), and was opened. Toward the end of September, she was obliged to travel with her master and mistress on the way to Bombay, but was conveyed in a palanquin. During her stay in Bombay, in November, while still very weak, she was exposed, in a tent, to wet feet during an entire day, in the discharge of her duties, and caught cold, which brought on, as she states, inflammation of the bowels; and being also at this time much occupied in the care of children, one an infant, and in the packing and lifting of trunks, her hernia (femoral) occurred at this time, on the same side on which the abscess had been shortly before. She continued in delicate health till her arrival in Malta, where she sought medical advice for the first time since the occurrence of the hernia in the end of February. She left her service early in March, being unable to carry the children, and went to Graefenberg, to place herself under the treatment of Priessnitz. She was very asthmatic at this time.

He commenced her treatment the first week in April, ordering her a leintuch every morning, to be succeeded by an abreibung, and this followed by a sitz bath; the abreibung and sitz bath to be repeated at 12 o'clock, and the leintuch, abreibung, and sitz bath, at 4 o'clock P. M. every day; to wear a wet bandage, night and day, round her loins, and to wear a truss upon the situation of the hernia, which was not to be removed night or day.

After having been a month under the fore-mentioned treatment, she complained of very severe pain in the region of the bowels; upon being informed of which, Mr. Priessnitz directed that she should have an abreibung every ten minutes until she should obtain relief, and to walk up and down the room wrapped in a dry blanket between each. Every abreibung relieved her; and when she had taken six, she became quite comfortable.

In the course of the treatment, the catamenia occurring, apprehension was entertained at the probable injury from continuing the treatment; in consequence of which, the advice of Priessnitz was sought, and he directed that there should not be allowed any interruption. The effect was, complete relief from the distressing pains habitually attending the performance of this function, the quantity of the discharge was much increased, but did not continue longer than the usual time, and no weakness was experienced. Upon the return of the periodical function, the same relief from pain was experienced; the quantity was not excessive, the interval was nearer to the natural period than usual, and the discharge did not continue. She now enjoys good general health and strength (May 24th), and no longer suffers from asthma. Her hernia also she considers decidedly better. The truss is still worn; but she has not noticed, as formerly, any tendency to the descent of the bowel.

NERVOUS DEBILITY FROM EXCESSIVE STUDY.

A gentleman, aged 25, tall and slight, had brought on debility by excess of study, attended with circumstances distressing his mind. For two years, suffered from great and almost continued pain in the head, chiefly in the back part; with pains of the teeth and down the cheek; constant noises in the ears. Was also generally weak, and in a very nervous state. Circulation irregular, with ice-cold feet. Bowels torpid. Had been at Graefenberg six months. The treatment: Leintuch in the first of the morning for half an hour, followed by the abreibung. Both repeated in the afternoon. Used also daily head bath and foot bath, the feet being well rubbed for half an hour. Was desired, in addition to the regular head bath, to rub the head very freely with cold water, whenever it was painful. Drank water as usual. In the first week, the functions of the bowels became quite regular, and he was released from his former necessity of taking one or other kind of medicine. This benefit arising from the water-cure treatment is one of the highest magnitude, and happens, as far as my inquiry went, almost without exception. This gentleman assured me that he found himself well at the end of three months, and only remained at Graefenberg longer in order to confirm the establishment of his strength. It was pleasing to hear him describe the altered state of his nerves for the better, the loss of all pains of the head and face, and the improvement of his circulation. He was no longer troubled with coldness of the feet.

INDIGESTION AND PAIN IN THE SIDE.

A gentleman, aged 40, arrived at Graefenberg, in a weak state, with bad digestion and constant pain in the right side. He went at once from the leintuch into the cold bath. He abstained from the douche when the weather was severely cold, and never took it more than two minutes. He was several months before he got a crisis, but was cured of his indigestion before that time. When the crisis came, it was on the opposite side, a large boil, very painful, accompanied by much irritative fever for near a week; but it has *cured* the pain in his side, for which he could get no remedy before.

GREAT SUFFERING FROM NERVOUS WEAKNESS.

The wife of this gentleman was an invalid in many respects—had pains in the loins and in one leg; had for years been a great sufferer from general nervous weakness. She is now quite well.

Until the crisis, which appeared in the form of several large boils on one leg, her treatment was—leintuch one hour, then cold bath; at eleven, abreibung and sitz bath; at half-past four, leintuch one hour; then, either the cold bath or abreibung, whichever she pleased.

When the boils were painful and discharging, she had tepid bath after leintuch, instead of cold bath. From being very debilitated, she has become strong enough for any exertion. This lady has returned to Graefenberg, out of gratitude to the place where she and her husband received the blessing of health. I saw him on the day of my departure. They will now use only slight treatment, to confirm the general strength.

GENERAL FEVER.

A gentleman, aged 44, of full habit, thus describes his case: "I was troubled and annoyed, four days or more, with pain of the left side opposite the heart. I met Priessnitz and informed him of it. He called the next morning at 9 o'clock; the pain still continuing, he ordered me, at 11, to take an abreibung for five minutes, that is to say, I was to be rubbed, and rub myself, that time in a wet sheet, standing upright. I was then to wait ten minutes, walking about the room; then take another abreibung for five minutes; then to walk half an hour and take a sitz bath for twenty minutes. All this I did. At half-past 3, I was ordered to do precisely the same things over again. However, after the morning operations, I found that I had taken a severe cold, or that the operations had made me ill. I had pains all over me; my limbs, my back, and my head were in pain; and I became very hot and feverish. The pains and feverish symptoms increased; at four o'clock I took an abreibung five minutes, then walked about half an hour; then I had a leintuch for one hour, then a tepid bath five minutes, at 68 degrees. All the pains soon left me. I walked out for half an hour, had supper, and went to bed. At five in the morning, my attendant came; and, as I had been feverish in the night, was so then, and had some pain in the head after the leintuch, which I took for an hour; I used a tepid bath at 64 degrees for four minutes, receiving also one cold affusion over the head. Without further treatment, I found myself next day quite recovered.

INDIGESTION AND SORE THROAT. (BY THE PATIENT, AGED BETWEEN FORTY AND FIFTY).

"I arrived at Graefenberg 15th July, 1842; my complaint, as described by my physician, being 'bad digestion and sore throat.'

"I have *always* been subject to irritation of the throat, more or less, from a boy: within the last eight years it has troubled me more, and given either real or fancied cause of uneasiness.

"For years previous to 1835, I was subject to *boils,* which gave me much pain and annoyance. Up to this period, my throat gave me little or no trouble; was generally, though relaxed, free from phlegm. The end of 1835 I began an aperient pill; I took one generally daily till 1842, up to the time of my coming here. Soon after I began to take this pill *the boils ceased,* and my throat gradually grew worse: though I felt more comfortable in my digestion, my throat grew worse—more and more troublesome.

"For nearly twenty years I had constantly taken wine and spirits *freely.* When I came here I was much more corpulent than I am now, and my whole system seemed deranged. I was nervous, and like a *barometer.* I could not venture, after exercise, into a church, or into any large cold building, for fear of taking cold, which I almost invariably did, and this always affected my *throat*—sometimes laid me up for a week in my bed-room. I attribute this sensitiveness to having taken, seven years ago, a quantity of mercury, which has come out here, making my mouth sore, and affecting my breath strongly occasionally. This, I believe, has now ceased. I am less sensible now to changes of temperature. For years I have been unable to take walking exercise in a week, equal to that which I can now take in a day. Previously to coming here, I always *rode* every where. I had pains in the stomach and in the feet, with redness in the hands and knuckles, and in the legs: in all these there is now no pain, having had crises in them. The arms are still painful, but I have had no boils or crises in *them* yet. My digestion is better, my throat is better, and progressively improving. I have no pain.

"Treatment commenced July 16, 1842. The first five weeks, leintuch, at five in the morning, one hour; then abgeschreckte (tepid) bath, 13 degrees Reaumur, three minutes; an umschlag round the body; then walk an hour; then breakfast; at eleven, abreibung; then wait a quarter of an hour, then sitz bath a quarter of an hour; then walk, then dine. The same at four P. M.; got better daily.

"For six weeks, all the operations, as above, were continued; and the douche at nine A. M. for two minutes, which was gradually increased to seven minutes, I took regularly for six months, and during the winter.

"The ninth week, in addition to the sitz bath, I took the cold bath every morning; then—leintuch one hour, tepid bath one minute, cold bath two plunges, then tepid again one minute. I have lately omitted the douche and cold bath, in consequence of having crises. When I was first enveloped in the wet sheet, a strong sour smell, like mellow apples, proceeded from me, and filled the room; and was of so subtle a quality, as to be with difficulty washed out of the blankets. I had never experienced this odor before. Priessnitz told me that it must all come out, for I could never get better till it was entirely removed. This smell has not been perceptible the last three days.

"I have daily, by order, taken 10 or 12 glasses of water, 5 before breakfast, the rest distributed at intervals. Before breakfast, much mucus has been rejected from the stomach, very sour and bitter, sometimes of a green color, sometimes yellow. I have still eructations of water before breakfast, but not sour; and now and then a little froth and phlegm. Upon the whole, I am quite satisfied, and consider my coming here providential; for, in England, I could find no certain remedy for one thing that did not cause inconvenience and disorder of some other kind.

"When I showed Priessnitz my throat, he said, 'This is caused by your stomach, which must be set right before your throat will be better; besides, your nervous system is all wrong; but I have hopes I can make a different man of you; you must get thinner, and then your digestion and throat will both get better.'"

He had pursued active treatment for ten months; a duration that may appear surprising. The throat has been his greatest trouble. The mucous membrane had long been diseased; and at one time the uvula had become so elongated, that a portion of it was excised. He might probably have desisted from such a regular proceeding as he was still pursuing, some time past; but his determination was to stay at Graefenberg, under treatment, as long as a vestige of complaint remained; so truly did he enjoy and estimate the great improvement which he had received. The odor of which he speaks was connected, I have no doubt, with the gouty diathesis. He had experienced occasional gout. He told me that, on his first arrival, he had scarcely the feeling of energy to cross the road. I saw abundant proof of his acquired activity; and he looked strong and well.

INFLAMMATION OF THE STOMACH AND BOWELS.

A fine, lively boy, aged three years, is generally well, yet subject to inflammation of the stomach and bowels.

He had an attack of inflammation of the stomach, accompanied by sickness, with strong fever and determination to the head. In the evening, the child was placed in a bath at 70 degrees Fahrenheit, in which he remained 20 minutes; cold water was added as the temperature rose. During this time, cold water was poured from a tumbler on his head, repeated at intervals of a minute; and, as usual, his whole body was carefully rubbed. He was then taken out and placed on the sofa, and covered with a sheet and blanket, with the back of his head in cold water for 10 minutes. By this time, reaction had taken place, and then wet compresses were applied to the head and back of the neck; and the body, from under the arms to the hips, was wrapped in a similar way. He slept quietly till three in the morning, when the previous symptoms having partially returned, the first treatment was repeated; after which the child was again placed in bed, where he slept till morning, and was then quite well, and went out as usual.

One month after this attack, he was taken ill in a similar way, but with symptoms much more severe—the fever running high, accompanied with delirium. The treatment was commenced by placing him successively in nine wet sheets, from which the water was but slightly wrung out. In each of these he remained about 5 minutes; toward the last, the heat being diminished, he was allowed to remain 10 minutes. The feet were cold; and, as long as they remained so, the wet sheet was only applied down to the knees; meantime, the feet and legs were rubbed strongly with the hands.

While the extreme heat continued, the wet sheet was covered by a thick, dry one, instead of a blanket, as is usual. After the application of the last wet sheet, he was placed in a bath of 70 degrees, where he remained nearly an hour; the same process of rubbing and pouring water over the head being practiced. The first day, the same process was repeated four times; the duration of the bath being not so long when the fever was not so high. During the night, the wet sheet was changed almost every hour. On the morning of the second day, the child refused to go into the bath, calling out himself, at intervals, for additional wet sheets. Orders were given that his inclination should be complied with. In the course of the morning, the child himself desired that he might be put into the bath, where he remained till the heat under the arms and on the back of the neck was the same as the rest of the body; this equality of temperature being the general guide for the duration of a bath. It is worthy of remark, that the more the fever was reduced, the more quiet the little patient became, till at last he remained in the bath perfectly tranquil. The same treatment, slightly varied, was continued four days, when the child was well, and was sent out to play with the other children. In eight days after this, a pustule appeared on the foot, containing matter, which discharged freely.

Observation.—This case might probably have passed into continued infantile fever had it not been in this manner promptly and successfully treated. When fever runs very high, as shown by the burning skin, delirium, and other symptoms, it is a good modification of the use of the leintuch to cover it with a dry sheet, instead of the blanket, and packing up in the usual manner.

NERVOUS DEBILITY, WITH FREQUENT CRAMPS.

A gentleman, aged 45, tall and stout, received two injuries of the head by a fall, one of which was in hunting, about seven years ago. The nervous system was much deranged, especially since the second accident, five years ago, when the spine received a strong contusion and shock. For a long time he had been very nervous, and unable to compose himself during any sedentary occupation; having also heavy and stupid feelings of the head; *muscæ volitantes;* constant singing in the ears; prickings and numbness of the limbs, with frequent cramps; unrefreshing nights, often sleepless, and in the morning more tired than when he went to bed. He neglected himself after the first accident; but after the second, having the use of the limbs so much impaired that it was with great difficulty he could walk half a mile, he went to Bareges: first used the baths at St. Sauveur, for two weeks; lay in them for an hour and a half to 2 hours: then, at Bareges, douched every day for 10 minutes; after which, was put into bed, where he had most copious sweating; and then, covered with a blanket, was carried to his lodgings. At the end of four months, his amendment was very satisfactory, and he quitted early in August. Relapsed at the end of the year, and passed a bad winter. Next year, he used hot sulphurous baths in Switzerland, with advantage, but remained a great invalid. He had several symptoms indicating a disposition to gout. He did not use any further treatment till coming to Graefenberg, nine months ago. He has had all the processes, and been on full treatment, without having received any decided benefit to his nerves. Yet his muscles have become stronger, and his digestion is improved. He found it necessary to douche very cautiously; for, if he received it with great force and much continuance, he found his head exceedingly disordered by it. It was his intention to give up the treatment and quit Graefenberg, if he did not improve in two months more.

It seems probable that more than functional error in the membranes of the brain and spinal marrow exists in this case, so persistent have all the distressing symptoms been. I do not expect that he will be benefited by the water-cure treatment, and think that he might receive advantage from undergoing a regular course of alterative and purgative medicine, to be followed by the use of the baths and douche at Buxton. It is probable that he may have recourse to such measures, should he be finally disappointed at Graefenberg.

NERVOUS DEBILITY AND SLEEPLESSNESS.

A lady, aged 27, had typhus fever, from which she dates her loss of health. Subsequently, she had a fall from a horse, causing concussion of the brain; and, on another occasion, a severe contusion of the head, with a wound by the falling of a beam. For a long while, she experienced intense sufferings, from which she never recovered; and she came to Graefenberg with the following symptoms: Frequent severe pains of the head, with a strong sensation of burning heat of the scalp; hearing and sight affected; altogether in a highly nervous state, and seldom sleeping more than an hour in the night; all the functions irregular; the feet almost constantly affected with icy coldness; with frequent pains and oppression in the hypogastric region. She had always received more benefit from cold water applications than any other means, and especially from using the *mer de glace* (a stream derived from the melting of ice and snow from the mountains), in Switzerland, as a bath. Very active medical treatment had been used at different periods; leeches and blisters to the spine again and again; and courses of medicine of various kinds.

On her arrival she was put on the following treatment: In the morning early, leintuch, tepid bath (Reaumur 14 degrees), and plunging bath in immediate succession. Abreibung and sitz bath in the middle of the day; a regular head bath once in the day; and whenever painful and heated, to apply cold water freely by the hand, and leave wet compresses on any heated part. The foot bath once or twice a day; rubbing the legs also with the water, for they were affected with weakness and swelling. An eruption of irritable pimples appeared, which was treated with wet bandages covered by dry. Priessnitz was glad to see this early crisis. The body-bandage was used. She drank a medium quantity of water, and was much in the air; but she could not take great exercise. At a particular period, the nervous system was greatly disturbed; and there was some hysteria, with much affection of the head. In these circumstances, Priessnitz directed four abreibungs in the morning and four in the afternoon, with intervals of half an hour, during which she went into bed, to gain composure and warmth. She did not complain of this troublesome treatment, and acknowledged the very sensible relief which it afforded her. On my quitting, I compared her state with what it was on her arrival, with great satisfaction. Her health was in every respect materially improved; and the head so relieved that she could sleep comfortably. There was every promise of the case proceeding to a favorable issue.

INDIGESTION, DISTRESS, AND DEPRESSION OF SPIRITS.

A clergyman and schoolmaster, aged 35, had too intensely exercised his mind and feelings, and brought on so distressing a state of nervousness, that, in preaching, he became painfully confused in a quarter of an hour. He had severe indigestion, with opposite states of the bowels, but most commonly inert; headache, with confusion, noises of the ears, and dimness of sight; as in the last case, heat of the scalp and extreme coldness of the feet; depression of spirits, with distress that he was incapable of any mental exertion, being an ardent student. He was much affected by every change of weather. His treatment consisted of leintuch and tepid bath, with plunging bath, sitz bath, head bath three times a day, foot bath twice a day, the soles of the feet being diligently rubbed; the body-bandage. He drank water freely; and he had abreibung whenever the head was more than usually uncomfortable. After about a fortnight, the use of the douche was added to the treatment.

He described, in glowing terms, the happy improvement which he received after ten days' treatment, and especially in his digestion and the state of his head; but when he had employed the douche for a week, he was apprehensive that it did not suit his nerves, for his head became painful and confused after using it.

In all these cases of morbid sensibility of the nerves of the head, it appears to me that the application of the volume douche, if ever used, should be much delayed; and that the jet shower bath, applied with only moderate force, continued from one to three minutes, is a more appropriate remedy.

It is very obvious that, in the management of all delicate and difficult cases, a good medical judgment is required to adapt the treatment to the many changing circumstances which must occur.

GOUT AND RHEUMATISM.

A gentleman, aged 44, of slight frame and delicate appearance, had received great trials to his constitution, from living in various climates under circumstances of immense exertion of mind and body; so that he incurred a severe liver disease, followed by both gout and rheumatism. His father had been a sufferer from gout and from tic-douloureux. He, therefore, had the hereditary predisposition. By treatment, his health was improved up to November, 1839, when, from exposure to wet in shooting, he experienced painful rheumatism or gout, for each name was given, in one knee-joint. It was so swollen and misshapen, that some thought it was dislocated. The frequent use of leeches; of iodine, externally and internally; of calomel, sarsaparilla, and other medicines, formed the chief treatment. The disease increased severely. He describes that "the leg wasted away; that the hip had the appearance of being dislocated; and that some inflammation became visible at the lower part of the spine, with frequent aching pain. The knee was so bent, from contraction, that the limb was drawn up almost to doubling, and quite useless; in addition to which, he was reduced to a skeleton, having lost all appetite and sleep." The actual cautery to the spine was proposed; but not having profited by any of the various means employed, he fell into despair, and was urged to try the water-cure at home. He here says, "I was so weak that I could only allow gentle measures. My diet was strictly regulated. I drank plenty of pure water; morning and evening had an abreibung and shallow tepid bath (66 degrees Fah.); in the middle of the day, free ablutions of the whole limb, and wet bandage covered by dry. From the commencement I began to feel differently. Sleep and appetite soon returned; and, my strength gradually improving, I was able to bear the use of the sweating blanket, followed by the half bath. Ere long, numerous boils appeared on the legs, which afforded great relief to the deep-seated pains." Had sitz baths. In one month he was so much improved, that he could use crutches for half an hour; and at the end of three months, he had gained sufficient strength to undertake the journey to Graefenberg. But still having a very large number of boils in a state of suppuration, his nerves were greatly disturbed, and he was rendered very ill by traveling five hundred miles; was much affected with cramps and hysteria. He arrived. Priessnitz told him he would recover, but a long time would be required. At first, his treatment was moderate, and afterward increased, with a cautious use of the douche. He drank water very freely. For a time, its early morning use was slightly emetic; but this relieved him of bile and phlegm. In October, 1840, he could walk a little with two sticks. The boils increased over the body. In November, the weather being unfavorable, he took cold severely from accidental exposure, and new symptoms arose. An abscess gradually formed between the bladder and the rectum, and at length broke, the matter being discharged partly by the rectum, and partly by the urethra. His cramps and pains of the bladder and bowels were so severe, that his life was in imminent danger. For a fortnight he was without sleep, could not take any food, and for ten days had water only to support him, if support it could be called. Cold water lavements, half and quarter baths, fomentations, and wet linen rubbings, all more tepid than usual (80 degrees), were freely employed. When the abscess found free vent, the symptoms so much abated, that a little sleep and the capability of taking some nourishment returned. He gradually improved, so that by the middle of January, 1841, he could again walk with two sticks about the house. Now more active treatment was resumed; and even the sweating in the blanket twice a week, and the cautious use of the douche. The progress of cure became very favorable. Before the end of summer, he was able to take exercise and enjoy the mountain air; and appetite and sleep returned favorably.

In April, 1842, he was sufficiently recovered to leave Graefenberg, with the use of the limb quite restored, all contraction being removed, and the general flesh, strength, and spirits quite regained. He was the wonder of Graefenberg! I saw this gentleman about 10 weeks ago. He was in good health and spirits, but felt the necessity of avoiding great fatigue; as in such case he was reminded, by achings, that his limb, although so happily restored, could not possess the vigor of one that had never been diseased. In a review of all the circumstances of this important case, infinite praise was due to Priessnitz for its management. He had been indefatigable in his attentions.

SYPHILITIC ERUPTION, HERNIA, SCIATICA, BILIOUSNESS, INDIGESTION, ETC.

A gentleman, aged 27, tall and stout, very muscular, came to Graefenberg nine months ago, having a cutaneous eruption of a syphilitic character, a hernia humoralis, enlarged tonsils, sciatica, and great disposition to general rheumatism, with a bilious countenance, much indigestion, and great nervousness and depression of spirits. Priessnitz at once told him, that his case would require a long period for the cure. The treatment was at first mild; but, without unnecessary delay, was made active; he sweated in the blanket each other day; and, after four months' douching every day, had two sitz baths every day, lasting an hour, the water being changed twice or thrice; with also abreibung, leintuch, head baths, and foot baths; for this patient was very liable to pain and congestion of the head, with great coldness of the feet. He was exceeded by none in his zeal in drinking water. His usual quantity was 16 pints daily; and one day he was ambitious to take four pints more; from which he had all the feeling of having drunk too much wine, attended with a vertigo; and being alarmed by these symptoms, he returned to and continued his former quantity without inconvenience. He had passed the last winter at Graefenberg, and was in the habit of taking his first morning walk before the rising of the sun, and in an atmosphere of from 6 degrees to 10 degrees Fah., much enjoying the sight of the glorious orb first appearing in the horizon. After breakfast, he used with great satisfaction the icy douche! for 8 minutes; but when I found him at Graefenberg, the duration was 10, and twice a day. He had been there nine months. He was the picture of health; and described himself as being strong and free from all inconvenience. His muscles were large and firm, and many remarked that his chest had considerably expanded. In the general history which he gave me, he stated that, in the first instance, he had been freely treated by mercury and iodine, sometimes with the effect of removing the immediate symptoms; but they recurred; and at length, feeling much incommoded by the medicines, and having some addition of complaint, after an interval he had recourse to the water-cure treatment. Under it, he had repeated severe crises of boils, from which he was persuaded that he had received most material benefit. In this case, the copious draughts of water certainly appeared highly useful, and particularly to the bladder, the mucous membrane of which had been so much affected, that in the beginning the urine was passed with great difficulty, and highly charged with mucus; but it must be observed that, when using these great libations, he took immense exercise, often walking 6 or 8 miles before breakfast.

INDIGESTION, RHEUMATISM, AND SPITTING OF BLOOD.

A gentleman, aged 40, tall and slight, appearing free from complaint, gave me the following account. When a boy at school in Germany, he was compelled, with the rest of the boys, to take a purgative every Saturday morning; and thinks that from this unfortunate and absurd practice he acquired the subsequent necessity, and that an increased one, of resorting to medicine. He was subject to great depression of spirits, inaptitude to exertion, rheumatic pains, shortness of breath on ascending a hill, and occasional spitting of blood of a scarlet hue. He had tried various medicines, and long persisted with a slight mercurial alterative; but, he says, without improvement. He was dependent on lavements for any action of the bowels. He went to an establishment near his home, where he was sweated in the blanket every day, had the plunging bath and other means; but he did not feel equal to the perseverance in such treatment, and went to Graefenberg, where he had been nine months when I first saw him, remaining, however, more from choice than necessity. His treatment had been leintuch in the first of the morning, avoiding the perspiring, followed by the tepid and plunging baths in succession; an occasional abreibung; two sitz baths every day, at first tepid, afterward cold; body-bandage.* He drank from 10 to 12 glasses of water. After two months, he used a douche daily. His recovery was perfect, and he was an excellent specimen of the good effects of the water-cure. In a few weeks after using it, his digestion became quite regular.

GOUT.

An Austrian officer, aged 47, tall and robust, had acquired gout in the ankle and side of the foot at 37, and since in various parts, never escaping a winter till the last, and having fits of from 6 to 9 weeks' duration. He had been at Graefenberg 11 months. On his first arrival, the limbs were very infirm, the ankles swollen, and the feet and knees severely affected with chronic pains, giving him a dread of attempting walking exercise. He had previously been treated with various medicines, and with calomel very freely. He began with the use of from two to four abreibungs daily; then two leintuchs, followed by the shallow bath; afterward by the

* In future this is to be understood, if not mentioned; the exception to its use being very rare.

plunging bath; next, the sweating in the blanket each other day, until crises formed extensively on the legs, when it was discontinued; and he had also a strong vesicular rash on the body, with a line of demarcation exact with the bandage.

He experienced immediate and very complete relief to the pains in the knees and ankles when the boils appeared. Afterward, they formed also on the knees, arms, and shoulders. When the crisis subsided, he douched twice a day for eight minutes, instead of using the plunging bath, as he thought it suited him better, and proved more favorable in producing good crises; for the chronic pains had returned occasionally, but were invariably relieved by the formation of boils. When I saw him, he was almost perfectly restored to health. He related that he had derived great strength to his ankles from the daily use of a cold foot bath, deeper than usual; that when he did use the blankets, he found the afternoon more favorable than the morning for the producing of perspiration; and this, he thought, especially as he had a quick digestion. For those who might have a weak and slow digestion, he considered it, from observations he had made, an unfavorable time. This gentleman was so well recovered, that he was about to leave Graefenberg.

GOUT AND RHEUMATISM.

A gentleman, aged 47, robust and plethoric, subject to regular gout, hereditary, for 10 years, the fits severe and very protracted, once had a rheumatic fever, and now often suffers from rheumatism, especially in the shoulders and the arms. He related that he had been regularly treated in his fits with mercurial purgatives and colchicum, with a sure control over the symptoms, but without lasting benefit; that the last fit, of two months' duration, had been left more to itself; and one knee had remained so much swollen, stiff, and painful, that locomotion was extremely difficult. The usual liniments and lotions being ineffectual, although in combination with the internal use of iodide of potassium, he had recourse to a part of the water-cure treatment, using wet bandage, covered by dry, constantly to the knee; and every morning, on first rising, a cold bath. This bold practice was so successful, that he soon recovered the power of walking. He had tried every kind of regimen as a preventive—meat without vegetables, and then a farinaceous diet without meat, total abstinence from wine and beer;

and yet his prudence was not rewarded by success. Since he had drank water freely, he had not found any necessity, as far as his feelings dictated, of being at all mindful in his diet, so perfect was his digestion, doubtless rendered better by the acquired power, from the improvement in the limbs, of taking free exercise. There were chalk-stone deposits in the fingers and elbows.

His treatment was as follows: In the morning, early, sweating in the blanket, followed by plunging bath; a walk and free drinking of water; at 11 A. M. a douche for five minutes, having begun with three; on his return from the long walk to and from the douche, an abreibung, which much refreshed him; at 5 P. M. two abreibungs, within half an hour of each other; umschlags to all the affected parts. I left him making very favorable progress toward his cure. I should observe, that this patient was not desired to make use of the body-bandage, as he had so regular and perfect a state of digestion.

HEREDITARY GOUT.

A gentleman, aged 50, of middling bulk and stature, had hereditary gout first 20 years ago, brought on by violent efforts in swimming, to save himself from drowning, on a winter's day; was for years subject to fits of great severity, and of six or eight weeks' duration; has chalk-stones in various parts, particularly in the hands and feet; disappointed by allopathic medicine, of which colchicum and mercury formed part, he tried homœopathic, with no other result than the longer staying away of the gout; and this benefit he attributed to the care in diet. The fits were of equal severity when they did return. For some time he adhered to a diet of fish and vegetables, and for several years has wholly abstained from wine. Five years ago, went to Toplitz and Carlsbad, without benefit, and afterward to Wiesbaden, going through a full course of treatment there, still without apparent advantage. He next proceeded to Franzens-bad, in Bohemia, and tried the mud baths for a month, sitting in the mud, up to his neck, at 97 degrees Fah., for half an hour, each other day, with no other good result than curing his lumbago, which has never returned. He came to Graefenberg three years and nine months ago, in a state of such lameness and continued suffering, that he felt himself fast approaching to a bed-ridden state. For the space of two years, with the interruption only of two months, he made daily use of the sweating blanket, with this frequency more by his own desire than the wish of Priessnitz, wishing to force crisis; but he is convinced that it was an error, and that he was weakened. In six weeks, he had boils on the insteps, which remarkably relieved the chronic pains; and, some time after, the urine deposited much substance, which appeared to him like wet chalk. In the beginning of the treatment, Priessnitz examined him, first at the half bath, then after the plunging, and told him his complaint would be cured in time, and even encouraged him to expect the recovery of the hands; but I am persuaded there was too much disorganization of parts to admit of it. In some of the joints of the fingers there was anchylosis, and here and there absorption of cartilage. However, much of the chalk-stone deposit had been removed by the treatment, and I doubt not he will obtain further improvement. After five months, he had an acute attack, which at first he left to itself, but afterward used rubbings in the shallow tepid bath, with tepid affusions and umschlags; all with much advantage. He remained the whole winter, but considers that the "winter-cure" did not suit him, the cold being often severe, from 4 degrees to 10 degrees Fah. for a continuance; but he says that the atmosphere was so clear and still, with often a full sun, that the cold was agreeable to those who could take very active exercise. When restored from the fit, he resumed treatment. His skin was with difficulty excited to perspiration; and Priessnitz had desired him to use two douches a day, and even advised three occasionally; but he continued with two, sometimes using a plunging bath also, and always, twice a week, after the sweating in the blanket. He quitted Graefenberg for a time, and returned. He has used umschlags always, and drank 10 or 12 half-pints of water daily. He related to me that the gout now very rarely and very slightly affects him, and that he can walk ten miles with more ease than one formerly. He looked well. He had not touched medicine since he had been under the water-cure treatment, which he extols in the highest terms.

CUTANEOUS ERUPTIONS AND UNIVERSAL PAINS.

A gentleman, aged 49, robust and rather corpulent, after syphilis five years ago, had a fever in Italy, for which he was bled so freely that his strength was exceedingly reduced. He kept his bed three months; was bled from the arm fifteen times, and had leeches, also, very freely applied to different parts. On recovering sufficient strength, he went to Graefenberg, then having universal pains of a doubtful character, with much cutaneous eruption; sweated in the blanket every morning for four months; and, instead of being weakened, gained strength regularly; always the plunging bath after it. At that time the leintuch was seldom used, except in fevers. He douched also occasionally, and drank from 12 to 15 glasses of water daily. He recovered perfectly, and remained well three years. By many acts of imprudence he lost his health again; had an inflammatory attack on the chest, for which he was freely bled, and with relief at the moment; but other evils followed—lumbago and sciatica, of the most painful description. Leeches and blisters were applied to the hip repeatedly, without relief. He consulted the most eminent physicians in Germany; and, by their advice, used leeches, blisters, and mercurial frictions; in opposition to which the sciatica increased. He went to a water establishment in his neighborhood, his convenience not permitting him to travel to Graefenberg. He used, first, a plunging bath, then the vapor bath for one hour, and next the plunging bath again; but this treatment much disagreed, causing particularly oppression of the chest. The sciatic pain still increased, and at length became so intolerable, that the actual cautery was extensively applied to the hip, of which I saw the evidence. He took mercurial purgatives frequently.

By these means the violence of the disorder was broken; but he got cold, and had inflammation of the larynx. After much interval, it was with great difficulty he could accomplish the journey to Graefenberg, where his anxious thoughts were directed. At length, he again presented himself to Priessnitz; then having severe sciatica; pain also of the femoral nerve; indigestion; hæmorrhoidal suffering; hypochondriasm, and general debility. At first, the treatment consisted of leintuch, shallow tepid baths, sitz baths, and wet bandages, covered by dry, to the affected parts. Afterward, he sweated in the blanket, and used the plunging bath, not finding any disagreement, as he had done with the vapor bath, etc. After three or four months, had general crises, but no boils in the affected limb till eight months had elapsed, when also the thigh was covered with a scaly rash. The pains were entirely relieved when the last boils had suppurated freely. He next used the douche very regularly; and, when I saw him, did so for eight minutes every day. The limb had recovered its size and power;

he could walk almost any distance without inconvenience. He remarked that, till within the last few weeks, the bad limb had never perspired when the other parts of the body freely yielded to the influence of the blanket process.

This was a very important case, and one that did infinite credit to Priessnitz and the water-cure means. It shows also the necessity of their being used with judgment; for, till he came to Graefenberg, he had been injured rather than assisted.

GREAT NERVOUSNESS.

A military man, aged 32, had used mercury for a long time, which created great nervousness eventually; and, in a state of much debility, with wandering pains, he went to Graefenberg. He began with two leintuchs, a shallow tepid bath, and sitz bath. Soon after, a plunging bath was added every other day. But his zeal led him into error; he would go far beyond his instructions in every thing. One morning, he drank eight large glasses of water, instead of the four prescribed, before breakfast; and, omitting the necessary walking exercise, went into the billiard room. The kidneys had not actively secreted. His feet became cold, and he was altogether uneasy. He went out for a walk, accompanied by a friend. He soon fell into incoherent conversation, and was got home with some difficulty. He did not quite lose consciousness, but was speechless; made signs for pen and ink, but could not write. He had violent headache. Priessnitz directed a tepid (62 degrees) foot bath, with free rubbing; sprinkled water on the face and head; and shortly after were applied three abreibungs in the course of half an hour, and wet bandages to the head: he was put to bed. Intense pain of the head ensued, with some general fever and extreme feebleness of the limbs. Priessnitz, at his next visit, a few hours after, ordered two abreibungs, with an interval of ten minutes; then a foot bath for an hour, the water being changed two or three times; next, a leintuch for 20 minutes, followed by the shallow tepid bath, in which he was rubbed for half an hour by two attendants, with occasional affusions of cold water over the head. He now vomited freely, and this gave relief. The whole treatment was so successful, that, in another hour, he recovered sense and speech, and lost the pain of the head. In a few days, general treatment was resumed, and continued with great regularity. He was now always careful to take free exercise before and after every process. Numerous boils formed chiefly in the upper part of the back, but also in the thighs, and they suppurated favorably. He was called away sud denly by military duty, but pursued treatment at home to a certain extent: and a letter from him to Priessnitz, a short time ago, announced the complete recovery of his health.

URINARY FISTULA, OR OPENING.

A gentleman, aged 18, slight and rather delicate, received a severe contusion in the perinœum and neighboring parts by a fall from a horse; to which was attributed the formation of a fistula, and one of a complicated nature, attended with much ulceration and very severe pain and inconvenience. The surgeons wished to operate, but his father determined on taking him to Graefenberg. Priessnitz directed an abreibung twice a day, and umschlags to the affected parts. In the progressive treatment were used leintuchs, plunging bath, and douche; and, at the end of a month, he obtained a perfect cure. The healing was complete.

This case cannot fail to interest the surgical reader. The symptoms had been of an urgent character; the bladder and rectum being affected with very painful irritation; and, at the commencement of the water-cure, the ulcerated parts appeared in a very unhealthy condition.

HEMIPLEGIA, OR PARALYSIS OF ONE SIDE.

A gentleman, aged 60, had suffered many years from dyspepsia and general debility of the nervous system, with often universal pains, which were called both rheumatic and nervous. He was seized with hemiplegia; the right side affected. He got better for a short time, but had a severe relapse: was sent, after a time, to Toeplitz and Marienbad, but became worse. The mind and body were equally prostrate; the digestion was languid; the bowels wholly inactive without medicine or lavement. In April, 1842, he went to Graefenberg, in opposition to the advice of his physicians. Priessnitz prescribed, at first, two abreibungs in the day, and a head bath for 15 minutes; and, as he became stronger, two leintuchs, omitting one abreibung, together with the shallow tepid bath. At the end of three months, boils formed in the head, arm, and leg, only on the affected side, from which evidently great benefit resulted. Neither plunging bath nor douche were used in this case. He received his health entirely at the end of seven months; nervous energy was restored; he had the power to climb the hills, to write his letters, and again enjoy his spirits in society.

CATALEPSY, OR TRANCE, GENERAL DEBILITY, AND INDIGESTION.

A Russian nobleman, aged 36, had reduced the vigor of his constitution by dissipation; and, on a severely cold day at St. Petersburg, 10 degrees below zero, paid a visit of ceremony insufficiently clothed. He had scarcely entered the room when he was seized with catalepsy, and appeared like a statue! The ladies who were present were at first amused, thinking that he was acting! but soon they took the alarm. He could not speak; but, retaining his senses, made signs that he wanted water. He was affused all over from buckets, soon drank freely, and in less than an hour recovered his power of moving. But from this day he became an invalid, suffering especially from pain and nervousness of the head, with general debility and depression of spirits, also having severe indigestion. He was under medical treatment for two years, and visited Carlsbad, Toeplitz, and other baths in Bohemia, without any marked benefit; then went to a water establishment near St. Petersburg. He used the vapor bath, as being considered preferable to the blanket, and after it the plunging bath for five minutes, followed by cold water lavement, all without taking exercise to produce reaction. The treatment was repeated, but so much disagreed that he soon left the establishment. He consulted an eminent physician, who advised another water-cure establishment, but that he should first go to Kissingen for a few weeks, to improve the state of the digestive organs. He followed this advice. He thought himself rather injured than benefited by Kissingen. In the second trial of the water-cure, the shower bath in a continuous mass was applied to the head for some minutes, eight days in succession; he also used the plunging bath. His expression was, that he thought he should have gone mad; and, in despair, he quitted for Graefenberg. Priessnitz gave him every encouragement, but thought mild treatment necessary at first: for two days, one abreibung and one sitz bath, then two of each; and in this manner for ten days, when he became stronger. He proceeded gradually to the use of active treatment, but never to the fullest extent: the douche, once a day, was the strongest part of it. In half a year, he perfectly recovered, and was again in possession of his spirits and the use of his faculties, which had become impaired by the disorder of his nerves. He said he owed his cure to the superior method of treatment pursued at Graefenberg, and to the fine mountain air.

SEMINAL WEAKNESS, WITH GREAT NERVOUS DEBILITY.

A superintendent of mines, aged 24, had found his nervous system much deranged by the unwholesome atmosphere in which he lived ; and at length experienced an involuntary discharge of prostatic liquor, and occasionally of seminal secretion from slight exertion, attended with pain in the spine and loins, occasionally severe. He was in a miserable state of nervous suffering, and went to Graefenberg. For a considerable time he could bear only very mild treatment; yet, after four months, the discharges ceased. The pain remained, and also his feebleness. He douched and received the water particularly on the spine and loins. Boils and "dartres" formed near the seat of pain, and immediately gave the greatest relief. His recovery was complete in eleven months. It is unquestionable that the crisis in this case was highly advantageous. The boils suppurated favorably; and the pain, which had been of long duration, gradually passed away, and has never returned.

DEBILITY, NERVOUSNESS, AND BALDNESS, FOLLOWING THE USE OF MERCURY.

A gentleman, aged 33, having used mercury with great freedom, and been careless in exposing himself in unfavorable weather, fell into a state of great debility and nervousness, and gradually became almost bald. He went to Graefenberg in this state, and was described to look more like a corpse than a living person. His first treatment was a sitz bath, two leintuchs, followed by a shallow tepid bath and free drinking of water. Afterward, he sweated in the blanket, and used the plunging bath every other day; douching also on most days, but omitting one leintuch, and not using any on the day of the blanket. He drank water freely, and took as much exercise on the mountains as his strength would allow. Soon after his arrival, the few hairs on the head which he brought with him disappeared, and the baldness was complete. Boils formed particularly at the nates, and suppurated freely, when the treatment was reduced to the use of two leintuchs and a sitz bath. Soon after, an eruption appeared over the whole body; first vesicular, and afterward scaly; also more boils. The linen was stained with appearances which were supposed to arise from mercury. At the end of six months, he gained some color of the cheeks, and became stronger; but also new shoots of hair appeared on the head, and which in two months more so increased, that when I saw him two months later, he had a fine head of hair! He was pursuing regular treatment, and evidently was quite in a fair way of recovery.

DOES WATER BRING MERCURY FROM THE SYSTEM?

During my stay at Graefenberg, I heard frequent mention of the stains of mercury and of iodine appearing in the leintuchs, either of blue or reddish color; but Priessnitz assured my friend, Dr. Buxton, that he had seen mercurial globules issue at the ends of the fingers after a continued course of the water-cure, in patients who had made a great employment of mercury, either internally or externally, or both, notwithstanding that they had desisted from all use of the medicine for even several years! This appears almost incredible. I cannot doubt the veracity of Priessnitz; and Liebig, with whom I discussed the subject, had no doubt of such a fact, and offered this explanation: that mercury combines with animal matter, and may remain so combined for an indefinite time; and that the quick change of matter which belongs to the water-cure treatment would tend to the separation of the mercury, which might appear in a globular, or other form.

I have witnessed examples of the latent stay of mercury in the system, and shall cite the following: I prescribed to a poor woman, afflicted with rheumatism of the wrist joint, threatening anchylosis, a mercurial ointment, which she rubbed in with only occasional intervals from January to the end of May. No mercury was taken internally; none used externally after May. In November following, she was seized with the most violent salivation that can be imagined.

DEFECTIVE HEARING AND SMELLING, WITH GENERAL DEBILITY.

A gentleman, aged 24, of healthy appearance, when 12 years old, had a nervous fever, which exceedingly weakened his constitution and rendered him very deaf; from that period, he had been weak and sickly, and unequal to much exertion. When he arrived at Graefenberg, four months and a half ago, such was his state, with a bad appetite and almost a loss of smell. His hearing always very defective. Began treatment very gently with abreibung, leintuch, and sitz bath; to drink water very freely and take abundant exercise. After a fortnight, his appetite and strength were improved; and treatment was increased to the use of the sweating blanket, followed by plunging bath twice a week. The douche on the other days; head bath twice a day; and to sniff water freely several times in the day.

There ensued a critical diarrhœa several times, after which the hearing improved. When this diarrhœa occurs, boils seldom happen also. The sniffing of water was at first disagreeable; but finding advantage from it, he persevered; and when I last saw him, his hearing and smell were both recovered. He was strong, active, and in good spirits.

HIGH FEVER, WITH DELIRIUM.

A young man, aged 21, on his way to Graefenberg, for the treatment of a rheumatic complaint, found himself unwell at Vienna, but traveled on, and, when he reached his destination, was in a high fever, with delirium. Until this was reduced, an abreibung was kept applied in the quickest succession, so immediately hot did the wet linen become. The delirium quickly subsided. When the fever was much abated, he was put into the leintuch, and this was followed by the shallow bath. Very soon a copious small-pox eruption appeared. Leintuchs were continued, according to the state of the skin. There was no return of fever; the appetite was natural. In ten days, he was able to walk out of doors. He had been vaccinated in his infancy; but, notwithstanding, the pustules were universal and of full size. No pitting ensued.

It is unquestionable that the water-cure treatment, applied at the beginning especially, is admirably adapted to the cure of eruptive fevers, small-pox, measles, and scarlatina.

DYSPEPSIA, SLEEPLESSNESS, AND NERVOUSNESS.

An Austrian officer, aged 60, had been very stout and remarkable for the goodness of his appetite; but by degrees he became dyspeptic, very nervous, and, above all, lost his sleep more and more by degrees, till at length he was not able to procure more than one hour of dozing in the twenty-four, for upward of two years. He had no regular sleep whatever: opiates would not succeed, and he was in a most wretched state when he went to Graefenberg. Three months passed away without any decided improvement. It was in the beginning of spring; the weather very cold, and he was not strong enough to take much exercise. Hence a slower improvement. Treatment: in the first of the morning a leintuch followed by a shallow tepid bath; an abreibung twice a day; usually a second leintuch, followed either by an abreibung or shallow bath. By degrees he improved, gained some appetite, and sleep returned, at first for an hour only; then more and more, till, by the middle of summer, he could sleep comfortably for seven hours; and he quitted Graefenberg recovered from every inconvenience.

RHEUMATIC NEURALGIA.

A gentleman, aged fifty, of the nervous temperament, yet appearing to have good muscular power, had lived many years in the West Indies, and become enfeebled in constitution by dyspepsia and complaint of the liver. On returning to England he contracted rheumatic neuralgia, which principally affected the thighs and legs. They were morbidly sensitive both to heat and cold, not being able to bear the heat of the fire even at some distance; and instant severe pains occurred in going into the cold air. The skin would not endure flannel. He wore wash leather. His whole nervous system was so deranged that he could not bear the least mental application; not even to write a letter. At successive periods he went to the two Wildbads in Germany, last to that in Gastein, and from both received benefit. The strong douche was used, and which acted so powerfully on him that he could not continue it. On his return home, he caught cold, and had a severe return of the pains. He was advised to go to Bath, and to use the baths of so high a temperature as 106 degrees! Instantly he found his head congested as if filled with blood; had singing of the ears, and a general distress. He left the bath quickly; afterward bathed at 102 degrees to 100 degrees, a few times, but thought himself much injured. On a subsequent occasion, he went to Buxton, and was much benefited. He was highly satisfied both with the baths and douche.

The water-cure treatment, however, attracted his notice, and he went to Graefenberg about a year ago. He has pursued very regular treatment, has had several crises, and is materially benefited, but still has some returns of neuralgia. He bears the douche and the plunging bath, and certainly is greatly improved in nervous energy; and is by no means so sensitive to heat and cold. For example, he bore the Graefenberg winter, and could, when I saw him, take exercise in the sun. Priessnitz expected his cure to be completed in three or four months.

GOUT.

An Austrian field-marshal, eighty-two years of age, had been a gouty martyr through a long life, and visited Graefenberg four years ago, when in such a state of infirmity that he could scarcely put his feet to the ground. Mild treatment was used, but it proved sufficient to produce boils, which formed near the affected joints. He gradually improved, and finally threw away his sticks, walking and riding on horseback with almost the activity of former years.

An old Polish general, nearly eighty years of age, also received equal benefit from the treatment of his gouty sufferings and infirmity.

MENORRHAGIA, OR EXCESSIVE AND DEBILITATING MENSTRUATION.

A lady, aged forty-three, of full habit, for a long time subject to menorrhagia to such an extent as to make her feel enfeebled, had much shortness of breath on exertion, with indigestion and disturbance of the head. A year ago had paralytic distortion of the face: this did not last. Had been upward of four months at Graefenberg. Treatment: leintuch in the morning early, followed by the shallow tepid bath. A sitz bath, at first tepid, afterward cold, twice a day, for twenty minutes, but not during the catamenia. At that period, the wet bandage around the body was to be changed every half hour; but at other times, only when it should become dry. Such, with moderate drinking of water, was the principal treatment. Crises (boils) formed on the legs; and the discharge from them was considerable and continued. She obtained a favorable recovery, and the periods became satisfactorily regular. When I quitted Graefenberg, she could ascend hills without difficulty, and was attentive to take regular exercise.

GREAT DEBILITY AND DEPRESSION OF SPIRITS, FOLLOWING NERVOUS FEVER.

A young lady, aged nineteen, having been strong and healthy, was reduced to a state of great debility by a severe nervous fever, and became the subject of intense headache, attended with great depression of spirits. She went to Graefenberg in October. First treatment: a leintuch twice a day, one sitz bath, and one head bath. Soon after, from exposure to damp evening air, she had a short feverish attack, for which eight abreibungs were applied on the first day, followed by a leintuch. In less than thirty hours the fever was quite removed. Ere long, crises (boils) formed in different parts, and from that time she scarcely experienced any headache. She drank water freely, and had umschlags, but never had stronger means used than I have mentioned; and she perfectly regained her health and strength. When she arrived, she appeared, as I learnt, pale and very weak. On quitting, after five months' sojourn, she had a nice color, and was cheerful, strong, and active.

INSENSIBILITY, FOLLOWING AN IMPROPER BATH.

A gentleman, aged twenty-three, not appearing delicate, of middling bulk, was undergoing treatment for deafness. After very slight preliminary means, he used the sweating blanket in the morning early. He was desired to go into the shallow tepid bath before entering the cold bath; but he was disobedient, and at once plunged into the latter, on a severely cold day, when the temperature of the water was little more than 40 degrees Fah. On quitting the bath, he fell down insensible. Priessnitz was called to him, who directed the most free rubbing of the lower extremities with cold water, and then the shallow tepid bath, with abundant and universal friction, together with moderate tepid affusion over the head. He was quite restored in about an hour. This example shows how careful the patient should be to obey instructions, and not attempt to judge for himself when using the active processes of the water-cure treatment.

INSENSIBILITY FOLLOWING OVER-DRINKING.

A lady, aged thirty-two, disposed to corpulency, and having a short neck, drank, on first rising, four pints or more of water, in a short space of time, taking only a slow walk in the garden. She was suddenly seized with an universal feeling of coldness over the chest and in the extremities, very quickly followed by insensibility. Her state appeared very alarming. Similar treatment to that mentioned in the last case was adopted, and with eventual success; but she was not quite restored till the expiration of twenty-four hours, and for a long time after, she was reminded of the shock from which she had suffered. This case is sufficient to point out the infinite importance of taking active exercise when much water is drunk. Here, the kidneys had not acted. There was a temporary plethora of the vessels; and some effect must be attributed to the influence of the cold water as a sedative to the nerves of the stomach and first intestines.

SECONDARY SYPHILIS. (A HORRIBLE CASE).

A gentleman, aged 34, was attacked, in the year 1828, with secondary syphilitic symptoms, having had primary disease seven months before, and which, he said, was very badly treated. He exposed himself carelessly during the use of mercury. Afterward measures were used with apparent success, for he got and remained pretty well for several years. At length, no fresh cause having existed, a swelling appeared on the forehead, painful, persisting, and resisting all treatment. He went in the summer of 1837 to Aix-la-Chapelle, and used the baths with only slight advantage. An abscess formed in the forehead, and was opened. No healing process afterward. He continually grew worse. Twenty months ago he went to Graefenberg; then having three foul ulcers, deep, and each the size of a sixpence, attended with deep-seated pains, and often prickings near the surface. He had also a painful node on the shin of the left leg. His constitution was much weakened, and I was told that his appearance then was alarming, from the signs of exhaustion and distress. He was without appetite, and procured but little sleep.

Priessnitz ordered a leintuch, followed by a shallow bath, morning and afternoon; a sitz bath for half an hour in the middle of the day; and wet cold water compresses, not covered by dry, to be applied to the ulcers, and changed ten times a day. Waist-bandage; and to drink water as freely as possible.

After three months' treatment, exfoliation of a large portion of the entire cranium, exposing the dura mater, took place. I am in possession of this. When I saw the patient, smaller portions were in process of coming away. Notwithstanding this, he appeared in a fair way of recovery, for he was improved in strength sufficiently to walk two miles; appetite and sleep were good; the granulations were healthy, and the whole complexion of the case was changed very greatly indeed for the better. It is one that renders a valuable testimony to the efficacy and simple character of the water-cure treatment. So much of the dura mater will be eventually exposed, that he will require some ingenious instrument to be worn for the protection of the brain.

INFLAMMATION OF THE BRAIN, WITH DELIRIUM.

A gentleman, between forty and fifty years of age, was suddenly seized with all the symptoms of inflammation of the brain; pain of the head, with urgent feelings of congestion appearing at the outset, a hot skin, great excitement, and very quickly strong delirium. The attack was met by active measures; the rubbing down in the shallow tepid bath, and small affusions of cold water for several hours in succession; and when the violent symptoms were subdued, leintuchs were used, followed by the further use of shallow bath and affusion. This was the chief treatment, and the recovery was quite accomplished in two or three days. By ordinary proceedings, it is not improbable that more than as many weeks might have been required. Both Captain Claridge and Dr. Wilson relate similar cases to this, treated in the same manner, and with equal success.

DYSPEPSIA, HEADACHE, AND FULLNESS AT THE HEAD.

A gentleman, aged 25, was affected from his earliest youth with dyspepsia, and attacks of headache from various exciting causes, attended with heat of the scalp, flushings of the face, and a distressing sense of the vessels of the head being too full of blood. He had been under treatment several weeks with advantage. One afternoon, his dinner not digesting well, he took a very long walk, and, during it, was seized with a strong pain between the lower ribs, affecting his breath. It was with great difficulty he could reach home, so urgent did the spasmodic pain become. Priessnitz saw him immediately, and directed the shallow tepid bath (60 degrees), with abundant rubbing for two or three minutes, instantly followed by the cold plunging bath (44 degrees), in which he remained longer than usual, in order that the cold might make more impression on the spasm ; but, also, this alternation of tepid and cold process was repeated no less than four times, till at length his limbs were quite benumbed, and to a degree of much suffering. The pain of the side was relieved. He was next exceedingly well rubbed; put to bed, became warm, went into a sleep; and, after an hour or two, awoke perfectly recovered. I know that this was a muscular pain connected with indigestion and intestinal flatulence. I have several times experienced it, and found it removable by simple means; as quietude in the recumbent posture, warmth, and a carminative in warm water. In this instance the treatment was out of proportion to the occasion. I suppose that Priessnitz apprehended internal inflammation. I take the liberty of thinking that it was an error in diagnosis, the knowledge of which is always so important in the administration of any kind of treatment. I saw this gentleman immediately after his recovery, and received from him a very minute account.

DEBILITY, SLEEPLESSNESS, DEPRESSION OF SPIRITS, ETC., FROM EXCESSIVE MENTAL APPLICATION.

A lady, aged 30, brought on a state of extreme nervous debility, with impaired digestion, headache, and confusion, with loss of sleep, depression of spirits, and many other nervous symptoms, by a course of severe literary application. She had the highest medical advice in London; but, although relieved in her most troublesome symptoms, she continued in a state of such great debility, that she could not walk across the room without assistance. She tried change of air and scene without success; and, as a last resource, went to a water establishment in England. An abreibung twice a day, and a sitz bath once, with body-bandage, and free drinking of water, constituted her treatment. In three weeks, her amendment was such as to enable her to walk out of doors; and after a few months, she was strong enough to travel. She felt convinced that her nervous debility required further and most skillful treatment. She arrived at Graefenberg shortly before I quitted; and she was in good spirits, with the prospect of her perfect recovery.

SCROFULOUS DISEASE OF THE KNEE JOINT.

Miss ——, aged five years, a child of nervous temperament, first suffered, four years ago, from a painful inflammation of one knee, appearing otherwise in good health. Leeches and evaporating lotions were applied freely; and afterward repeated blisters. At a later period, malt and hop baths at 88 degrees Fah. for one hour at a time, two or three times in a week, in alternation with warm salt water. She had been at Graefenberg about fifteen months. When she first arrived, she could not put the foot to the ground, and used crutches with difficulty. The knee was painful in stormy weather. I examined the joint, which was evidently diseased from scrofula. There was still enlargement; but I was told by the nurse it was very much reduced in size; and this indeed was manifest from the loose state of the skin. It was almost free from tenderness. There was some motion in the joint. She could walk very nimbly without a stick or any assistance; first moving on the heel, then on the toe. The limb was shortened and the tendons of the hams were contracted; but the improvement was very satisfactory. She had been delicate and weak: she was become strong and healthy. The case is so important that I shall particularize the treatment.

At six A. M. the leintuch for an hour, followed by a shallow bath at 64 degrees for five minutes; wet bandages to the waist and around the knee, covered as usual; to go out before breakfast, and drink three small glasses of water. At nine, the knee was rubbed for five minutes with the wet hand, and wet applications were again put on. At 11, repeated, and a sitz bath for 10 minutes. At one P. M. the local treatment and waist-bandage. At half-past two, same treatment. At four P. M. sitz bath for 10 minutes; temperature at a later period reduced to 60 degrees; the knee again rubbed with cold water, and a bandage reapplied. At five P. M. leintuch and shallow bath, which also was reduced in temperature by degrees to 60 degrees. Local treatment repeated. Since last June she had douching at 11, and omitted the sitz bath; but when the weather proved unfavorable, this treatment was reversed.

SCROFULOUS ENLARGEMENT OF THE KNEE JOINT.

A little boy, aged five years, of calm disposition, when two years old had a fall, by which the knee was injured. This, like the last, was a scrofulous enlargement of the knee joint. He was just arrived at Graefenberg. The leg was drawn up two inches from the ground. Priessnitz observed that the tendons were so contracted and rigid, that a division of them by the surgeon would become necessary, but he would treat the enlargement of the joint. The treatment directed was, a leintuch for half an hour three times a day, followed by shallow tepid bath with local application of water, and the drinking of water, as in the last case.

Having related, I believe, a sufficient number of cases to display the powers of the water-cure treatment, I shall only add to their number by alluding, in a cursory manner, to a few other examples, the details of which would require more space than I can afford on the present occasion.

I witnessed two cases of incipient inflammation of the lungs, with much inflammatory affection of the throat, and of the mucous membrane of the trachea, promptly and successfully treated by abreibungs, leintuchs, tepid shallow baths, and umschlags.

In a case of hœmoptysis, it was evident to me that the free drinking of the water had proved injurious; although in other respects the general treatment had been very useful. I am convinced that in this disorder the patient should be even painfully restricted in the quantity of drink. I should prescribe iced water, in very small quantities at a time, as almost the only beverage; and the same principle of management I should observe, in any case of arterial hæmorrhage.

SKIN DISEASES.

I witnessed many urgent cases of disease of the skin, various in their nature. They were chiefly impetiginous or herpetic. *Dartres* is the common name assigned by the foreign patients to most of the eruptions.

LEPROSY.

One of the worst examples of lepra that I ever saw, presented itself to me in the case of a gentleman, 23 years of age. It was universal from head to foot. He had been at Graefenberg one year; and for a long time had been on full treatment, using the douche every day, and sweating in the blanket three times a week, with other processes. He considered himself to be very materially improved; the patches were much less scaly than formerly, and in various parts the skin had assumed a healthy cicatrized appearance. Priessnitz told him that in these cases the water treatment prospered most during the spring. He expected to be successful in the cure. There is no description of cutaneous malady in which, according to my experience, it is so difficult to be effected. This patient had formerly taken various mercurial and other alteratives; had been at Carlsbad; at Gastein, in Tyrol; and at Kreuzenach, a celebrated place for diseases of the skin.

I believe that the water treatment is more adapted than any other to the relief or cure of obstinate diseases of the skin. The continued frictions, ablutions, perspiring processes, douches, etc. must have a powerful influence in exciting an entirely new action of the vessels of the skin; but in any case in which, after a fair trial, the water means did not seem competent to meet the evil, I should not hesitate to add the use of some mild alternative. I saw many cases of scrofula, some of which were materially benefited. In others, it was doubtful whether any improvement had been effected.

TETANUS AND HYDROPHOBIA.

In the melancholy diseases of tetanus and hydrophobia, I should consider the employment of the most active of the water-cure processes well deserving a trial. Priessnitz assured me that he had cured a dog of hydrophobia by incessant douching with the coldest water. Many years ago, one of my horses was seized with locked-jaw, and the poor animal appeared to be fast approaching to a hopeless condition, the farrier having exerted all his skill in vain. The late Professor Coleman by chance arrived at the time, and advised repeated affusions of the spine with the coldest water from buckets. After about an hour, according to my recollection, the spasms of the jaw, and of the several affected muscles, became relieved. A complete recovery ensued. I have thought it not unbecoming to relate these comparative cases.

CHAPTER XIV.

THE GRAEFENBERG TREATMENT OF DISEASES.

General Remarks on Fevers.—Boerhaave's Theory.—Ill effects of the Heating, and good effects of the Cooling modes.—A great Change has been wrought within a few Years.—Animals instinctively go to Water in Feverishness from whatever Cause.—Curious cases of Fever, from Dr. Baynard, one hundred and fifty years ago.—Water the best of all Remedies in Fevers and Inflammations of whatever kind.—Water the Invigorator of Nature.—Remarkable Facts from Howard the Philanthropist.—A singular case of Resuscitation of a Child supposed to be Dead.—Priessnitz's Modes.—Typhus, Jail, and Ship Fever.—Priessnitz is never known to fail in curing Fevers of whatever kind, if he commence at first.—Detail of the Treatment of Ship or Typhus Fever.—Advantages of pure fresh Air.—The great general Principle of treating all Fevers.—Ague and Fever.—Prevention always better than Cure. Detail of Treatment in this Disease.—The Cold Stage.—The Hot Stage.—The Sweating Stage.—Object of the Treatment in each Vapor Bath recommended in the Cold Stage.—Cold Water at the beginning of the Cold Stage.—Treatment on the "Well Day."—Diet.—Fasting and Water Drinking.—Their probable Effects.

GENERAL REMARKS ON FEVERS.

Boerhaave, the most learned physician of his time, held as a theory, that fever was caused by a *lentor* (something cold) in the blood. This theory—for it was only a theory—caused, for about two centuries, one of the most erroneous modes of practice that ever crept among the already multiform and barbarous jargons of the medical art. Alas! what erroneous theories and practices which the human mind could by any possibility invent, have not been put forth to torture human nature with! Every one of you that has arrived at adult age, can well remember how, a few years since, no fever patients—none with inflammatory disease of whatever kind—could touch a drop of cold water, at the peril of life. "It will be the very death of you," exclaimed the practitioner. The anathemas against no poison could not be more imperative than this against pure cold water in fever. Now and then, however, there were those who, spite of physicians, nurses, and attendants, broke over all bounds in their frenzy, and betook themselves to this best of all remedies. And what was the result? Were these patients killed by the dreaded element? Every one knows the proper answer to the question. And now, thanks to Priessnitz, the temperance reformation, and the light of advancing science, this horrible practice of which I have been speaking, is consigned forever, I trust, to be remembered only among the things that were.

Whenever a general feverishness, from whatever cause, is brought on in animals, they not only instinctively drink water, but immerse themselves in it, if it is possible for them to do so. It is said that in some countries wild pigs become violently convulsed by eating henbane, and that by going into water and by drinking it, they recover. And when animals become feverish from mutilations or mechanical injury, they seek lying upon the damp ground in the cool air, and even in mud and wet, and go not unfrequently into the water.

Rats, all housekeepers know, go at once to water, when they have swallowed arsenic that had been set for them; and hence, too, it is well known that water must be kept out of their reach; otherwise they are very apt to recover from the acute gastritis caused by the poison. Domestic animals, as cats and dogs, when poisoned by arsenic that had been set for rats, take at once to lapping down great quantities of water, and are thus sometimes apparently saved. I knew a fine old pointer dog in the city of New York, that, after he had been nearly beaten to death by the barbarian dog-killers, went for days without food, but lapped often large quantities of water, and was thus saved.

Dr. Edward Baynard, an able and very amusing writer on water one hundred and fifty years ago, gave the following cases: "A Turk (a servant to a gentleman), falling sick of a fever, some one of the tribe of treacle conners being called in, whether apothecary or physician, I can't tell, but (according to custom), what between blister and bolus, they soon made him mad. A countryman of his, that came to visit him, seeing him in the broiling condition, said nothing, but in the night-time, by some confederate help, got him down to the Thames' side, and soundly ducked him. The fellow came home sensible, and went to bed; and the next day he was perfectly well. This story was attested to by two or three gentlemen of undoubted integrity and worth; and I doubt it not, but believe it from the greater probability; for I'll hold ten to one on the Thames' side against treacle, snake-root, and all that hot regimen which inflames and exalts the blood, breaks its globules, and destroys the man, and then, forsooth, the doctor sneaks away like a dog that has lost his tail, and cries, it was a pestilential, malignant fever, that nobody could cure; and to show his care of the remainder, bids them open the windows, air the bed clothes, and perfume the rooms for fear of infection; and if he be of the right whining, canting, prick-eared stamp, concludes, as they do at Tyburn, with a mournful ditty, a psalm, or a preservative prayer for the rest of the family. So exit Prig, with his starched, formal chops, ebony cane, fringed gloves, etc."

"In the year 1665," says Dr. Baynard, "I very well remember that it was the talk of the town, that a brewer's servant at Horseleydown, in Southwark, was seized with the plague, and in his delirium ran into a horse-pond, first drank his fill, and then fell fast asleep with his head upon the pond's brink, where he was found in the morning. How long he had been in the pond nobody knew, for it was in the night he went into the water, and had no nurse then with him; but he recovered to a miracle."

But a more singular case is given by this amusing old author, as follows: "My worthy and learned friend, Dr. Cole, showed me an account from an apothecary in Worcestershire, whose name (I think) was Mr. Mathews; the substance of which was, that a young man, delirious in small-pox, when his nurse was asleep, jumped out of bed, ran down stairs, and went into a pond. The noise awaked the nurse, who followed with an outcry, which outcry raised the posse of the family, who surrounded the pond; but he parleyed with them, and told them, that if any body came in he would certainly drown them, and that he would come out when he saw his own time. He accordingly did so, and walked up stairs, and sat (in his wet clothes) upon a chest by the bedside; in which posture Mr. Mathews found him when he came into the chamber. *Note here,* that the apothecary lived three or four miles distant from the place, and he was in the water and on the chest during all that time, in his wet clothes, that the messenger was gone for him. The apothecary asked him how he did? He answered, pretty well. He asked him if he would have a clean shirt, and go into his bed? He said, by and by he would, which accordingly he did. When in bed, he asked the apothecary if he had nothing good in his pocket, for he was a little faintish? He said that he had a cordial, of which he drank a good draught; so went to sleep, waked very well, and in a little time fully recovered. Now, as Dr. Cole observed very well, 'A man,' quoth he, 'would not advise his patients in such a case to go into cold water, though this man escaped without injury; but it gives good occasion to reflect on the many mischiefs that attend the small-pox in the hot regimen, since such extravagant and intense cold does so little or no harm.' "

Water, rightly employed, is as much better than all other substances for curing fevers and inflammatory diseases, of whatever name or kind, as it is better than all other substances for quenching fire.

Water is nature's great invigorator—the most genial and yet most powerful of all tonics. There is nothing in all the world beside to compare with it in giving life and energy to the frame. It has been said poetically of that vast expanse of water, the ocean, "It is the breath of God condensed on what were otherwise a cold and barren mass of rock—a breath which has communicated fertility, and beauty, and life." When struck down with severe disease, the strength all exhausted, and the individual unable to move, there is not in all nature beside, any substance, or any combination of substances, that has a tenth part the vivifying and life-giving power of water.

"I might mention," says Howard, the philanthropist, "as an evidence of the advantages of baths in prisons, that I have known instances of persons supposed to be dead of jail fever (*typhus gravior*, or malignant typhus), and brought out for burial, who, on being washed with cold water, have shown signs of life, and soon after recovered." And when at the county jail of Hertfordshire, Howard was told of a prisoner who, on being pumped upon in the yard when in a state of apparent death from jail fever, recovered; and he afterward declared he had known other instances of a similar kind. When he was in Turkey, a young man was shown him in one of the prisons, who had been bastinadoed so severely, that his body was swollen from head to foot in a most shocking manner. He desired the people to bathe him in cold water; and this, with some other simple means, such as a cooling diet, effected his recovery, contrary to the expectations of his keepers.

A few months since, an account was published in the papers of a singular case of resuscitation, by means of water, in the state of

Wisconsin. The account was as follows: "Captain Hood, a well-known citizen of Beetoa, Dame county, had a little child taken sick, which, after much suffering, and with all the usual indications of the final struggle with death, received its parents' parting embrace in the presence of other friends. The glazed eyes of the little sufferer were closed, and a bandage was applied to support the under jaw, as is customary. After the lapse of some twenty or thirty minutes, a woman in attendance, who was aiding in ablution and laying out the corpse, commenced by sprinkling cold water in its face. Strange to tell, the child opened its eyes, began to recover, and is now in the enjoyment of full health."

During a second visit at the fountain-head of hydropathy, so called, in the winter of 1847–8, I was at the pains of writing down, on the spot, the treatment as recommended by Priessnitz for the principal, I may say all the worst forms of disease to which human nature is subject. I would here express my obligations to Mr. Priessnitz for the information he has so willingly communicated to me. If I am successful in persuading others to follow these modes, I shall in some degree have rewarded the great founder of the new system, his great and all-absorbing object being to benefit his fellow-creatures.

I proceed to speak first of

TYPHUS, JAIL, AND SHIP FEVER.

Those who have been at Graefenberg a sufficient length of time to enable them to become acquainted with the facts in regard to the treatment there practiced, know that Priessnitz *never* loses a patient in fever of any kind, provided he is applied to in season, and before the ordinary means have been resorted to, which means are, for the most part, only destructive in their tendency, helping the patient the more rapidly toward his grave.

PRIESSNITZ'S DIRECTIONS.

1. Envelop the patient in one or more heavy wet linen sheets, according to the heat and strength, the sheets not much wrung out, and to be frequently renewed, as often, at least, as they begin to grow dry. There must not be much covering over the sheets. In severe cases the patient should be kept in the wet sheet the most of the time until the fever is broken up. As much fresh air

as possible is to be admitted into the room. The sheet should always be doubled, and wet towels applied to such parts as the arm-pits, between the limbs, and wherever one part comes in contact with another.

2. The cold bath is given three or four times in twenty-four hours, and even oftener, should there be much heat. If the patient is very weak, the water is used tepid, but never higher than 20 degrees Reaumur (77 degrees Fah.), and this should be diminished from time to time, until it can be borne cold. The bath should, if possible, be administered to the patient in a reclining posture. At the same time, the back of the head and neck should be bathed in water of the same temperature as the general bath, ending always with the water cold. The surface of the body should be rubbed constantly while the patient is being bathed, and the bath continued until the temperature of the arm-pits is the same as the rest of the surface.

3. As the patient becomes able to take nourishment, give cold milk, fruit, and farinaceous food, in small quantities, always cold, and at intervals of the usual meals. Great care is necessary in the food. Water at all times to be drank according to the dictates of thirst.

4. Wear the umschlag, or wet girdle, all the time when the patient is not in the wet sheet.

5. Injections, or clysters, of pure water, are to be given, if the bowels do not act naturally without; the water cold, if the patient is not very weak, one pint at a time.

The object of the whole treatment is to supply the body amply with sufficient coolness and moisture, in order to counteract the tendency of the disease to dry up and consume the natural juices.

The above are the directions that Priessnitz gave us for publication in English and American papers, with the hope that some good might thereby be done. The ship fever, so called, is neither more nor less than severe typhus fever. Were he called to such cases as have been treated a length of time already by other modes, his directions would, of course, be somewhat different. If a patient has been all but killed with drugs (a thing often done), or if the disease has been allowed to go on until the strength is exhausted, and the patient has become delirious, then the treatment is modified. But even in such cases, let the surface be sponged over with tepid water, as at 85 or 90 degrees Fah., and see what relief will follow. Get permission of your doctor to do this. No one will object, only he will want a little vinegar, or spirits, and the like, put with it; whereas the pure thing is the safest and best, for the surface as well as the internal parts. Put also the great wet fomentation about the body, to act as a soothing poultice. This no physician will object to either. Have a mattress for the patient to lie upon—never a feather bed; and use the hair or straw pillow instead of the heating, debilitating, and in every respect injurious feather pillow which is in universal use. There is truth in the old maxim, "keep the head cool." Instead of worrying and irritating the delicate internal organs with cathartics, administer daily, if need be, clysters of pure tepid water. I repeat, no well-informed physician will object to any of these things. Get thus what water treatment you can, in the absence of such practitioners as understand the new mode thoroughly. Nature and good nursing have cured many; drugs very few.

The advantages of fresh air in fevers is wonderful. I was told by the learned Dr. M. Barry, of Edinburgh, that during the past summer, in that city, the hospitals were so filled, that it became necessary to erect tents in the open air, to accommodate patients having the ship fever; and it was found the mortality was much less in these airy, out-door places, than in the more comfortable hospitals. Could all fever patients be, from the first, kept perfectly clean, have constantly a full supply of cool, fresh air, pure soft water to drink as the thirst indicates, and be nourished in the most careful manner, how few would die with fever. But the sad truth is, as patients are treated nine times in ten, if not ninety-nine in the one hundred, we might be led to suppose that men were putting the old saying into practice—"If any man sin, let him fall into the hands of the physicians."

"I have just returned home from a passage in the London packet ship American Eagle, Captain Chadwick. There were nearly two hundred persons on board. Although a most excellent ship, with a very able and experienced commander, we had a very long passage. I had the care of all such as needed medical advice on board. We had a considerable number of cases of sickness, some of which were incipient ship fever, yet through prudent care, and depending almost wholly upon the hygienic means, we had not a single death—a thing very uncommon in so long a passage, and with so large a number of persons; and there were but very few days in which we could not have mustered every soul on deck, had it been necessary to do so.

"In the very midst of the past summer, when ships were losing patients by the hundred, Capt. Watts, of the ship Emma Watts, sailed from London to New York, with a large number of passengers, and lost only one little child, a day or two from London, and which was nearly dead when it was brought on board. Capt. Watts had just been cured of the fever in London, by water. He therefore took the hint, required every passenger to bathe or be bathed regularly, by means of an apparatus which he had prepared for the purpose; and thus, with other well-regulated hygienic means, he accomplished what probably no other ship sailing during the past season between England and the United States did—not to lose a single case by ship fever."*

The treatment of fevers of any kind, without regard whatever to the name, is to be conducted on general principles. KEEP DOWN THE FEVER is the great law. Administer wet sheets, ablutions, water to drink, injections, etc., etc., as often as there is need, five, ten, or twenty times in the twenty-four hours—AS OFTEN AS THE HEAT rises above the natural standard. It is the incessant heat that takes away the strength; therefore this should be always prevented. Persevere also as many days and nights as may be necessary. In the old modes persons often lay many weeks in fever; in the new mode a few *days* at most is all that is required, if the case is taken at the first and managed properly.

AGUE AND FEVER.

In ague and fever, as in all other diseases, it is by far better, when possible, to *prevent* rather than *cure*. It would doubtless be saying too much to affirm that ague and fever could in all cases be prevented, as for instance, where the air is so very impure as in some marshy sections of our country. But I have known more cases than one, in which persons have to all appearance warded off the disease, by observing a very plain and frugal diet, water drinking, and daily bathing. No doubt in those parts of the country where intermittents are the most common, many, to say the least, could by proper management keep entirely free of the disease.

* The Author's Note-Book, 1848.

Priessnitz's treatment for this, as for all other diseases, is very simple. The directions he gave me were as follows:

1. In the first or cold stage, use the rubbing wet sheet perseveringly until the paroxysm is quelled; or use the hip or sitz bath, with much rubbing of the abdomen and the whole surface with the wet hand; or the half bath, long continued, the water being somewhat tepid, may be had recourse to.

2. In the hot stage, the packing sheet often changed, so as to reduce sufficiently the abnormal heat, the cold half bath, or affusions of water—in short, the general means of reducing feverishness from whatever cause.

3. In the sweating stage employ the tepid half bath only. This may be well enough administered in a common wash-tub, the patient sitting with the feet outside of the vessel.

The tendency of this treatment in the first stage, is to promote circulation toward the surface, thus relieving the internal organs of the abdomen, which are always congested, or, in other words, have too much blood in this stage. It also tends to either mitigate or wholly prevent the *second* and *third* stages.

The treatment in the second stage reduces the fever, and thus saves the patient's strength. It also mitigates or wholly prevents the *third* stage.

In the third stage, the treatment acts to prevent the debilitating sweats, thus supporting the strength, and thereby giving the individual the best opportunity for speedy recovery.

The vapor bath, properly managed, would no doubt be an excellent means at, or probably better a little previous to, the coming on of the chill. But there is another method which would seem to be the opposite of this, and which has done good, as I have proved by actual experiment, viz., to place the patient in a cold hip or shallow bath, just before the cold paroxysm is expected. A good deal of friction should be practiced, to cause circulation toward the surface. The chill arising from cold water is a different thing from the chill of the disease. The one strong impression takes the place of the other apparently, and with good effect. I spoke to Priessnitz of this mode which I had adopted; he thought favorably of it, and pronounced it good. But in order to determine precisely what mode would prove generally best in ague and fever, a large number of cases should be subjected to the treatment; more, probably, than any one has yet had either in this country or the old.

Priessnitz recommends that on the "well day" of ague and fever, the patient should have a wet sheet packing early in the morning, and a cold bath; one or two hip baths during the forenoon, and the wet sheet and plunge again in the afternoon; the wet girdle to be worn all of the time. A wet sheet, three double, worn about the trunk of the body during the night would be well in most cases. The diet should be of the simplest possible kinds, and spare in quantity.

Vomiting by means of warm water at the beginning of the chill, or indeed at any time during the paroxysm, would I think be an excellent means; certainly it would in all cases where the stomach is foul, and I think it is hardly possible to have any thing but a foul stomach in this disease.

Perfect and entire fasting from all food and drink except pure soft water, for two, three, and even five or six days, if necessary, with a moderate amount of bathing, would probably be one of the very best modes of treating ague—perhaps the *best* mode.

CHAPTER XV.

THE GRAEFENBERG TREATMENT OF DISEASES—(Continued.)

Priessnitz's Views of Small Pox. —Vaccination.—This often fails of its Object.—It is often very Injurious to the Constitution.—Priessnitz's mode of treating the Small-Pox.—Fresh Air and Diet.—Malignant Small-Pox.—A Case at Graefenberg.—Thirty-six Cases at Sea cured by Captain Johnston.—Testimony of Dr. Hahn in 1738.—John Hancock, D. D., 1700.—Dr. Baynard, 1706.—Dr. Currie, 1797.—Scarlatina, or Scarlet Fever.—Remarkable success of Dr. Corson, of Pennsylvania.—General Remarks on the Treatment of this Disease.—Dr. Elliotson quoted.—Dr. Burns.—Dr. Dewees.—Dr. Currie.—Measles.—Remarkable success of the Water Treatment.—Priessnitz's Mode.—A Case.—Cases from the Water-Cure Journal.—Skin Diseases generally.

THE SMALL-POX. (WRITTEN AT GRAEFENBERG.)

Priessnitz himself had the small-pox, and his face is quite badly marked, showing the effects of the disease. This happened before he understood the water treatment. Could he have been subjected to the benign influences of the new mode, he says he would not have been disfigured by the disease. Having thus experienced in his own person the effects of the terrible malady, and carrying its mark as he must to the grave, it is to be presumed that he has thought seriously concerning the modes of its prevention and cure. What, then, in the first place, are his views of the advantages and disadvantages of vaccination?

Will it be credited that Priessnitz objects strongly to this far-famed prophylactic means? "Introducing poison into the system," says he, "is not good. Vaccination sometimes kills the child, often does serious harm to the system, and always, even in the most favorable cases, renders the system much more liable to take on diseases of other kinds. It moreover fails to prevent the disease. It is better, even in large cities, to rear children as healthfully as may be by a judicious regulation of the diet, by bathing, exercise in the open air, and cleanliness, and then run the risk of their having the disease, than to vaccinate. If children are thus managed, the disease, should it be contracted, will be comparatively a trifling matter—easy to cure by the water treatment, and that without leaving any marks. I object decidedly to vaccination." These are Priessnitz's views as he gave them to me, both at this and my former visit to Graefenberg. I myself have had some experience in treating the small-pox, and I may say my success has been very satisfactory—in truth, wonderful, compared with that of the ordinary modes. Those who desire, can refer to a part of my experience, published in the Water-Cure Manual, page 183.

PRIESSNITZ'S TREATMENT OF THE SMALL-POX.

This is as follows: In the early stages of the disease, treat the fever according to the general principles for feverishness of any kind; apply the wet sheet one, two, four, six, or more times in the day, as the symptoms may demand, with plunge baths, half baths, or the rubbing sheet, accordingly as the patient may have strength to endure them. A good treatment, I will remark, and one that Priessnitz would follow in ordinary cases during the more feverish stages of the disease, is, morning, noon, and evening to give two wet sheets, one immediately following the other, with light covering, so as to communicate a good degree of coolness to the system, each sheet to continue only for ten to fifteen minutes, and the bath, according to the patient's strength, following. The tepid half bath at 70 degrees F. would be a mild means for a very feeble person, or an ablution by means of the rubbing wet sheet, the person remaining in a reclining position if very weak. But this seldom happens in the earlier stages of the disease. If the fever should run very high, many sheets might, and indeed should be applied in the twenty-four hours, the patient remaining in them, as in cases of bad typhus, most of the time. But in all these cases, care must be taken that the patient does not become too warm in the sheet. Better not apply it at all. Manage to keep down the feverishness, and the acrimony and severity of the disease will be greatly mitigated. The wet girdle is also to be used constantly when the patient is not in the wet sheet. Water drinking, of the purest and softest cold water that can be obtained, is to be encouraged, and at all times practiced as freely as the patient desires. The diet must be cooling and very spare. In severe cases, it is better when the fever is the worst, to pass two, three, or even more days, without any nourishment whatever.

I will remark, also, that there is no need at any time of going to excess in chilling the system. Do not cause prostration by the cold. The sheets and ablutions should revive and refresh the body. This is the normal effect of cold when judiciously applied. But if the cooling treatment be carried too far (which is very rarely the case), depression and prostration would be the result. This would follow immediately, and the cause is easily traced. The exercise of a little common sense will guide us in all this matter. I will mention, that patients often dread the cold, and feel a reluctance to enter the baths, when they find on entering them they are refreshed and invigorated. It must be remembered, therefore, that the feelings are not always the true guide.

We should not forget that in this, as in all febrile diseases, that a supply of air, as free and fresh as possible, should at all times, both by night and day, be admitted into the patient's apartment. In the summer time, Priessnitz has had patients in fever taken out to remain all day in the open air and shade.

TREATMENT AFTER THE PUSTULES HAVE COME OUT.

After the pustules have come out well, there is no need of so much of the cooling treatment as before. But the sheets should be yet freely used, so also the baths, to moisten and soften the skin, and by the diluting effect of the water (for water is absorbed by the skin), to render less acrid the corrupt matter of the disease. Thus will the marks be much modified, or wholly prevented.

In cases of a malignant character, in which the disease is confluent, the sores running together, so that the whole surface becomes as it were one complete sore or scab, it is a serious matter to the patient; and the practitioner, if he have any conscience, will be solicitous as to what is the best mode of treatment in that stage of the disease. The face, neck, and head, are so swollen that the nearest friends cannot possibly distinguish the features. That, of itself, is a terrible thing. Then, as the scabs come off, the horrible smarting that takes place, because of the contact of the air—how can this be prevented? I confess, I do not know. Oil, or some unctuous substance, has been the means used by some to shield the part from the air. But this Priessnitz objects to, on the ground that the natural diminution of morbid matter is thus hindered; the same being necessarily, in consequence thereof, thrown inward, or retained in the system. I have had cases in which we used wet cloths much over parts of the body, and in which it seemed as if it would have been impossible to have used the entire wet sheet, so great was the soreness over the whole surface of the system. But Priessnitz says, "Persevere: it is difficult at first, but you will find the entire wet sheet the best." I cannot think of such cases of small-pox as I have witnessed, without experiencing a sense of most painful dread for years after they have happened, and I could desire most earnestly that no human being should ever be attacked with so dreadful a malady as the malignant, confluent small-pox.

CASES OF THE SMALL-POX.

Priessnitz has often treated cases of this disease. I have not heard of his losing any. Many of these cases have been among the poor and peasants of these mountain parts; and be it said, to his everlasting praise, he always attends such cases as faithfully as if they were among the most noble and rich, *and that without fee or charge.* Noble generosity, of a most humane and noble heart!

My bathman (at Graefenberg) tells me, that some three years ago he had the small-pox severely, and that Priessnitz cured him thus: "two wet sheets, in succession, and bath in the morning; the same at noon; also at night; wearing, and often wetting, the body-girdle, with all the drinking he desired. Then, the most days, he took no food of any kind." In two weeks he was quite over the disease, and in three weeks was about his business as usual. He had the disease badly. Those people about Graefenberg who have the means, do not live near as plainly as they should, and are accustomed to greatly overheated rooms. Hence their diseases are often of a violent character.

The good effects of the water-cure, as well as the apparent disregard of danger from acute disease at Graefenberg, may be seen from the following case, related by Mr. H. C. Wright:

"While at Graefenberg, we had a case of malignant small-pox, and the patient lay in the main building, near the passage, through which we all passed to and from our meals three times a day. The bathman who attended him attended other guests, and we visited him without fear, each knowing that if we should take the infection, the disease was entirely under the control of the water-cure. The patient was confined to his room fourteen days, covered with the pustules from head to foot. I saw him while in this state, and a more loathsome object I never beheld. When he recovered sufficiently to leave his room, he mixed freely with the other guests, and, in about three weeks, almost every trace of the disease had passed from his face. Wet sheets and tepid and cold baths were the only remedies employed, and a constant supply of pure cold air was admitted, by day and night, through the open windows of the chamber. The woman who washed the wet sheets and bandages used by this patient, took the disease, but it was soon conquered by the cold water remedies."

Captain Johnston, the able commander of the steam-ship Washington, informed the author, that a few years since, in a passage between Havre and New York, thirty-six of his passengers in the steerage were attacked with small-pox, all having it at the same time. Being well aware of the good effects of the cooling treatment, he had the sick persons placed in as cool a part of the ship as possible; extra wind-sails were arranged to give a free supply of fresh air; they were allowed to take, as freely as they desired, of cooling drinks; were kept as cleanly as possible, and very sparing nourishment only was allowed during the disease. No medicine was used, and in a few days every one of these persons recovered. This is a striking example of the beneficial effects of the cooling treatment in that terrible disease, and nothing but the best and most judicious management, amid the disadvantages of a medical treatment in the steerage of a ship at sea, could be the means of bringing about such a salutary result.

Dr. John Sigmund Hahn, of Schweidnitz, Silesia, Germany, in 1738, remarked, that "it (water) is equally beneficial in measles and other rashes. Scarcely any one of them died; and in small-pox not one fourth of the number die that usually perish under the hot regimen. Of 156 small-pox patients which a neighboring physician had treated in this way, only eight died, although the disease raged at the time in a virulent manner. In 1737, during the prevalence of a malignant epidemic, accompanied with *petecchiæ*, very few died who were submitted to this treatment, although they were washed until they became very cool, even during the continued and debilitating sweats."

Elsewhere this author observes: "In exanthematous diseases, as small-pox, measles, scarlet fever, and other rashes, we may freely wash with cold water from first to last, during the whole course of the disease, in order to prevent the fever from becoming too violent. The skin is thus rendered more soft, so that the acrid matter can the more easily pass through it. In small-pox, the corrosive quality of this acrid matter, so that it does not eat into the skin, leaves no scars behind; and very few patients who have been treated this way have been marked by the disease. The Africans wash all their small-pox patients. A captain having a cargo of slaves among whom this disease made its appearance, treated them after the European mode, putting the patients between two mattresses, and otherwise heaping bed-clothes upon them, with the view of bringing out the disease. In great distress, they cried and begged to be allowed to treat themselves according to their own method; upon which the other slaves tied ropes around the bodies of the sick, and dipped them frequently during the day into the sea, drying them afterward in the sun, and in this manner they were cured, and scarcely one died."

Dr. Baynard, in 1706, gave the following cases: "Dr. Yarborough told me that his kinsman, Sir Thomas Yarborough, sent him a letter from Rome, wherein he gave him an account of a footman of his, who, when delirious in the small-pox, got from his bed, and in his shirt ran into a grotto of a cardinal's, where there was water, in which he plunged himself, but was presently got out. The small-pox seemed to be sunk and struck in, but upon his going to bed, they came out very kindly, and he safely recovered.

"But my worthy and learned friend Dr. Cole, showed me an account from an apothecary in Worcestershire, whose name, I think, was Mr. Mathews, the substance of which was, that a young man, delirious in the small-pox, when his nurse was absent jumped out of bed, ran down stairs, and went into a pond of water. The noise awaked the nurse, who followed with an outcry, which outcry raised the *posse* of the family, who surrounded the pond; but he parleyed with them, and told them that if any body came in he would certainly drown them, and that he would come out when he saw his own time; and accordingly did so, and walked up stairs, and sat (in his wet shirt) upon a chest by the bed-side, in which posture Mr. Mathews found him when he came into the chamber. *Note here,* that the apothecary lived three or four miles from the place, and that he was in the water and on the chest all the while, in his *wet shirt,* that the messenger was gone for him. This apothecary, Mr. Mathews (for so I take his name), asked him how he did. He answered, pretty well. He asked him if he would have a clean shirt and go into bed. He said by-and-by he would, which he accordingly did. When in bed, he asked the apothecary if he had nothing good in his pocket, for he was a little faintish. He said he had a cordial, of which the patient drank a good draught, so went to sleep, and awaked very well, and in a little time recovered. Now, as Dr. Cole observed very well—'A man,' quoth he, 'would not advise his patients in such a case to go into cold water, though this man escaped without injury; but it gives a good occasion to reflect on the many mischiefs that attend the small-pox in the *hot* regimen, since such extravagant and intense cold does so little or no harm.'

"Dr. Dover, of Bristol, told me of a vintner's drawer in Oxford, that, in the small-pox, went into a great tub of water, and there sat at least *two hours*, and yet the fellow recovered and did well.

"A gentleman, delirious in the small-pox, ran in his shirt in the snow, and knocked them up in the house when he went, they being all in bed; the small-pox sunk, and yet by the benefit of a looseness, he recovered.

"I remember about two years since a learned gentleman, a divine, told me that in the country where he was benefited, in a small town not far from him, many died of a malignant small-pox. A certain boy, a farmer's son, was seized with a pain in his head and back, vomited, was feverish, etc., and had all the symptoms of the small-pox. This youth had promised some of his comrades to go a-swimming with them that day, which, notwithstanding his illness, he was resolved to go, and did so, but never heard more of his small-pox. Within three or four days the father was seized just as the son had been, and he was resolved to take Jack's remedy. His wife dissuaded him from it, but he was resolved upon it, and did immerge in cold water, and was after it very well. The worthy gentleman who told me this story, promised to give me it in writing, with the persons' names and place, but I neglecting it, he went out of town in two or three days, so I lost the opportunity of being better informed.*

* It would not probably be safe to infer that in these cases the eruption of the small-pox was actually prevented by the immersion in cold water. Yet such might have been the case. Such treatment in the very beginning of a disease, sometimes has a most wonderful effect, as was proved by Dr. Currie in his fever cases. I have known a number of persons who had all been daily exposed to the small-pox, to have, in due time, all the premonitory symptoms of the disease, and yet pass free from the eruption. These persons every one bathed often, and lived nearly fasting while the symptoms were upon them. But in a still larger number of cases where persons have

"Mr. Lambert, brother to my worthy friend, Mr. Edmund Lambert, of Boyton, in the county of Wilts, told me that when he was at school in Dorsetshire, at least thirty or more of the boys, one after another, fell sick of the small-pox, and that the nurse gave them nothing but milk and apples in the whole of the course of the disease, and they all recovered. There was but one dissenting boy from that method, who by command went another course, and he had like to have died; nay, with very great difficulty they saved his life. And since, another gentleman told me that himself and divers others were cured by the milk and apples, and buttered apples, in the worst sort of small-pox."*

OF THE USE OF THE AFFUSION OF COLD AND TEPID WATER IN SMALL-POX, WITH CASES.

Dr. Currie, in 1797, gives the following cases: "The singular degree of success that on the whole attended the affusion of cold water in typhus, encouraged a trial of this remedy in some other febrile diseases. Of these, the small-pox seemed more particularly to invite its use. The great advantage that is experienced in this disease by the admission of cool air, seemed to point out the external use of cold water, which being a more powerful application, might be more particularly adapted to the more malignant forms of small-pox. The result corresponded entirely with my expectation. Of a number of cases in which I witnessed the happy effects of the affusion of cold water, I shall give the following only:

CASE I.

"In the autumn of 1794, J. J., an American gentleman, in the 24th year of his age, and immediately on his landing in Liverpool, was inoculated under my care, the prevalence of the small-pox

practiced the same prevention, the disease has come out, but usually in a very mild form. J. S.

* Apples are a very watery, cooling regimen. The old-fashioned mode of giving scraped apple tarts, as one of the first things of nutriment, I have always practiced. Milk, although composed mostly of water, must be given cautiously in inflammatory diseases. As for the butter mentioned by Dr. Baynard, it were better avoided, although the article used fresh, as it generally is in the old country, is a very different thing from that so much impregnated with salt, as is generally used in this country. Salt is very heating and inflaming in its nature. J. S.

rendering it imprudent to wait till the usual preparations could be gone through, or indeed till he should recover from the fatigues of the voyage. He sickened on the seventh day, and the eruptive fever was very considerable. He had a rapid and feeble pulse, a fœtid breath, with pain in the head, back, and loins. His heat rose in a few hours to 107 degrees, and his pulse beat 119 times in the minute. I encouraged him to drink largely of cold water and lemonade, and threw three gallons of cold brine over him. He was in a high degree refreshed by it. The eruptive fever abated in every respect—an incipient delirium subsided, the pulse became slower, the heat was reduced, and tranquil sleep followed. In the course of twenty-four hours the affusion was repeated three or four different times at his own desire, a general direction having been given him to call for it as often as the symptoms of fever returned. The eruptions, though more numerous than is usual from inoculation, were of a favorable kind. There was little or no secondary fever, and he recovered rapidly.

"In situations where the eruptive fever of small-pox is clearly distinguishable, and where it does not abate sufficiently on the admission of cold air, the affusion of cold water may be resorted to with confidence and safety, regulated however in this application, as in every other, by *the actual state of the patient's heat, and of his sensation of heat.* In the confluent small-pox, however, after the eruption is completely formed, this remedy cannot perhaps be used with advantage. The following case will illustrate this position.

"H. A., aged 23, an American mariner, fell under my care (*Dec.* 7) on the third day of the eruption of the small-pox; that is, on the sixth day of the disease. His pulse 114, and feeble, his heat 109 degrees. His head, back, and loins, ached severely—thirst great—skin livid—small-pox confluent.

"He was put on a milk diet; gentle mercurial purgatives were ordered from time to time, and an opiate every night at bed-time. Lemonade was given largely at first by itself, and afterward mixed with wine, and the affusion of cold water was directed in the usual way. In ten minutes after the affusion, the pulse was 96, the heat 98 degrees; the livor of the skin was much diminished, but the pains were not relieved.

"*Dec.* 8.—Noon.—Pulse 96, soft and regular—thirst gone—respiration slow and natural—heat 97 degrees. The affusion was ordered to be repeated; ten minutes after, pulse 84, and feeble—heat 84 degrees.

"*Dec.* 9.—Noon.—Pulse 88, heat 93 degrees—the cold affusion was not repeated in this very reduced state of heat; the decoction of bark was ordered, and a pint of wine daily in lemonade.

"*Dec.* 10.—Noon.—Pulse 116, and full—heat 98 degrees—respiration still easy—expectoration considerable, and viscid—thirst less—eyes quite closed—head swelled—a complete union of the pustules on the face. Bark and wine continued, with the opiate at night.

"*Dec.* 12.—Pulse 118—heat 96 degrees. A bucket full of water of the temperature of 92 degrees was poured over him. He appeared refreshed at the moment; ten minutes after, pulse 112, heat 94 degrees. Complained of being chilly. Respiration still easy—free of pains, and his face less swelled. Complained of his throat. A blister was applied to it all round.

"*Dec.* 13.—Noon.—Pulse 118—heat 96 degrees—respiration still free, but his throat very sore. Medicines were continued, but the affusion of tepid water was not repeated.

"*Dec.* 14.—Noon.—Pulse 138—heat 100 degrees—respiration had now become laborious, and the expuition difficult. The throat was much swelled. He was frequently sponged with tepid water, and the medicines continued.

"*Dec.* 15.—Noon.—Unfavorable symptoms increased.

"*Dec.* 16.—Noon.—Vomiting came on, which was relieved by opium. His senses and his intellect remained acute till within an hour of his death, which happened at eight o'clock in the evening of this day.

"If this case be more detailed than seems necessary, let this be excused, as it is the first in which the actual heat in confluent small-pox has been recorded. It is here given accurately from the period when the disease came under my care.

"In regard to the effects of the cold affusion, it may be observed, that this remedy was not used during the eruptive fever, nor till three days after the eruption had appeared, and the character of the disease was decided. In the stage in which it was employed, the fever and the heat were abating, as is usual after the eruption; and in all cases in which the heat is sinking, the application of cold must be made with great caution, as has already been mentioned. After the second affusion (on the 8th) the heat sunk below its natural standard, and continued below it for some time; so that this remedy became inadmissible. The disease went through its usual course. The tepid affusion on the eighth day of the eruption (*Dec.* 12) was used in part to wash off variolous matter, and in part to produce refreshment. The heat which was before 96 degrees sunk two degrees, so that it could not with safety be continued, for experience has proved, that the tepid affusion is a powerful means of diminishing heat. The heat rose again with the secondary fever, and the patient died of the affection of the throat, as I believe is general in the confluent small-pox.* It will be at once perceived, on the principles already laid down, that in a disease like this, the affusion of cold water could only be essentially useful during the eruptive fever. It is during the eruptive fever that the quantity of the assimilation is determined, as well as its kind. This is, I believe, invariably found to bear an exact proportion to the eruptive fever, and whether we consider the eruptive fever as the cause or effect of the assimilation, there is every reason to expect from the laws of the living system, that the diminution of this fever will diminish the quantity, and meliorate the quality of the variolous eruption.

In the case just related, the heat during the eruptive fever (judging from trials in similar situations) had risen to 106 degrees or 107 degrees;† but it had sunk to 100 degrees before the cold affusion was employed. It may easily be conceived that this remedy could have been employed to a much greater extent, and that its effects would have been far more salutary, if it had been used throughout the previous fever. That it would have essentially altered the character of the disease, I presume not to assert. This, however, I can declare, that in all the cases in which I have used the affusion of cold water during the eruptive fever, however severe the symptoms may have been, these symptoms instantly abated, and the disease assumed a benignant form. The case of Mr. Johnston (Case I.), already given, will illustrate this observation; and six or seven others I might adduce to the same purpose. As yet my experience extends no further.

* See Zoonomia, vol. ii., page 237.

† 1803. I now believe that the heat does not rise so high in any stage of confluent small-pox. See the *Additional Reports*.

SCARLATINA, OR SCARLET FEVER.*

The following letter of Dr. Hiram Corson, of Conshohocton, Montgomery county, Pennsylvania, is published by Dr. J. Forsyth Meigs, of Philadelphia, in "A Practical Treatise on the Diseases of Children," under date 1848. The facts given by Dr. Corson are presented in a clear and lucid manner, and illustrate well the remarkable power of water in this formidable disease. He speaks as follows:

"Scarlet fever is a disease that has prevailed very much in our region during the last seventeen years, and has caused me much thought and anxiety. It will give me much pleasure to make you acquainted with the *results* of a plan of treatment, which I owe mainly to Dr. Samuel Jackson, formerly of Northumberland, now of your city, who first put me in the way of treating the disease successfully. In 1832, I treated the disease, which, however, was not malignant, very successfully, with iced drinks, moderate purges, and slight irritation externally upon the throat, and thought the practice peculiar to myself, but afterward saw, in the May and August numbers of the American Journal of Medical Sciences, the communications of Dr. Jackson. Encouraged by these, I prepared to try the cold externally; when a most unfortunate trial by a neighboring physician, so alarmed the people about the application of cold, that I could not prevail upon them to suffer the trial. From 1838 until within the last two years, we have annually had the scarlet fever for some months, and my treatment, with the exception of iced drinks sometimes, and cold to the head occasionally, was like that in general use, until August, 1844. At that time I was called to a child eight months old, that had been sick two days. There was great swelling of the glands both sides of the neck, hot skin, frequent pulse, but no eruption; slight discharge from the nose; the glands not easily seen upon the inside, but the drinks came back through the nose sometimes, and it could not take more than one draw at the breast without dropping the nipple, because of the obstruction of the nostrils impeding respiration when the mouth was closed. I stated candidly to the mother that I had never saved a child in that condition, and of that age, by the old treatment, and recommended *ice internally*

* Published in the Water-Cure Journal of March, 1849. Fowlers & Wells, New York. Joel Shew, M. D., editor.

and externally, cold water to the head, and no medicine. I could urge nothing on the score of experience, but she agreed. Lumps of ice were folded in linen cloths, and held night and day upon the two sides of the throat; while a small thin piece, inclosed in white gauze, was held in the mouth. In less than three hours improvement was manifest in the ability to swallow. The swelling of the glands, the heat, and the frequency of the pulse all regularly diminished; and in two days the child could nurse well, and was out of danger.

"The next severe case occurred in about two weeks. It was one of the most intense scarlet eruption, with tumefaction and ulceration of the tonsils, vomiting, coryza (running at the eyes), great frequency of the pulse, excessive restlessness, and swelling of the external glands. The heat was intense: there was heaviness amounting to stupor. My treatment was a kind of half-and-half; emetics, purgatives, cold externally and internally. But half satisfied with myself, my course was vacillating and inefficient, and I at length called in a friend, who turned the scale in favor of irritating gargles, and our patient died. I was mortified and provoked, and determined to act out my convictions at the next opportunity. A few days after I was called to two boys, of five and seven years of age, who had been blistered upon the throat, legs, and arms, and had had hot drinks, calomel purges, etc., and who were discharging copiously from the nose, and were almost dead. Their countenances were sunken, the throats gangrenous, pulse above 150; their appearance was that of persons in typhus fever. I expressed my fears of the blisters, predicting that they would all be gangrenous in twenty-four hours, and that they would be likely to destroy the patients. I had cloths dipped in iced water wrapped round the neck, ice was put in the mouth, and cold water upon the heads, which were much affected. The throats were filled with ropy mucus, which was expelled through the mouth and nose during the coughing which attended efforts to vomit. The palate was literally destroyed by gangrene. A few hours produced no amendment. The blisters mortified extensively, and though both children recovered from the disease, one died two weeks afterward from the sloughing of the throat and neck from the blisters.

"I now treated all that occurred with cold externally and internally, moving the bowels with cream of tartar and jalap. The cases were seen early, and easily subdued; and it seemed to me as though the remedy was very efficient, or that my patients had a mild disease. That the latter was not the case, however, I thought probable from the fact, that in my region many cases differently treated died; while in Norristown, only four miles distant, children from one to twelve years or more were swept off, after an illness of only two or three days, the deaths being evidently produced by disease of the brain.

"On the 16th of July, 1845, I was called to see a little girl, four years and nine months old. She had been sick a day or two. The case began with vomiting. The eruption had been out from morning till 6 P. M.; sickness the most intense all over that I had ever seen: pulse as rapid as it could be, to be counted. The mother had been alarmed during the last few hours, in consequence of delirium and jerking, which she feared was the prelude to convulsions. There was tumefaction (hardening) of the sub-maxillary ganglions; tongue furred with projecting red points, breath hot and offensive. When she found some one holding her wrist, she started from her dozing state, and being somewhat afraid of the 'doctor,' went off immediately into one of the most terrific convulsions that I ever saw. It lasted, in spite of ice to the head, or rather iced water *constantly* poured upon it, almost half an hour. I stayed with her, had her undressed, and placed two nieces of mine (her mother being one) by her side. A large tub of water, with cakes of ice, at least a peck, floating in it, was brought into the room, and during the *whole* night, these two persons bathed her from head to foot with the water from the tub, applying it by means of large sponges. It was to me a most painful case (independent of the convulsions), but in order to be certain that I had a case fit for the trial of the ice, I had my brother (a physician practicing at Norristown, where the disease was very fatal) brought at 10 P. M. to see the case, and say whether it was the same as those that had for a few weeks been carrying off some of the finest children of Norristown, and carrying terror into every family. He assured me that it was one of the most violent character, and that she would in all probability not live till morning. She was at this time free from convulsions, but in a muttering delirium. As I had perfect control in the case, I assured him that she should live, if I could quench the fire that was burning out her vitals, by the use of ice. Not a moment did the attendants whom I had placed by her intermit their labors. Before midnight reason had returned, and her mother said she was more herself than she had been during the whole day. I had gone away, but returned at sunrise, and found her cooled off perfectly. There was scarcely the least appearance of eruption, the skin was cool, the head cool, the intellect clear, and the pulse moderate in frequency and force. She had been unable to drink for many hours, and her tongue, which had been very much cut during the convulsion, was so swelled and sore, that I could obtain no view of the throat. I now directed the mother to intermit the sponging, doing it only once in every two hours until I returned. My return was delayed until 4 P. M., when I found that the heat of the skin, frequency of pulse, eruption and delirium, had all returned. She was moving her hands as if feeling for something, slowly protruding and withdrawing the tongue, and muttering. She did not notice her mother's questions, and was apparently unconscious of all that was going on. We threw on the water, ice cold, in the utmost profusion, and lapped cloths, dipped in the water, around the neck, changing them every minute or two. We poured it upon the head constantly, holding a large basin under to catch it. In one hour reason returned. We continued it until the eruption almost disappeared, until the child shrank from it, and until she was ready to shrink from cold. I now gave her cream of tartar and jalap, directed the water to be used just as was needed to keep down the heat, and had no farther trouble with her. I forgot to say, that so soon as she could swallow, cold drinks and ice were kept in the mouth. She took no more medicine. The wounds in the tongue healed up kindly.

"There were two younger children in the family, both of whom were attacked a few days after, while apparently in good health, with vomiting, and the same symptoms as in the first case. The throats were red, swelled, etc. Cold cloths were wrapped around the neck; they were purged with jalap and cream of tartar; as the heat of the skin and eruption appeared, ice water was profusely applied to the whole body, so as to keep down the heat, and allow but a very moderate eruption to show itself. They were well in a few days, without a bad symptom. It was now midwinter. The cases followed each other rapidly. I treated them all in the same way, and *all* with like happy results. The disease had a wide range, extending from the Schuylkill across the highlands, between Norristown and Doylestown, and was in that range very destructive in many families. There was much alarm, and I was called two miles back of Norristown to a girl about eleven years old. The eruption had been out about twenty-four hours. The throat was swelled, and covered with white patches (generally called ulcers), tongue dry, hot, and red, skin hot as skin could be, and what to me characterizes the most malignant cases, the eruption, instead of being a bright scarlet, was of a purple-red, like the congestion sometimes seen in the faces of old drunkards. There was great oppression, not *difficulty* of breathing, but a state like that which exists when a person is deathly sick, but cannot vomit, with extreme restlessness and jactitation. The disease had been so fatal, that the mother thought the case almost beyond remedy; but when I told her that the cold had proved successful, she was eager to try it. It was 8 o'clock A. M. The girl was stripped, and the ice water applied all over. Ice was lapped around the neck, and positive directions given to continue the application without intermission until I returned. It was about four miles from me, and I did not return for seven hours. The moment my eyes rested upon her, I knew that we had done *too much*. She was white as the sheet upon which she lay. The neighbors had been in and desired the mother to desist, that 'she would kill her,' but she had been true to her trust. The child was apparently bloodless, covered with 'goose skin,' and shivering with cold. Her pulse was *small*, and much less frequent, but not weak or fluttering, and she was sensible. (I forgot to say, that in the morning she was quite flighty.) I told the mother we had used rather more cold than was necessary, but that if we left it off now, she would probably do well. I omitted it for two hours, and gave nothing. At the expiration of that time, the heat, and with it the eruption, showed themselves, so as to cause me to direct the sponging to be used just so as to keep them in check. The ice was kept constantly on the neck, and water poured frequently over the neck. I had no more trouble with her, although the skin desquamated (peeled off) from head to foot.

"Six other children in the same family took the disease. Five of them had the ice and ice water used upon them, and all did well. I gave none of them any medicine, except a little cream of tartar and jalap, to move the bowels moderately. I gave this combination, because it is pleasant to children, and easily swallowed. The sixth case was a very mild one, so that the mother merely gave it a little castor-oil, and it did well, and seemed perfectly recovered in a few days. Indeed, the attack was so mild, that it would not have been detected as scarlet fever, if it had occurred at any other time. It was attacked with dropsy and an affection of the lungs about two weeks after, lingered several weeks, and finally died of pneumonic (lung) disease.

"I suppose I have attended more than a hundred cases of scarlet fever, of every grade, since I began the cold treatment. In no instance where I had it fairly applied did it fail. Indeed I have lost but two patients since.

"In every variety of sore throat and quinsy, in summer and in winter, my treatment is ice around the neck; or when the nurse is faithful, iced cloths, renewed as soon as they approach the heat of the neck.

"In no single instance have I seen dropsy follow scarlet fever that had been treated by cold affusion. I have never seen it occur except after the mildest cases of the disease, those that had probably only needed a mild laxative."

Those who understand the water treatment, know that the laxatives are better supplied by water injections, bandages, etc. We have in the above, certainly, very strong evidence of the good effects of cold water in scarlatina. The great effect of the treatment was, as it should be, that of constantly and perseveringly keeping down the heat.

Dr. Elliotson, of London, in his Principles and Practice of Medicine, remarks of cold affusion in scarlet fever:

"The disease has certainly been cut short, by taking a patient out of bed, and pouring cold water upon him. The heat of the body is so great in this disease, that no danger is to be apprehended from the cold affusion. It is true, there are cases in which the patient is more or less chilly, but if, in this affection, the general rules I laid down in the case of common fever be followed, there is no danger whatever, but the greatest advantage, in taking the patient out of bed (however hot he may be) and pouring cold water upon him. These rules are, that the temperature is steadily above 98 degrees (Fah.); that there are no profuse general sweats; that there is no chilliness, and no inflammation of the chest or abdomen. I presume this would be done oftener than it is, were it not for its appearing a violent measure to take a person in fever out of bed, put him into a washing-tub, and souse him well with cold water. It is a great comfort to the individual, and as long as it is comfortable, it should be had recourse to. Sponging the hands, arms, face, and trunk, with cold water, is grateful to the patient, and is an excellent practice in the disease."

I remark on these directions of Dr. Elliotson, that as few non-professional persons can be expected to have a thermometer suitable for measuring the animal heat (and even among physicians hardly one of a thousand ever has any such thing), some other rule must in almost every case be adopted as a guide. The thermometer is not strictly necessary, for it requires no more than ordinary judgment for a person to decide as to whether the heat is above the natural standard merely by the sensations of the hand. This rule is sufficient for all practical purposes.

As to profuse sweating, it is to be remarked that this is of itself a cooling process. The tepid washing is then very comforting and salutary. But the sweating seldom happens in scarlet fever at all.

In the *beginning* of fevers and inflammations there is often chilliness to the feelings, while at the same time the skin is hotter than is natural. The cold bath is then beneficial; and what may appear singular, it makes the patient feel warmer. The half bath and the rubbing wet sheet are excellent means in the stage of which we are speaking. In the later stages of fevers and inflammations, if chilliness is experienced the same rules do not apply; that is, there cannot be so much cold water borne. Indeed, under any circumstances, whenever the system is *really* chilly, do not make it more so with cold water or any thing else. True, the rubbing wet sheet is often serviceable in such cases, but this excites a better circulation toward the skin, and thus helps in the end, even if used cold, to prevent the sensation of chilliness.

I controvert Dr. Elliotson, and various other authorities, by saying that in inflammations of the chest or abdomen, or any other internal organ, attended with general feverishness, which is generally the case in the active stages of these diseases, the same general rules of practice apply as in any other case of fever. This we have proved from oft-repeated experiments. Any thing which tends to reduce feverishness in the general system, must also tend to reduce the fever of any local part; and it is upon this very same principle that bleeding, calomel, and other remedies that act upon the system generally, are administered.

Dr. Burns, author of a work on Midwifery, regarded affusion

with cold water as a remedy of utility in scarlatina. It is, however, but justice to him to remark, that he did not advocate the affusion in cases where internal inflammation existed in connection with the disease in question. He says of the affusion :

" It is of consequence to use it early, if it is to be done at all; and whenever the skin feels steadily hot, the shivering having gone off, and the skin feels very warm to the hand of another person, it is time to put him into an empty tub, and pour over him a large ewer full of cold water. By this I have known the disease arrested at once, the eruption never becoming vivid, and the strength and appetite in a few hours returning. Even where it is not arrested, it is pleasant to observe the change which often is produced. The patient, from being dull, languid, and listless, feels brisk and disposed to talk or laugh ; the skin becomes for a time colder, and refreshing sleep is frequently procured. The repetition must depend on the degree of heat, and the effect of the application. If that have done no good, it is useless to try it again. One application is sometimes sufficient, but it may be necessary the first day to use it twice, and once the next day. It is seldom requisite afterward, for although the disease may continue, it is mild, and laxatives complete the cure. If the fever be mild, and the heat not pungent and great, we do not employ the affusion. We keep the patient cool, or have the surface cooled frequently by a sponge dipped in cold water, and, indeed, this seems now in most instances to have superseded the use of the affusion."

In reference to the above principles laid down by Dr. Burns, we remark :

First, that where internal inflammation does exist in connection with scarlatina, the cold affusion is not contra-indicated if there is general pyrexia or feverishness of such degree as would warrant the use of the remedy in cases where the internal inflammation does not exist. The same general principle in regard to cold affusion or cooling means externally of whatever kind, holds good in all cases of general feverishness.

Second, where one application is not sufficient to arrest the disease, as it seldom would be, the remedy should be applied and reapplied as often as the heat and feverishness demand it, no matter if every hour, although this could seldom happen ; and if in any case there is doubt as to whether the patient's strength will admit of the cold affusion, the tepid, as with water at 70 degrees or 80 degrees Fah., may be employed. The tepid bath is cooling in effect, and will in every case of increased heat be certain of doing at least some good and no possible harm. It would be hardly possible for a patient to die of scarlet fever, if he have cold water enough to drink, cool fresh air in abundance, and the tepid affusions, washings, etc., enough to keep down the inordinate heat. Thus people of good common sense and judgment may proceed cautiously and safely, without coming at once to affusion with the coldest water.

Third, the use of laxatives, either with or without water, is by no means so salutary as fasting, and injections two or three times a day repeated. These may be cold or tepid if the patient is very weak. They may also be repeated two or more times in quick succession, and are certain of doing much good.

Dr. Dewees, in Practice of Medicine, says of the treatment of scarlet fever, "In the early or inflammatory condition of scarlatina, when there is considerable arterial action, and vast augmentation of heat on the surface, cold ablution or sponging gives great relief to the symptoms, and is a most comfortable process. * * * Some, however, are afraid of these cold applications because the throat is sore; but this forms no exception; for it is not accompanied with cough, or other pneumonic symptoms like measles, and the sponging or even affusion has checked the sore throat most evidently."

Dr. Currie, a very able writer on water fifty years ago, spoke of the results of his practice, after much experience, as follows: "The plan that I follow, if called in at this early period (namely, when the heat is great), is to strip the patient, and dash four or five gallons of the coldest water to be procured over his naked body. This produces its usual cooling effects; but these are less permanent than in typhus. In one or two hours afterward the heat is often found, on examination, as great as before. The affusion is therefore repeated again and again, as the obstinacy of the heat may indicate. It is necessary to use it ten or twelve times in the twenty-four hours. At the end of this time, but commonly earlier, the force of the fever is broken, and a few tepid affusions, at longer intervals, are sufficient to subdue it entirely. During this time cold water and lemonade should be used as drinks, and the bowels opened, if necessary, by calomel. In a few cases, I have thought it advisable to assist the affusion by the diaphoretic (sweating) power of a solution of tartarized antimony. If left to myself I use no other means."

I have thus extracted from medical authorities on the treatment of scarlet fever at greater length than I at first intended. In some regions of country where our journal goes, scarlatina of malignant form is now prevailing. This we trust will be taken by our readers as some apology for the great length of our article.

MEASLES.

In all febrile and inflammatory diseases, whether upon the surface or otherwise, the same great principle, KEEP DOWN THE FEVER, always holds true.

I have known no cases of measles lost in which the water treatment was applied—not a single case. I have known of a great number of cases treated on the new plan, many of which were managed wholly by the parents or friends of the patients, and without the aid of a physician. There is no need of people being at the expense of running for the doctor in every little emergency. Better study the principles of health and disease, and thus be ready for the coming on of physical ills. With good treatment and nursing, we do not believe that one case out of five hundred need be lost of measles.

I may here repeat what we said years ago in the "Water-Cure Manual," concerning the treatment of this disease: "It is to be treated on the general principle of all inflammatory diseases. The wet sheet, properly managed (that is, so as to keep down the general feverishness), has a most salutary effect in bringing out the eruption. So also the tepid bath. Keep down the fever; give little nourishment; keep the bowels open, and allow an abundance of fresh air. Keep up the treatment for some days to prevent bad consequences of the disease."

The following is the treatment that was employed by Priessnitz in a case that happened while I was last at Graefenberg: The case was that of a little lad from New York, five and a half years old. He had enlarged tonsils, and was a feeble, delicate little fellow. He had had croup and inflammation of the lungs repeatedly, and at one time, after having been calomelized and blistered according to rule, was given up by a council of four physicians to die.

The treatment Priessnitz put him under for his general condition of swelled tonsils, debility, great susceptibility to cold, etc., was the wet sheet twenty minutes on rising, followed by the plunge in cold water (it was in the midst of winter); rubbing wet sheet before noon; packing and plunge in the afternoon, as in the morning; the wet bandage about the throat constantly night and day, and also the wet girdle about the abdomen both night and day.

After three months of this treatment, which benefited the little patient materially, he was attacked with measles. For this, Priessnitz directed the wet sheet packing as before, in the morning, but to be followed by a tepid half bath (about 70 degrees Fahrenheit), instead of the cold plunge: also in the afternoon. This treatment was continued through the rash. Then came a diarrhœa. For this, in addition to the other treatment, cold rubbing sheet, followed by a cold sitz bath twenty minutes, forenoon and afternoon, but no packing in the latter. When the diarrhœa appeared worse either night or day, the cold sitz bath was to be given thirty minutes at a time. This had evidently a very salutary effect in checking the looseness. The treatment altogether did remarkably well in the case.

I published in 1847 the following cases of measles, one of which was combined with a very dangerous attack of croup:

"*March 12th*, 1847.—Went to attend the little son, three years old, of Mr. Osborne, of 444 Grand street. He had been exposed to the measles, and the parents daily expected the coming on of this disease. For three or four days, the little boy had been coughing, and had the symptoms of a considerable cold. The day before, there had been some sneezing and slight affection of the eyes, which symptoms usually precede an attack of the measles. In the evening came on an attack of the croup. The nursery room, or one in which the children generally were, had a close coal stove, and was, therefore, as is a common thing throughout the city, most of the time too warm. Mr. Osborne's children seem also to have a predisposition to colds and the croup. Two have been lost under the ordinary modes of treatment the preceding year—one of croup, and the other of inflammation of the lungs.

"In this case of the little boy Homer, Mr. Osborne called for me in the night, but was unable to find me. Consequently, he went home, and himself and wife concluded to do what they might toward arresting the disease. They had some knowledge of the water treatment, but concluded to give some of Cox's hive syrup, an antimonial preparation, for the purpose of producing vomiting. There is a great error among many with regard to the giving emetics in croup, and, by a wrong explanation, physicians often promulgate it. In croup, as is well known, there is always a strong tendency to the formation of a false membrane in the throat. Whether this membrane comes in the larynx that goes to the lungs, or whether in the œsophagus, or meat pipe, that lays back of the breathing pipe, is not at all considered. The emetic, it is supposed, causes the throwing up of the phlegm and false membrane by actual contact with the part affected. But it should be remembered, that the medicine passes only in the œsophagus. Every one knows how much difficulty is experienced, if a little of any substance is swallowed the 'wrong way.' It is admitted, however, that vomiting does cause some apparent relief in the croup, and also, by that process, there is caused some expectoration from the throat. Yet the harm done the system by the poisonous drug far exceeds the good. Mr. and Mrs. Osborne had also made water applications to some extent. Cloths wet in cold water were kept upon the throat and chest; the body had been washed, but not in very cold water. Water, as much as was desired, had also been given to drink. All that was done with water was well, and had, no doubt, done considerable good. He was allowed food as usual, and this was an unfortunate thing.

"At 12 o'clock, noon, I arrived at Mr. O.'s. It was now sixteen or eighteen hours since the first appearance of the croupy symptoms. I at once told the parents that I did not believe the little child could live. There was that deep, hollow, stridulous or barking cough, which every one fears so much who has had to deal with the croup. I had seen cases apparently as bad as this, perhaps worse, that had, under water treatment, resulted favorably But in cases as bad as this appeared to be, cures would be the exception, and not the rule. It was then understood that I would, of course, prefer not treating a case of the kind, especially as the medicine mentioned had been given. I said, however, to the parents, 'It is for you to decide. You have called me, and now, after giving you my opinion, you are to determine who is to treat your child. If you desire it, I shall be the last to give up, as long as any thing can be done.' After considering the matter a few minutes, they determined to rely exclusively on the water, and trust for the result.

"First, then, the child was to have no more food for twenty-four hours at least. He was to be encouraged to drink a little water often, and the bowels were to be kept open by injections. He was to have a bath immediately (not in water entirely cold, as the previous applications had kept the fever down very much); wet bandages were to be kept about the neck, and large, wet towels about the whole body and lower limbs, nearly to the feet; and these all were to be changed every hour. Thus, substantially, a wet sheet, the whole of the time, was to be used. If the general fever should by any means come on, a thorough ablution would be practiced, and then again, immediately, the wet cloths. The child was, of course, wrapped up sufficiently to induce a comfortable degree of warmth. A general bath or affusion was to be performed about three or four times in the twenty-four hours.

"Returned at evening. The feverishness was much reduced, and, on the whole, the symptoms a little better. Still the croupy cough was decidedly bad. We had hoped that the measles would soon appear upon the surface, and thus some relief would be brought. One object of the constantly wet cloths was, by their poultice effect, to bring out the eruption. Those who have witnessed the water treatment in measles, must have observed the truly wonderful effect of the wet sheet in bringing out the eruption. Often a single application, with a bath, serves to bring out a complete rash. Now, at evening there were some appearances of very slight eruption about the face and neck, but nothing of any account. As the tendency to fever was now less, the cloths about the neck and body would be changed once in two hours. A bath (the extreme chill removed from the water) to be given late in the evening, and if toward morning the symptoms should grow worse, still another.

"In the morning we found the little boy had passed a better night than the one preceding. The eruption now began to appear more distinctly, but was yet very tardy. Keep on precisely the same treatment. Allow the little fellow to taste of apple, a small portion, if he chooses, at the regular meal time, but nothing else. The first day the appetite was most imperious; but this always takes place in fasting. The first day is the worst to bear.

"This same treatment, continuing the wet cloths over the greater part of the surface the whole of the time, changing them every two hours, and giving three or four baths, by affusion in the wash tub, small quantities of water frequently to drink, tepid injections daily, admitting constantly fresh air to the room, and giving a very small amount of nourishment, was kept up for three whole days, reckoning from the noon of the first day in which I saw the little boy. Not more than a half ounce of food was given in all this time, and the little fellow grew better and better every hour. It was not until this time that the measles were fully and in perfection over the whole surface. I had never seen a case any thing near so tardy under water treatment as this. We would now give a little more nourishment, but yet only a little at a time, and but three times in twenty-four hours. Keep on the wet envelopment precisely the same as before, the sooner to poultice away the eruption. The croupy cough had diminished constantly, as the eruption came more and more out.

"The fourth twenty-four hours I was away from the city. On returning, I found the wet cloths had acted like a charm. It seemed as if in that time almost every trace of the eruption was literally bleached away. Some cough, of course, remains.

"Now, for the fifth day, and onward, the wet cloths will be applied two hours forenoon and near evening. Sponging the surface will be performed after these applications, and the mild bath, by affusion, in the morning, before breakfast, and on going to rest; more nourishment will be given, and yet but a small quantity at a time, and this amount of treatment at least is to be kept up for one week.

"Toward morning of this fifth twenty-four hours, the little fellow became restless and coughed. The wet cloths were put upon the chest, and he then became quiet and went again to sleep.

"The lungs and throat, it will be recollected, are very liable to become more easily affected after the measles. With this treatment Mrs. Osborne will practice upon her little boy. I am now confident no ill result will follow, and he will grow more and more vigorous and strong. It should be remarked, the face and eyes were frequently washed, and light was admitted freely into the room. Darkening the room is injurious to the general system, and causes weakness of the eyes. Wash the parts, and accustom them to the light.

"This case, I confess, has thus far resulted very differently from the manner in which I felt almost certain it would.

"OTHER CASES OF MEASLES.

"A few days since, two or three children of Mr. H. P. Osborne, of an adjoining house of the above, had the measles. I was called but once to one of the children. Mrs. Osborne has studied the water treatment considerably. She gave the wet sheet, and thus brought out the eruption quickly. She repeated it daily, gave baths, kept down the fever, and dieted, and all went on well. These were good instances of domestic water treatment. The little girl I saw had passed through the worst part of the time; but Mrs. O., not having seen the measles treated by water, wished to know from me whether she was proceeding well.

"ANOTHER CASE.

"Some days since, Mr. Joseph Allen, of McDougal street, called and wished to know what to do for his little girl. She seemed to have a cold, and was coughing. I told him to give her the wet sheet and an extra bath per day, to have her diet plain and spare, and if the cough yet proved at all troublesome, to have the wet bandages upon the chest. The sheet and bath brought out the measles. I directed that the sheet be given twice a day, an hour each time, and a tepid bath as often as the fever rose; wet bandages constantly upon the chest, and injections to regulate the bowels. Every thing went on favorably.

"ANOTHER CASE.

"My friend, Mr. Perry, 115 Orchard street, tells me he has just been treating a child of his with the measles. Friends, relations, and the doctor, have expostulated, but all without effect. Mr. P. tells me he is succeeding well."

SKIN DISEASES GENERALLY.

In all skin diseases, whether acute or chronic, the water treatment is a sovereign remedy. In itch, ring-worm, salt-rheum, scurvy, in short, in skin diseases of whatever kind, the water treatment managed according to the demands of the general health, is a most valuable means.

CHAPTER XVI.

TREATMENT OF DISEASES CONTINUED.

Erysipelas.—General erroneous Notions concerning this Disease.—The great principle of Treatment to be observed in this Disease.—Great success of the Treatment.—Case of Mrs. Goss.—Case of Mr. Wetmore.—A second Case.—The great benefit of Fasting in this Disease.—Scalds and Burns.—Different classes of Scalds and Burns.—Principles of Treatment to be followed in Scalds and Burns.—Blisters cannot rise under Cold Water.—Danger from Burns.—Treatment of extensive Burns.—Treatment in sinking, or collapse from Burns.—The soothing effect of Warmth and Moisture.—Advantages of Water, even in fatal Cases.—Injurious effects of Opium in Burns.—Deformation caused by Burns.—Common remedies for Scalds and Burns.—Convulsions.—Frictions with Cold Water Priessnitz's main reliance in this Affection.—Hippocrates and the earlier Physicians.—Dr. Currie's Mode.—Cases.—Dr. Elliotson.—Hysteria, or Hysterics.—Cold Water a famous Remedy for this Disease.

ERYSIPELAS.

There is a very general impression that cold water is a dangerous remedy in erysipelas. This disease is attended with perhaps greater heat than any other to which the system is subject. From this fact, no doubt, the delusion arose. So in high fevers, it was long believed that no remedy more dangerous than cold water could be used; and the greater the heat, the more danger there was supposed to be. The best authorities in the healing art now all agree that the treatment of erysipelas, as well as of all other inflammatory diseases, should be of the cooling kind; and that cold applications, to arrest both the general and the local fever in this disease, are always entirely safe, provided they are made in accordance with well-ascertained principles. The more heat there is in the system, or any of its parts, the more salutary and grateful are the means. Common sense, as well as science, dictates, that any means, however good, must not be carried to extremes. A medium is always to be observed. If there is any where a sensation of too great heat, unattended with fatigue, use the cooling means sufficiently often and long to remove that condition; not, however, to cause much chilliness, which, if protracted, might end in harm.

The author has repeatedly cured cases of erysipelas of the face and head by water treatment. He has failed in no single instance. In one case, a medical man took upon himself to affirm, *that the lady's constitution must have been one of a thousand, or she would have been killed.* Some have not sense enough to refrain from judging of a matter before hearing it; and we find this truth verified in the opposition so often set up to the water-cure by those who know not the first lesson concerning it.

In 1845, I treated the following cases of erysipelas:

CASE OF MRS. GOSS.

About one year ago we had the honor to prescribe for our friend, Mrs. Goss, of 26 Vesey street, then suffering from a severe attack of erysipelas of the face and neck. The heat and swelling had gone on to a very considerable extent before we commenced. We directed that the face and neck should, as far as practicable, be immersed in cold water, and this as frequently as was agreeable. By kneeling at the side of a chair, and having upon it a large bowl of water, the object could be tolerably well effected. At other times, wet cold cloths were to be kept upon the parts. Two general baths per day were to be taken. Only a little water gruel, and perhaps an apple or two, daily, were to constitute the food. By these means, perseveringly carried out, a radical cure was effected in about three days, so that Mrs. Goss was about as usual. Awhile after, a friend of hers had the same disease. She recommended her to have water treatment, as she had done. Her physician, learning what treatment Mrs. Goss had had, said, very confidently, that her constitution was one of hundreds, or she could not have endured it; but the fact is, Mrs. Goss has naturally a feeble frame. The treatment was the safest possible that could be adopted.

CASE OF MR. L. WETMORE.

In the month of September, 1845, Mr. L. Wetmore, a gentleman residing in the boarding-house kept by Mrs. Goss above mentioned, was violently attacked with erysipelas of the head. The general fever had already become very high, and the swelling large and very hot. By the use of wet sheets, baths, cold applications, and immersions of the parts affected, together with fasting, Mr. W. was enabled to walk out each day, and quite cured in four days

He was directed to take a thorough cold bath as often as the fever came up, even if it were twenty times in a day. The night in which the disease was the worst he took four long continued Croton shower baths, between ten at night and six in the morning. The fever raged; he took a thorough cooling in the shower, slept soundly then awhile, and as the fever again rose, repeated the bath, and thus obtained a tolerably good night's rest, and was quite himself in the morning. Such are the modes of treating this often dangerous affection, erysipelas. It is a disease attended with great heat, and always the more there is, the more charm-like the cold water acts.

On the 25th of October, 1848, in the night, Mr. Wetmore was again attacked, and much more severely, by this disease. I saw him first this time at midday on the 27th instant. He had been bathing, using wet bandages, the wet sheet, etc., but not to so great an extent as the case required. He suffered rigors, or chilliness at times, a circumstance common in the beginning of severe inflammatory attacks. This circumstance deterred him somewhat from persevering with the water, and led him to wrap up too warmly in bed. In his case, the chilly sensation was caused by the skin being too hot.

At half-past 10 A. M. the next day, the 28th, saw Mr. W. again. He had used according to direction, the cold wet cloths constantly, with frequent washings of the face and parts affected; and during the last sixteen hours had gone to the bath (a liberal shower, with little fall, as mechanical force would be ill in such a case) seven times, taking, from the top of the head to the sole of the feet, a thorough drenching at each time. He had used the wet sheet, three double, about the trunk of the body nearly all the time, to keep down general feverishness. He had eaten nothing, or next to nothing, since the commencement of the disease.

He was doing so well on this day, I consented that he might go out and take the fresh air. He went in the afternoon to his store, there became much excited in business, and was made much worse. He became delirious in the night. I had gone out of the city, and could not return before Monday, Saturday afternoon being the time of his going out. With good aid he persevered in the treatment, going to the bath about every hour for some twenty-four hours, taking yet, according to my directions, no nourishment other than water. By Sunday night the fever was quite quelled.

The next morning, on seeing him, I found him doing well, but yet extremely excitable. He took a little nourishment this day, avoided company and business for three or four days, following up a moderate treatment, and thus recovered very rapidly.

The power of entire fasting was a great help in this case, the patient having taken no food for about five days. His going to the store and becoming excited in business, was an unfortunate occurrence for the time. However, in the end every thing went on well, and he recovered admirably, and in a very short time, from a most dangerous attack.

In no disease is the good effect of cold water more clearly shown, than in acute erysipelas. Keep down the general fever, as well as that of the local parts. Eat no food until it is quite subsided. Avoid company and all excitement, and thus every thing will go on well.

SCALDS AND BURNS.

Scalds and burns differ by being caused in different ways, the former being always the effect of heat applied through the medium of a fluid. A scald is generally more diffused in extent and more equable in severity than a burn.

The most useful division of burns, is the very ancient one, that of three kinds: 1st, those causing mere redness or inflammation; 2d, those causing vesication or blistering; 3d, those causing actual death or destruction of the part.

1. The first class are attended with mere superficial inflammation, and are not at all dangerous. They are, however, sometimes very painful. Homeopathically—that is, on the principle that like cures its like—the treatment is to be by hot applications, holding the part to the fire, etc., etc. Hydropathically, cold is to be constantly applied until the inflammation subsides. Allopathically, they are treated according to the fancy of the practitioner. The application of cold water is the best means we know of—the most comfortable, as well as the most effectual. There is not the slightest danger of taking cold, which some fear so much, as long as cold is agreeable. Nor is it true, as has been so generally believed, "that although the application of cold was most pleasurable, and continued to be so as long as it was employed unremittingly, still that if it were discontinued for a moment the pain returned with infinitely greater force."

2. From what we have seen, we doubt whether blistering would ever be caused if the part could be suddenly immersed in very cold water, and there kept, provided this is done before the blister is raised. When blistering has been caused, it is well to draw off the fluid collected. This is best done by piercing under the blister through the live skin a little way from the part; smarting is thus prevented. The elasticity of the live skin caŭses the hole to close, and air, the cause of smarting, is thus excluded. If there is need of any further treatment, wet cloths covered with dry ones, continued according to the feelings of comfort, are the local applications to be used. Large blisters will of course need treatment. The wet bandages should be so arranged and kept constantly wet, that the *air* is entirely excluded.

3. The third class of burns, those in which the part is destroyed, are sometimes exceedingly troublesome and dangerous. When of considerable extent, the constitutional symptoms are severe—those of collapse, or great prostration of strength, coldness of extremities, quick and feeble pulse, paleness of surface, repeated and violent shiverings, and severe sensations of cold. These symptoms are sometimes soon succeeded by difficult breathing, coma, or sleep-like insensibility, from which with difficulty only the sufferer can be aroused, and finally with death. In other cases, dissolution is preceded by a kind of imperfect reaction, or a general feverish excitement in the system, attended with delirium and distress.

Burns of apparently small severity, when extending over a large surface, should always be considered dangerous—they are really so, and more particularly if the skin has been removed. Of equal extent, burns on the extremities are always less dangerous than those upon the body. Infancy and old age are the periods most unfavorable. When burns are extensive, and there is little or no apparent suffering, this must be reckoned as indicative of most urgent peril. Severe pain, comparatively, is a favorable symptom; yet this may prove a symptom of danger, since it may so exhaust the vital powers, that death will be the result. "The early subsidence of complaint, unwillingness to be disturbed, apathy approaching to stupor, as if the scale of sensibility had sunk below the point of pain, is invariably a fatal symptom. Constant shivering is an ill omen. The failure of the pulse, and the consequent coldness of the extremities, with a livid hue of the transparent skin of the cheeks and lips from congestion (accumulation of blood) in the capillaries, drowsiness, with occasional muscular twitchings, are sure prognostics of death." The subsidence of swelling is likewise a most unfavorable symptom.

The treatment of severe burns, of the second and third classes, requires great skill and good judgment on the part of the physician, and patience and perseverance on the part of patients and nurses. Good nursing has been said to be the best part of "doctoring." If there is collapse, coldness of extremities, and shiverings, certainly we must husband to the greatest possible extent what little of heat and strength the sufferer yet has, and excite healthfully the vital organs to action. If we understand the capabilities of the human system, this is not best done by diffusible stimulants, as hot brandy and water, ether, ammonia, or hartshorn. In common practice, these are the first things resorted to. If the patient lives at all, he lives in spite of these remedies, if they are used. Warm applications, as heated bricks, or bottles of warm water, are often made to the arm-pits, between the thighs, and to the feet. These are good, but the best part at which to apply warmth so as to cause it to be diffused through the body quickly and generally, is the "pit of the stomach;" and this is the best done by *bladders* of warm water. The other applications mentioned should be used, if no better can be had. Next to the pit of the stomach, warm applications to the feet are probably best; but, if necessary, applications can be made to all of the parts mentioned. The wrapping the whole body also in an abundance of warm clothes, should by no means be neglected. Of this we shall speak hereafter.

To allay *vomiting*, which sometimes takes place in great collapse, it has been common to give a large dose of calomel and opium, or to give an opiate clyster. But these agents, though they often arrest vomiting, do a great amount of mischief. Pure soft water, taken, if necessary, little by little, as much as the patient can bear, is a far better means. Hickup, which sometimes occurs in such cases, and is severe and troublesome, is more effectually arrested by free drinking of water than by any other means. Both in vomiting and hickup, rubbing briskly the surface of the body with a wet towel, and then also with a dry one, is good in connection with the drinking.

In cases of great collapse, or sinking of the powers of life, whether caused by heat or cold, or other injuries, a very ancient remedy has, from time to time, been recommended and resorted to. It is, in principle and effect, a good one,—we mean the application of the warm skin of a recently slain animal, the skin being taken off immediately after the animal is killed, and then applied. Persons, too, have been placed in a carcass from which the entrails were quickly removed, the carcass being yet warm. The soothing and vivifying effect of the warmth and moisture in such treatment is most astonishing. All the good effect thus caused, with little inconvenience, can be readily obtained by means of the wet sheet, or cloths wrung out of water as warm as can be borne, and applied in the ordinary way, with the warm non-conducting blankets wrapped closely outside the wet cloths. All suitably arranged, the warmth of the cloths and the warmth of the body, which is always generated, and passes off as long as life remains, will be retained by the woolen blankets, and thus thrown back upon the body, which, together with the moisture, produces a most soothing effect over the *whole* body, the same as that of a warm poultice upon any *part* of the body. The great surgeon, Baron Larry, saw the warming remedy by means of the warm skins, used with great benefit, by certain humane Esquimaux, upon a company of Frenchmen who had been shipwrecked, and who were suffering greatly with cold, and fatigue, and hunger, and himself afterward put the same remedy in practice with good success, in the case of a distinguished marshal, during one of Napoleon's Spanish campaigns.

If in any such case of sinking, the best remedial means fail, and death takes place, still such means should be most industriously used. Life will be at least prolonged, pain will be rendered by far less severe, and death, to which all must submit, will be rendered less violent. It will thus be more like the gradual dying away of embers, than like the sudden extinction of a fire. Indeed, the writer has so much confidence in the application of warmth and moisture to soothe the system and relieve pain, that he believes that in all cases, if the means are rightly used, however violent the disease, death will take place, comparatively only like the sinking into a quiet sleep, almost without a struggle or a groan.

But to return: in these cases of severe scalds and burns there is sometimes, also, a feverish excitement or general fever throughout the whole system, attended with great restlessness and pain. To reduce the pain, most persons would at once say, "A good dose of opium, or some of its preparations, must be given without delay."

But still among the best medical authorities, there is discrepancy of opinion concerning the effects of opium. Larry, of whom Bonaparte said that he was the most humane man he ever saw, says, "Opium is injurious, whether used internally or externally. Externally, it stupefies the parts, instead of exciting them to a salutary inflammation; internally, if used in considerable quantity, it enfeebles all the organs, after producing a momentary stimulation." Another writer of considerable note, Travers, says, "In small doses it is ineffectual, and in large ones injurious." But how are we to proceed? The pain should be quickly removed. Pain should ever be regarded as the truthful admonition of nature, that something must be done—it should be removed. To personify, nature is attempting to accomplish the object, but asks assistance at our hand. In these cases, then, *locally*, we must use the wet cloths of temperature to suit the feelings; constitutionally, we must resort to wet sheets, clysters, drinking, etc., as in any similar case of general fever. As in all inflammatory cases, the greatest caution is necessary in diet. By the use of clysters the bowels should be kept freely open.

The ulcers resulting from burns are often very slow in healing. It is also not uncommon for a second inflammation to be set up by exposure to cold or cold moisture: a cold is taken in the burn, as it is said. People are in general too careless and inconsiderate when once the pain has ceased. The ulcer following a burn should be guarded, and the greatest care should be exercised that it be not exposed. It should be moist and comfortable, and the part of equable temperature. No possible application will cause it to heal as quickly as water, rightly applied.

It is best not to remove the dressing very quickly in case of a running ulcer. The part can easily be kept moist and agreeable by removing only the outward dry covering, and with a soft sponge, the part can be wet according to the feelings of comfort.

Most serious deformities are sometimes caused by scalds and burns. A limb may become obstinately bent; large and unsightly scars may be formed, and sometimes the chin may become fixed to the breast, and the eyelids become incapable of closing. These difficulties have often been augmented by the patient being allowed too full a diet. This, it is often believed, is necessary to support the strength under the weakening effect of the profuse discharges that often take place. The diet should be mild and unstimulating, and what would be termed low.

If the fingers or toes are badly scalded or burned, and the skin removed, care must be taken they do not adhere and grow together. Lint, or better, very fine cloths, will suffice to prevent an accident of this kind.

Flour frequently sifted upon the surface of the running ulcers, as also very finely carded cotton perpetually strewed upon the part, is a favorite remedy with some. The good effect of these substances is to exclude the air, to form a covering, and to maintain the part at an equable temperature. These applications are certainly good in many respects, yet they are apt to become dry, hard, and irritating, and are sometimes converted into a loathsome mass of putridity and worms. A liniment of linseed oil and lime water, or the soap liniment, have frequently been used. White paint is dangerous. Properly managed, we like pure clean water the best. In no case is skill and good judgment more needed than in scalds and burns.

CONVULSIONS.

In cases of ordinary convulsions, Priessnitz's main reliance is active frictions upon the surface and extremities, by means of cold water applied by the hand. A number of persons should aid in the operations, and the frictions must be carried on perseveringly, and in some cases for a long time. It is safer to chill the system much, than to allow the convulsions to go on.

The mode of treatment adopted by Priessnitz in convulsions, is certainly not so severe as that which has been sometimes adopted by others. At different periods of time, the regular cold immersion has been in vogue. Hippocrates, and other of the earlier physicians, used the cold bath in convulsions that were not caused by wounds or local injuries. That estimable writer, Dr. Currie, who used water so faithfully and perseveringly in his practice, says, that in the convulsions of children, he found the cold bath a most useful remedy, whether the disorder originated from worms or other causes. He seldom knew it to fail of arresting the paroxysms, at least for some time, thus giving an opportunity to employ other means for removing the particular irritation. In patients of early infancy he employed the remedy with caution, generally in such cases by affusion instead of immersion, tempering the water also, in very cold weather. These modes are all certainly more severe than the frictions used by Priessnitz.

After having employed the cold bath in convulsive diseases for fourteen years, Dr. Currie gave the following as his conclusions: "*That the benefit derived from the cold bath in convulsive diseases, depends on its being used in the paroxysm of convulsion; that its efficacy consists in resolving or abating the paroxysm; and that when this effect is produced, the return of the paroxysm is greatly retarded, if not entirely prevented.*"

TETANUS, OR LOCK-JAW,

Is a form of convulsions, and often a terrible disease to manage. Others besides Priessnitz seem to have had better success with water, than any other known means. Priessnitz's mode is the wet frictions energetically applied, and the half bath slightly tepid. He regards that in severe spasms, of whatever kind, it is not well to use very cold water: the temperature should be a little moderated. He places great reliance upon the frictions, perseveringly practiced.

Others have used more severe means in tetanus. Professor Elliotson, of London, in his large and able work on the Practice of Medicine, gives the following cases to illustrate the good effects of the cooling means in this disease:

"There is a case mentioned by Sir James McGregor, in the sixth volume of the 'Medical Chirurgical Transactions,' and also in his reports of the diseases of the Peninsular war. It proceeded from a slight wound in the finger. The patient (a soldier, of course) was carried in a bullock-car after the battalion to which he belonged, in a state of severe tetanus, in the midst of pouring rain, which completely drenched him in the early part of the day—the heat being fifty-two degrees; and then they ascended the highest mountain in Gallicia, the snow on the summit of which was knee deep! And there the temperature was only thirty degrees. He was exposed in this condition from six o'clock till ten o'clock at night, and arrived at his journey's end half starved from cold, but perfectly cured of his tetanus. Whether such a mode would succeed, if it were put into practice intentionally, I do not know. I stumbled on a similar case, published in 1827: a horse, which was in a state of tetanus, happened to be in a wet park, and was drenched with rain—precisely as was the case with this unfortunate man—and the horse also did perfectly well. Whether the depressing power of cold and wet, regularly kept up for a certain number of hours, has a tendency to cure the disease, I do not say; but I think that, in a disease of violent excitement as this is, the constant—not sudden, but constant refrigeration (by means of a low temperature, united with moisture), is likely to be of great service. There are at least two such cases on record, and it is surprising to find a soldier, so exposed from morning to evening, recover, and especially in so short a time as one day."

Some two years ago I wrote in my note-book as follows: "I have at this time (Feb. 22d, 1847), a case like this: Mr. Perry, of Orchard street, cut his hand one week ago. He is a machinist by occupation, and thinks his health has been injured by gases, and by verdigris flying off from copper in the form of dust. He has taken colds very easily. He took a cold in the wound, and it swelled prodigiously. He used poultices of different kinds, but it grew worse and worse. Very severe pain was experienced in the hand, and up the arm (a nerve was no doubt wounded), and there was also constant pain in the back. He was very feverish, and could get no rest. Last evening he had himself placed in a wet sheet, put on a large wet girdle, wet bandages all about the arm, and the hand in water. This stopped the pain completely in the hand, and he appeared better in every respect. He sent for me, and I directed him to use, in addition to the hand bath and wet girdle, the half bath quite cold, but not the coldest, to renew his bandages often upon the arm, take the elbow bath, drink water very often, eat no food for some days, or at most not until all pain and fever has subsided, and to take the half bath as often as the pain in the back returns. The hand to be kept in cold water most of the time, enough to prevent all pain in that part. This morning, I find Mr. Perry decidedly better, the pulse at 80 instead of 100, as when I first saw him last night. The hand is yet much swollen, and some days will be required for this to be removed."

In cases of considerable debility, when there is danger of lock-jaw, or when the disease is already present, we must be careful not to make too short and sudden an impression by means of cold. This caution is particularly needed when powerful medicines have been given. Warm baths which have been recommended, it is now acknowledged do harm. The half bath is an invaluable means, and must be persevered in. If we conclude to dash on the cold water, we must be sure that the patient has considerable strength, and that the paroxysm is at a high pitch, otherwise we may do harm."

Dr. Currie also mentions cases of this disease, in which he obtained strikingly beneficial results from the affusion of water. In some cases the cold bath, in this way, was used as the paroxysms came on, many times in the twenty-four hours, and for days in succession. In some cases, when other and the most powerful means failed, the affusion of water proved successful.

I will state, that I regard the free use of injections of water in this disease good; cold, if the patient is not too weak; tepid, if there is any doubt as to the propriety of the cold.

HYSTERIA, OR HYSTERICS.

It is pretty generally understood, that cold water is the thing for this disease. The cold bath and dashing of cold water at once cuts short the fit in many cases. The half bath is one of the best means. Fear, and the dread of being plunged into cold water, or of having cold water dashed over the body, has been known to prevent these unpleasant attacks. Persons thus affected, should do all in their power to fortify and invigorate the general health; for with such attacks such a thing as good health cannot possibly be. I very much pity the person who is thus affected.

CHAPTER XVII.

TREATMENT OF DISEASES CONTINUED.

Apoplexy.—Value of Cold applied to the Head, and Frictions with Cold Water over the Surface generally in this Disease.—Cold Injections in the Bowels.—Many are killed, doubtless, in the old Practice in this Disease.—Best means of applying Cold to the Head. —Inflammation of the Brain.—This is to be treated on the same great Principle of all Inflammations.—Cold to the Head.—General Treatment, etc.—Quinsy, and other acute Inflammations of the Throat.—Croup a very dangerous Disease.—Prevention better than Cure.—How to prevent the Disease.—How to treat it.—Inflammations in the Chest, Lung Fever, and Pleurisy.—How to be treated.—Case of Priessnitz's Daughter. —Sore Throat, Weakness of the Chest, Lungs, etc.—Priessnitz's Advice.—Remarks on Consumption.

APOPLEXY.

THE treatment for this disease is the free application of cold to the head, while at the same time a very brisk rubbing of the surface of the body generally is practiced with the hands wet in cold water, over the rubbing wet sheet, etc. There is too much blood in the brain in this state of the system. Hence the good effect of cold water in that part. Cold, continuously applied, repels the blood from the part. The frictions over the surface aid in driving the blood thereto, and thus the brain is also relieved of the too great quantity of this fluid.

Cold injections in the bowels have a good effect in rousing the patient in all states of stupor and unconsciousness, and consequently in apoplexy.

Many a person, doubtless, is destroyed in this disease, by the enormous bleedings that are sometimes practiced. Cold water, perseveringly applied, is a more effectual, as well as incomparably safer means.

Pounded ice applied to the head by means of a bladder, has been recommended by all authors, as one of the means to be resorted to in apoplexy. Ice, however, cannot always be obtained. If the head, extending somewhat over the edge of a bed, is supported (and it should be also somewhat elevated) by an assistant, cold water may be constantly poured upon it, letting it run down into a tub; thus the part may probably be as effectually cooled as by means of ice.

INFLAMMATION OF THE BRAIN.

This is to be treated on the same general principle of all severe inflammations. Keep down the general fever, and at the same time use cold applications to the head without stint. It is hardly possible to do too much. There is no need of shaving off the hair, if enough cold water is poured upon the part. Very cold and oft-repeated fomentations, wet cloths with ice between them, pounded ice in bladders, etc.—these are the local means.

QUINSY, AND OTHER INFLAMMATIONS OF THE THROAT.

These are also treated on the same general principle of all inflammations. The wet bandages, etc., about the throat, are here as useful as cold applications to the head in apoplexy and inflammation of the brain.

CROUP.

This very dangerous disease, which carries off every winter great numbers of children, is doubtless generally manageable, if taken at the very beginning of the attack. But it is far better to rear and manage children in such a manner, as to render them proof against the disease. Children that are not dosed with medicine, and are kept on food of the right kinds—that are bathed regularly each day, and are not subjected to the air of over-heated rooms, to feather beds, feather pillows, and the like, and that, on the other hand, are not subjected to too great extremes of cold—are not at all liable to croup. This, then, is the better philosophy—AVOID THE DISEASE.

TREATMENT OF CROUP.

As soon as possible—the sooner the better—after croup has commenced, let the patient be at once well washed over with cold water. It may be poured over the body, or the rubbing wet sheet may be used, or the general washing in a tub. Do whatever is done quickly. A good thorough cold bath will often cause a child to breathe with entire freedom at once—in a moment, as it were. Wet bandages should be placed about the throat and chest, and be frequently renewed. So also repeat the ablution as soon as the symptoms return. Meantime, if it is in the night, the child should be placed warmly between two persons in bed.

For the treatment of a very dangerous case of croup and measles, see account of the latter disease.

INFLAMMATIONS IN THE CHEST, LUNG FEVER, AND PLEURISY.

Priessnitz's great dependence now in the treatment of these diseases, is the sedative effect of the cold bath. This, with much frictions upon the surface generally, cold, or moderated a little if the debility requires, is the mode. Keep down the inflammation in the general system, and in these, as all other inflammations, we give nature the best possible chance. Between the times of bathing, the wet sheet should be applied about the whole trunk.

Priessnitz informed us one day at his table, that during the past year (1847), his eldest daughter was attacked severely with inflammation of the lungs. She was at the time three or four months advanced in pregnancy. He treated her by the cold bath and frictions. *Twenty-five* cold baths were given in succession within a space of less than four hours. Each bath was continued about five minutes, the body was then rubbed dry, and after resting a very few minutes she was again placed in the bath. By these means thus persevered in, the pains and inflammation were completely subdued, and the next day she was able to go about quite as usual. Her case, it must be remembered, was taken in season, and thus it was nipped in the bud.

SORE THROAT, WEAKNESS OF THE CHEST, LUNGS, ETC.

On returning from Graefenberg in the spring of 1848, I published the following article on these complaints in the Water-Cure Journal:

"The modes of treatment recommended by Priessnitz, in cases of colds, difficulties in the throat and chest, from whatever cause or causes, are exceedingly simple, and at the same time effectual for good. We have before us a work entitled "Six Months at Graefenberg," by Mr. H. C. Wright, of Philadelphia (published in England), a very accurate writer and observer. This author had himself been for years afflicted with serious difficulties of the above-mentioned kinds. He had, likewise, been in the habit of much and long-continued public speaking. He tells us that for years before going to Graefenberg, he was, as is the custom, wont to eschew the fresh air as much as possible. Flannel shirts and drawers, and a closely fitting shirt-collar and a neckcloth, were worn, and, whenever the weather seemed to require it, a fur muffler, or a large silk or worsted handkerchief, over the chin and mouth, to exclude all fresh air from the back of the head and neck, the throat, and lungs. He was exceedingly sensitive to cold, and though long accustomed to general ablutions of cold water, the exclusion of cold air, with a view to the preservation of health, had become an object of very particular attention. Heavy clothes and overcoats were worn to protect the body from the air and its free circulation over the surface. He continues: 'I now look back with astonishment at my folly; and the more so, because the days of my childhood and youth were chiefly spent in the open air, in the backwoods of western New York. Calm and storm, cold and heat, rain and sunshine, were all alike to me then; and many times since I attained my twentieth year, have I slept with my windows open, in the severe winter nights of New England. But for the last three years, since my lungs began to be affected, I changed my habits entirely, and, by the advice of medical friends, took every precaution against exposure to the air.'

"Mr. Wright further tells us, that, when he went to Graefenberg, away went the flannel shirts and drawers, and silk, worsted, and fur mufflers, and Priessnitz advised him to be in the open air as much as possible, like the other patients. We have ourselves seen at Graefenberg poor, weak bodies, who had for years been wedded to those 'comfortable' things, mercilessly stripped in the manner described by Mr. Wright. And what may appear strange is, that probably nowhere in the world can there be found the same number of persons as at Graefenberg, with less of coughs and symptoms of cold in the throat or lungs. The freedom from coughs and colds among Priessnitz's patients is notorious. Be it remarked, also, that there is there in the winter season much of damp, fogs, and winds; so that, according to the popular notions on this subject, persons would be much subject to the difficulties in question. But there is among the profession, as well as the people, much error in reference to the effects of wind and damp. We find that one of the best possible things for cough and cold is to go to sea. Consumptive persons, even, are recommended often to go sea voyages, and there appears in cases generally, whether curable or incurable, to be a manifest improvement in so doing. We have known persons, repeatedly, to have a severe cold, attended with cough, on going to sea, to become very soon cured. Now, it should be understood that there is, besides the winds at sea, a great deal of moisture. The atmosphere is, in consequence of evaporation, at all times completely loaded with humidity; and this is not *saltish*, as many suppose, but fresh; for we know that salt is of great specific gravity, and does not rise. In the manufacture of salt, by evaporation in the sun or by boiling, the mineral is left behind, while the pure water passes off. We see, from the above facts, that wind and moisture are not necessarily so deleterious as is generally supposed; but, on the contrary, that they are, under certain circumstances, extremely favorable to health.

"If a person has an incurable disease of the lungs, Priessnitz would, of course, be very careful in reference to changes of whatever kind. The cases we have referred to he regarded as curable. Such persons can make much greater changes with safety, than is generally supposed. Even in cases of incurable disease of the lungs, people are perpetually injuring themselves by too much clothing, confinement in close, overheated, and illy ventilated rooms, sleeping upon feather beds, down pillows, etc. Now in these, often great good may be done in the way of mitigating the disease. But all changes should be made with proper caution, and according to the dictates of an enlightened experience. Inasmuch as the water means, diet, etc., are the best possible for cure, so also, properly managed, are they in mitigating the sufferings arising from incurable disease.

"Before leaving Graefenberg, Mr. Wright prepared, in writing, a list of questions, which were proposed to Priessnitz, the answers to which were taken down upon paper at the time. Some of these questions were as follows:

"*Wright.*—In cases of severe cold on the lungs, attended with much coughing and expectoration, what should be done?

"*Priessnitz.*—Rub the chest and throat with cold water, holding, at the same time, some water in the mouth. In cold climates, the wet bandage around the throat would be of service occasionally. In warm climates, washing and rubbing alone are better.

"*Wright.*—In cases of inflammation and soreness of the throat, attended with hoarseness and difficulty in speaking?

"*Priessnitz.*—Friction, washing, and the application of wet bandages.

"*Wright.*—In cases of long attendance and speaking at public meetings, in hot, close, crowded rooms, and then going out into the chilly night air?

"*Priessnitz.*—The rubbing sheet, washing and rubbing the head and throat well, and the use of the foot bath.

"*Wright.*—When troubled with shooting pains across the chest, occasioned by long speaking at a time?

"*Priessnitz.*—Take rubbing sheets, and rub the throat and chest with water.

"In regard to friction, Mr. Wright judiciously remarks, 'that it is worthy of special notice that Priessnitz never orders the rubbing to be done with brushes, flannels, or even linen towels. He never applies flannels and brushes to the skin for any purpose; linen is only used for wiping the surface dry, and, even in this process, the rubbing should be gentle. He wishes to have the skin kept as smooth and soft as possible; and hence his disuse of flannels next the skin, and of brushes and hard substances in rubbing. He recommends that the hand only should be used; and it is not possible to be long under his treatment, and to enjoy the delicious sensations resulting from a clear, smooth, soft skin, the almost invariable result of the cure, without being convinced of the correctness of his practice in this respect.'"

CONSUMPTION.

The foundation of this most formidable disease is usually laid before birth. It is admitted on all hands that it is seldom cured. There are, however, exceptions to this rule. Just as ulcers heal in any part of the body, so they sometimes do in the lungs. As yet, comparatively but little has been attempted in the treatment of this disease by means of water-cure. Priessnitz has had all that he could do with more favorable cases than those in consumption. To a person in an advanced stage of this disease he would say something to this effect: "You cannot expect to be cured by any means; but by the proper use of water, with suitable attention to air, exercise, clothing, and diet, you can be much benefited. Your life can be prolonged, and rendered more comfortable."

Dr. Billing, senior physician to the London Hospital, a man of experience second to few, if any, in speaking of consumption, says, "Some years ago, a gentleman by the name of Stewart adopted a rational mode of treatment, with which he had considerable success; but because he could not work miracles, his plan was unjustly depreciated. His method was entirely tonic, and *especially the cautious use of cold and tepid ablutions of the skin,* a modification of cold bathing—a remedy which is found *so universally beneficial in promoting the resolution (cure) of strumous (scrofulous) tumors.*"

"One thing of which I am convinced," says Dr. B., "is, that the true principle of treating *consumption,* is to support the patient's strength to the utmost." This can best be done by water-cure. All will agree that the means used in the treatment by water are very powerful to promote strength, if the patient can bear such treatment. But the treatment, we contend, can be managed with perfect safety, even to the last hour of life; *and will always positively do some good, and no harm,* when rightly used, which is more than any one can claim for drugs. The action of drugs is always doubtful, and sometimes dangerous, and every dose, however small, acts only by virtue of its power to produce diseased action in the body. Furthermore, the indication of treatment is the same in all cases of the disease in question, and for all others that are not unfrequently mistaken for it; that is, to support the strength to the greatest possible degree. It is true, different cases always have different symptoms, so that the treatment must be varied accordingly; but it is the right way to support the strength by all possible means, so that the system may be better able to resist the disease.

In the early stages of this disease, much can be done by way of preventing an increase of its symptoms. All the daily and hourly circumstances which go to affect the health should be most scrupulously attended to. The strictest regularity and correctness in meals, bathing, exercise in pure air, sleep, etc., etc., if rigidly observed, will be found to prove highly salutary. But all this requires knowledge possessed by few. It is very common for persons in this disease to be greatly injured by the food they take. Even in the advanced stage of the disease, persons are told that die they must, and that it matters little what kind of food they take. It is not uncommon to find persons in the far advanced stages of this disease indulging freely in the use of rich pastry, and toast well saturated with butter, one of the worst dishes that well persons even can take; and all this is done because the patient has a good appetite, and because the *stomach* does not *appear* to suffer. The disease is concentrated upon, and spends its violence in, the lungs, so that the stomach cannot feel the injuries it receives; but the lungs and whole body suffer just as much from such improprieties, as if the stomach or any other important part was the seat of disease. In food, *we must always make the weak part the standard of what the system can bear.*

In this disease, as in all others, we believe it better that the patient take no animal food, other than preparations of milk, or cream, which is generally better and less feverish than flesh; and these, even, in many cases, it is believed, are better omitted—for they are more feverish and exciting than the mild preparations of farinaceous food.

In the more advanced stages of this disease, the early morning sweats, which are so weakening, can be much mitigated, if not entirely prevented, by judicious sponging, or wet cloth-rubbing the surface of the body. The hectic fever, which wears down the patient's strength, can also be much relieved. By bandaging and the wet sheets to soothe, great good can also be done to the last

CHAPTER XVIII.

TREATMENT OF DISEASES CONTINUED.

Inflammations of the Abdomen generally.—These are all to be treated on the same genera. Principles.—Enteritis, or Inflammation, with obstinate Stoppage of the Bowels.—How to be treated according to Priessnitz.—This very dangerous Disease sometimes needs much and powerful Treatment.—Colic.—Priessnitz's Mode of Cure.—Dysentery, Diarrhœa, and Cholera Morbus.—How to be Treated.—Erroneous Notions as to the Effect of Water.—Causes of these Diseases.—A Case of Dysentery, with Remarks.—Chronic Diarrhœa, Dysentery, etc.—How to be Cured.—Nausea, Vomiting, and Pains of the Stomach.—Curious Remarks of John Smith.—How to allay Vomiting.

INFLAMMATIONS OF THE ABDOMEN GENERALLY.

All inflammations within the abdomen are to be treated on the same general principles.

ENTERITIS, OR INFLAMMATION, WITH OBSTINATE STOPPAGE OF THE BOWELS.

Long-continued shallow bath, with much rubbing of the bowels; the water to be cold, and changed often, if the patient is not too weak. If there is much debility, the water to be used tepid. In either case, the treatment must be persevered in, otherwise the disease may pass very speedily to a fatal termination. Injections, full and oft-repeated—cold or tepid, according to the strength—are also to be used. These form a very important part of the treatment.

Drinking also to be practiced more or less. After the pain dies away or becomes subdued, and the bowels are made to act more or less, the treatment above mentioned is to be diminished. The wet girdle about the abdomen, or still better, the folded sheet wet, and placed about the whole trunk of the body, should be used while the person rests from the baths. Once the pain and inflammation are subdued, little bathing more will be needed. But the wet girdle should be worn for days, to tonify or invigorate the weakened parts which have been diseased.

Persons will be more likely to fail in the treatment of this disease from not persevering sufficiently. Many of these cases are among the most obstinate and dangerous that a medical man has to deal with. Patients often die of the disease, in spite of bleedings, calomel, and opium: so, if now and then one should be lost by water (which can at most very rarely happen if any thing is well done), it need not be said, "Oh, water killed the patient!"

If I had an attack of this disease, I would rather remain in a bath or tub of water for many hours, than allow the dreadful pain to go on wrenching one as it does to the very vitals. I would prefer to remain in the water and die there, if I must, than to quail under the racking tortures often caused by this disease. Cold water, rightly used, is more powerful than any or all other agents combined to remove pain.

COLIC.

In this very painful and sometimes dangerous disease, Priessnitz's treatment is as follows: Prolonged cold sitz bath, rubbing the abdomen with the wet hand at the same time, and cold injections to the bowels. Persevere in all these applications, and relief will generally very soon follow. If there are spasms, or if the colic is what may be termed spasmodic, apply the rubbing sheet briskly, repeating it as often as there is need.

Vomiting by means of water, which Priessnitz has not been in the habit of resorting to, is a very excellent collateral means in many cases of colic.

When all ordinary means have failed, dashing some buckets of cold water upon the abdomen has been found successful.

ACUTE DYSENTERY, DIARRHŒA, CHOLERA MORBUS, AND OTHER DISCHARGES FROM THE BOWELS.

The treatment Priessnitz recommends in all diseases of this kind is very simple. Suppose it a bad case of dysentery in a child. The great reliance with him is the hip bath, always cold if the patient is not already very weak. No time should be lost, and the treatment should be persevered in until the discharge is arrested. Cold injections he also uses if the hip bath does not readily arrest the discharge. The wet girdle about the abdomen is to be kept on constantly during the intervals when the other means are not used. As much water as the patient desires is to be taken, and at frequent intervals.

As to general ablutions, sufficient daily for cleanliness is all that he recommends in these cases; no half baths, no wet sheets, or means of that kind as a general thing. The sitz bath, injections, wet girdle, and the drinking, with spare and cooling diet—these are the means which Priessnitz has found in his great experience to be the best. If the patient is very weak, the water should be moderated a little in temperature, as at from 60 degrees to 70 degrees Fah.

In the house where I lodge at Graefenberg this winter (1848), there is a little boy five or six years of age that has been under the treatment for some weeks. He has just had the measles. As the disease passed off, a severe diarrhœa came on. He was of scrofulous tendency, often had the croup, and also chronic tonsilitis (inflammation of the tonsils). Priessnitz's directions for the diarrhœa were hip baths cold, every three or four hours during the day, for twenty minutes each time; and if the discharges come on in the night, the hip bath was to be given the same as during the day. There was also practiced in the case a light general treatment, such as would be suitable in any case where the measles were passing off, viz., slight general ablutions once or twice a day, with water at about 70 degrees Fah. The sitz bath had evidently a very marked effect in arresting the discharges.

Priessnitz holds that almost every conceivable case of acute disease of this kind may be readily cured by the simple processes we have here described, if it is treated in season and with sufficient perseverance. There must be no half-way work in the matter, and there is as much need of a doctor who understands his business, or of an old woman, or some one who is perfectly competent to take charge in the matter, and see that it is properly carried out; and how many foolish, ignorant persons, wise enough in their own conceit, do we have to encounter in almost every case of water treatment in acute diseases. The mode we have described will seem a harsh and dangerous one, no doubt, to many, and there will be doctors, wise men enough, who, if they take the trouble to investigate these things at all, will declare that such a mode would be perfectly hazardous—quite certain to kill. Let these ignorant pretenders (and they are plenty enough in our country), I say let them first learn the A, B, C of the water treatment before they assume to pronounce so sagely concerning the opinions and well-earned experience of the noble philosopher of

Graefenberg. I myself have been annoyed not a little in the city of New York, by having my patients told by these would-be wise men that the water-cure would be certain to kill them. "Yout system has not the power of *reaction*," that convenient word as little understood as it is common to use; "you will surely get your death by the water." Such are not unfrequently the expressions of those miserable specimens of humanity who know not yet the first principles of the laws that govern the human system, or of the water-cure as practiced by its founder.

But to return. In our cities, our hot, unhealthy American cities, where, in the summer season, such multitudes of infants and children drop off suddenly with these bowel complaints, I fear that in many cases death will be the result of such attacks, in spite of all that the best skill and judgment can dictate. So unhealthy is a great city like New York in the hot season, with its ten thousand filthy and pestilential emanations, from streets, gutters, privies, butcheries, and the like; and so unwisely, too, are children reared, starved now and then, but generally over-full, crammed, as people do with their housed geese and turkies before Thanksgiving or Christmas; dosed with paregorics and other poisonous compounds from the first hour of life onward; swathed and girted up so that they could scarce exist, even if all other things were right about them;—I repeat, any practitioner that has to deal with such cases, and under such circumstances, will have trouble enough, and if I am not mistaken will often be tempted to flee forever from a calling which is by most people so thanklessly appreciated and yet more thanklessly rewarded.

But in the practice of the water treatment, I have often been astonished at the results obtained in these unfavorable cases, and sometimes when the patient has been given over to die, when dosing and poisoning had been carried to the full extent.

If a child of my own should be attacked in a dangerous manner with dysentery, or any of the bowel complaints, I presume I should use a more powerful and energetic treatment than I should dare to use elsewhere, so great is the prejudice of the people against water, and so ignorant are physicians of its use. Why, suppose a man loses a patient and is sued for malpractice. It might have been the best treatment that could possibly be, yet the patient is lost. Now come the wise gentry of the profession to testify. The child was killed—and then comes the indictment, or, to say the least, a heavy fine; for the value of human life is often measured by money in this world. Thus it is; if we of the water system lose a case, no matter of what kind, ten to one if we have not killed the patient. But in the calomel and bleeding practice, it is another thing. A man may kill a score of patients in as many days, and so that each one be well crammed with poisons, and sent hence with the last repeated dose undigested on the stomach, all is well; the patient died *scientifically*. There is a charm in that; but we of the new practice, believing honestly and truly in what we do, and that the system is the greatest of all improvements that have yet come to man—we will undertake to teach people to die as well as to live by the water treatment. Let future times determine whether we succeed.

I must mention a fatal case of dysentery I had in the past year, 1847. A very worthy friend was the father of a second child, an only daughter, which he worshiped. It had been reared with great difficulty to seven or eight months by hand. It was not my patient at first. Being taken ill of dysentery, medicine was given. Then I was called upon. We practiced the water treatment, and then again some medicine was given. At last the child died; and now this friend, who is theoretically tired enough of the old mode, can never forgive himself that other means were not used. "Why," says he, "when one thing fails, we should try something else." This perpetually "trying" something else! Alas! how many are tried upon until they are sent to the grave.

The following case was furnished by our pupil, Seth Rogers, last summer, 1848:

"OYSTER BAY, 8th mo. 7, 1848.

"At this season of the year, when thousands are dying with the diarrhœa and dysentery, it seems proper to state a simple method by which these diseases can, as a general fact, be readily cured. By the proper use of water, immediate relief is almost invariably afforded.

"While in the city of New York a few days since, I found a married lady of my acquaintance suffering very severely with the last-named disease. The irritation and pain had been increasing for two days, and during the night before I saw her, the discharges consisted principally of blood. Her strength was fast failing, and it was evident that something must immediately be done. She had too much confidence in the power of water to listen to those kind friends who advised her to use other remedies; yet she did not understand its rightful and full application. But I have heard some one remark that '*water*, even if not very well applied, is far better than *drugs*;' so in this case, the more alarming symptoms were soon arrested by a very slight use of it.

"It was toward evening when I saw the lady. I recommended her to have the lower part of the body and limbs thoroughly rubbed in the half bath ten minutes. The water was nearly 70 degrees Fah., summer or rain-water temperature, and four or five inches in depth. The bath gave considerable relief. She then used injections of water at the same temperature, in quick succession, until the pain entirely ceased. Gallons were used. That night she slept as soundly, and was as much refreshed, as in ordinary health. The night previous, she did not rest at all. The next morning I advised her to commence very moderately with diet, but her appetite was excellent, and she partook quite freely of plain food and berries during the day. She walked considerable in the open air; her strength gradually returned, and she found no further difficulty. On the following day she experienced some nausea, occasioned by over-eating, but it was remedied by omitting a meal. S. ROGERS."

"EDITOR'S REMARKS.

"It will be seen that the treatment in the above case was somewhat different from that uniformly adopted by Priessnitz in such cases. The patient was a good deal weakened by the agony she had suffered, and the loss of blood. Still Priessnitz would have used water much colder. For persons of little experience, such as are not thoroughly versed in the heroic modes, the more moderate course is the better one. Every family should have first-rate injection instruments, for clysters are of great service in all these complaints.

"Fasting has a great power over diseases of this kind. We have cured many a case of bad dysentery at sea, depending principally upon entire abstinence from all food and drink other than pure water. A patient may be kept for days, a week or more, without any food, and yet run no risk of injury on that score. Many a person is killed by a relapse brought on by improper diet in such cases.

"Those who will, may refer to an account of the successful

treatment of a very dangerous case of dysentery in a colored boy, reported in the Water-Cure Manual."

CHRONIC DIARRHŒA, DYSENTERY, ETC.

Whenever these affections of the bowels become chronic, that is, of long standing, the treatment should be such as is best calculated to fortify and invigorate the general health.

NAUSEA, PAINS IN THE STOMACH AND BOWELS, AND VOMITING.

As regards the treatment of nausea, and pains of the stomach and bowels, arising from improper food and drink, I could not do better than quote the following remarks of a truly sensible writer, John Smith, whose work, "Curiosities of Common Water," was published in England, 1723:

"VOMITING BY WATER.

"By means of water all sickness at the stomach may be cured, which is done thus: Take four quarts of water, make it as hot over the fire as you can drink it; of which water let a quart be taken down at several draughts; then wrap a rag round a small piece of stick, till it is about the bigness of a man's thumb; tie it fast with some thread; and with this, by endeavoring gently to put it a little way down your throat, provoke yourself to vomit up again most of the water; then drink another quart, and vomit up that, and repeat the same the third and fourth time. You may also provoke vomiting by tickling your throat with your finger, or the feather-end of a goose-quill; but the cloth round a skewer maketh one vomit with most ease, which is done with no trouble when the stomach is full. And by this way of vomiting, which will be all performed in an hour's time, that vicious and ropy phlegm in the stomach, which causeth the sickness, will be cast up, so that the party in that time will be free from all that inward disturbance, if you use the remedy at first; but if the sickness hath continued for a time, it will require the same course once or twice more, which may be done in three or four hours, one after another, without any other inconvenience besides that of being a little sore in the breast the next day, which will soon go off by the force of nature. Which remedy, by forty years' experience, I look upon to be infallible in all sickness at the stomach, from what cause soever, and for all pains in the belly which seem to be above the navel; for these are all in the stomach, as by long experience I have found: which pains are generally counted the colic; but it is not so; for true colics are always below the navel, in the large intestine or colon. And by this means I have eased very great pains, caused by eating muscles that were poisonous; and it is also a certain cure for all surfeits or disorders that follow after much eating; so that the lives of multitudes might be saved by this means, who, for want of expelling what offends, do often die in misery. For, by thus cleansing the stomach at the first, the root of diseases proceeding from surfeiting, or unwholesome food, or any vicious humors from a bad digestion, are prevented; the stomach being the place in which all distempers do at first begin. No man was more subject to sickness than myself before thirty years of age; but since I found out the way of vomiting with water, which is now above forty years, I never have been sick for two days together; for when I find myself ill to any great degree, I betake myself to this way of vomiting, which, in an hour's time, restores me to ease, and perfectly removes my illness. And the same benefit all my family find in it, as do others also, whom I can persuade to try the experiment; which is such, that no physician whatever can advise a better to the king himself, should he fall sick. For, in the first place, it is not a nauseous remedy—it does not make the patient sick, as the best of all other vomits do; and then it is a vomit which is at our own command, since we can leave off when we please; and it infallibly works a cure to all sick stomachs.

"Some few, indeed, pretend that they are not able to vomit by this means. Now, if they cannot vomit, let them take a pint of water, when they find themselves ill from eating, and do so every three or four hours, eating no more till they are hungry; and they will find the water digest and carry off what was offensive. The ingenious Dr. Cheyne, in his Treatise of the Gout, doth affirm, that warm water drank freely in a morning, fasting, and at meals (and I say cold water is as good), hath been a sovereign remedy for restoring lost appetites, and strengthening weak digestions, when other more pompous medicines have failed. And he adviseth gouty persons, after excess, either in meat or drink, to swill down as much fair water as their stomachs will bear, before they go to bed, whereby they will reap these advantages: either the contents of the stomach will be thrown up, or both meat and drink will be much diluted, and the labor and expense of spirits in digestion much saved. And indeed I have found, by long experience, that nothing causeth so good a digestion as fair water; but this requires time to free us from the uneasiness that an ill digestion causeth, whereas vomiting is an immediate remedy, and frees a man from it upon the spot."

IN EXCESSIVE VOMITING, CAUSED BY IMPROPER FOOD, ETC.,

There should be practiced first a thorough cleansing of the stomach, as above explained; after which, small pieces of ice, or small draughts of cold water will be found very useful in arresting the symptom. This treatment is certainly very simple; but all who have occasion, may easily test its efficacy.

CHAPTER XIX.

TREATMENT OF DISEASES CONTINUED.

Meaning of "Cholera," "Contagion," and "Infection."—Is Cholera contagious?—Causes of Cholera.—Manner of an attack of Cholera.—Symptoms of Cholera.—First Stage.—Second Stage.—Stage of Collapse.—Nature of Cholera.—Orthodox Practice unsuccessful.—Water Treatment of Cholera.—Ice and Water Drinking.—Vomiting by means of Water.—Rubbing Wet Sheet in Spasm.—Priessnitz's mode.—Rationale of the Processes.—The Persian Treatment of Cholera.

CHOLERA.*

CHOLERA signifies a flow of bile; "cholera morbus," a morbid flow of bile. The term cholera, then, as used in modern times, is not correct, because, in the disease proper, there is no flow or discharge of bile whatever. The entire absence of bile in matters vomited and passed by the bowels, is a characteristic feature of the disease. Cholera, like many other medical terms, is used in a sense directly the opposite of its true and original signification. The term, however, is well understood, and that is sufficient for all practical purposes.

* For a more full exposition of the causes, symptoms, nature, and treatment of Cholera, the reader is referred to "Lectures on Cholera," by Joel Shew, M. D. Fowlers & Wells, New York.

Meaning of "Contagion" and "Infection."—The word "contagion" (from *contango*, to meet or touch) signifies, properly, the application of some morbid or poisonous matter to the body, through the medium of touch. A contagious disease is taken by a person coming in contact with another diseased, or by his being, in some mode or other, subjected to the morbid matter passing from the diseased body of the one affected.

An INFECTIOUS disease is one the principle of which exists in the atmosphere, without any relation or reference to the bodies of the sick. An infectious disease, then, is taken as easily without coming in contact with the sick as it may be with. If a disease is infectious and not contagious, all quarantine regulations are useless; and, in this case, there is no more danger in attending, nursing, or being with the sick, than in not doing so. This is an important PRACTICAL distinction between contagious and infectious diseases.

Is the Cholera a contagious Disease?—This is a difficult question to determine, if indeed that be possible at all. It is a "vexed question." Much proof may be brought on both sides. It is very certain, I think, that cholera is not contagious in the same degree as small-pox, and some other diseases. If it were strictly contagious—or, at least, contagious in the same degree as small-pox—it would live perpetually in a city like London, Paris, or New York, and not of itself soon pass away, as it always has done. Besides, many persons have been much among cholera patients—physicians, nurses, and attendants—and yet have not received the disease. Persons have slept with those having the cholera, dressed blisters for them, and nursed them in all manner of ways, remaining constantly with them night and day, and yet have not suffered an attack. We know, therefore, that cholera cannot be contagious in the same degree as small-pox, measles, scarlatina, and the like. Probably all epidemic diseases—diseases that rage, or come upon great numbers at the same time—are, to a greater or less extent, contagious. The bodies of persons suffering with such diseases, doubtless throw off matter that has a tendency to produce the same form of disease in others, whose systems are in a low condition of health.

Causes of Cholera.—Whether cholera is, or is not, a contagious disease, we know that certain classes of persons are far more subject to it than others; and investigations of this kind are far more useful in a practical view, than those concerning the question of contagion and non-contagion.

Judging from all the facts of cholera, we may lay down the following axiom: *that whatever tends in any way to depress or deteriorate the general health of the individual, must necessarily render the system more liable to an attack;* and, growing out of this, another axiom, *that whatever tends to fortify and establish the general health of the individual, is a natural means of enabling the system to ward off the disease.*

These are self-evident principles, and cannot be too well remembered or acted upon—not only with reference to cholera, but every known malady, and especially diseases of epidemic kind.

Manner of an attack of Cholera.—If it is impossible to arrive at the true nature of cholera, we may know and treat it by its effects. Mark well one thing: in its beginning it is in general a MILD disease. People are not struck down all of a sudden, as we have been often told, and without any premonitions of an attack. There must be a pre-existing disease. If a person is in all respects well, and practices uniformly good and regular habits, no attack of cholera can come upon him. There are people, however, who are thought by themselves and the many to be perfectly well, who are yet among the subjects most liable to cholera. Corpulent men, with red faces, high livers, the very personification of health, as people say, are very liable to diseases of the bowels, and consequently to cholera. The truth is, such persons are never well, and carry constantly within them the seeds of disease. Facts abundantly prove that no really healthy person can be attacked with cholera.

There is, then, preceding the real attack of cholera, a diseased condition of the stomach and bowels—a state of things which it is possible, in almost every conceivable case, to manage safely, and thus prevent the final invasion of the terrific disease.

Symptoms of Cholera—first stage.—The symptoms of cholera, as authors give them, are many and various. As in all other severe diseases, there will be much variation in the manner of the attack. The disease has been by some divided into three stages. After the mild diarrhœa, which has been generally for some days present, there occur griping pains in the stomach and bowels, nausea, tenesmus (or a bearing down and desire to evacuate the bowels, and without any effect); at other times there are watery discharges from the bowels; sometimes there is a thin, slimy discharge, streaked with blood. But generally the discharges are not attended with pain, as in dysentery, but take place with ease, almost without the consciousness of the patient. It is said that "in the debilitated, and especially in the intemperate, the evacuations from the bowels are, from the first, often extremely copious, whey-like, and produce a sense of extreme exhaustion, a faintness, or even fainting; and that in such cases, in a very few hours, the most terrible cramps, vomiting, and collapse come on." Any improper exposure, and especially any imprudence in eating, drinking, or the taking of medicine, will in such cases accelerate the coming on of the second and third stages. In the first stage the appetite is diminished or entirely gone, and the desire for cold water is proportionably increased. There are also shooting pains in the extremities, particularly the calves of the legs. Patients describe their symptoms as of all the blood rushing to the interior of the abdomen; sometimes feeling as if electric shocks were passing through the bowels, accompanied with very great and unendurable heat.

Second stage.—In what may be termed the second stage, there is almost constant vomiting and purging of what has been denominated "rice-water fluid." This turbid, whitish liquid, "pours again and again from the bowels in streams, and is spouted from the mouth as if from a pump." The vomiting itself is generally easy, and comparatively without effort, and appearing to give momentary relief. Again, there are violent pains of the stomach and bowels, and of the head and back, with violent spasms of the muscles, and more especially of the extremities.

The pain, we are told by those who have seen much of the disease, often causes the most courageous to make noisy outcries, and to roll themselves about as if frantic. The agony about the heart often experienced in cholera, is believed to be as great as that of any which mankind are ever brought to endure. In consequence of this agony, there comes on necessarily such extreme weakness, that the patient cannot move; the trunk of the body in particular becomes powerless.

The pulse may be full, or small and contracted. The skin is bathed in a clammy perspiration, and has a peculiar FEEL, like dough. Some have compared the skin in this state to a wet hide. The countenance is expressive of great anxiety and distress, although the mental faculties remain unimpaired. Already in this stage the secretion of the kidneys often entirely ceases; the thirst is inordinate—so great, in some instances, that the patient gets out of bed, goes to the pump, or wherever he may obtain water, and sometimes even drinks the fluid which he has before vomited. In no disease is the thirst so great as in cholera.

Stage of Collapse.—Next comes the stage of collapse, as it is called. A remarkable change takes place in the appearance of the patient. The surface becomes cold, and in many instances blue; the lips are purple, the tongue cold, and of the color of lead. The wrist becomes pulseless. The breath is also cold; the eyes are sunk deep in their sockets, and the whole appearance has changed and become ghastly as that of a corpse. In many instances so great a change takes place in a few hours, that near friends cannot recognize the sufferer. The peculiar appearance of the physiognomy in confirmed cholera, is so expressive of extreme anguish, that the name "triangular face" has been used to designate it. "It bears a striking resemblance to the appearance of AGE; and seems to arise from the paleness, wasting, and shrinking of the features, and the depressed and disturbed state of the mind, conveying into the countenance a strong expression of care, anxiety, and alarm." —*Orton, as quoted by Dr. Jas. Johnson.*

There is cold, profuse perspiration, which seems to exude in large drops from every pore; and, notwithstanding this coldness, the patient complains of the burning heat at the stomach, and craves more than ever cold water, and the cool fresh air. The watery discharges from the bowels continue; "the hands and fingers are shriveled, white, corrugated, and sodden, like those of a washerwoman after a long day's work. The voice is very peculiar, husky, and faint. At last the patient is free from pain and vomiting, and remains apparently tranquil; not willing to make the least exertion, and as if quietly awaiting the approach of death." Such are the symptoms constituting what is termed a state of collapse. The symptoms will, of course, vary greatly in different cases; sometimes coming on very suddenly, almost without any warning; at other times lingering for days.*

* Broussais thus describes the "exterior" symptoms of cholera:

"The muscles are strongly marked under the skin; the eyes are hollow, dry, and sunken; after some hours, the consistence of the eyeball seems to be dissolved; and one would say the eyes were turned inward by means of

If reaction or return of warmth and circulation appear in collapse, there is more hope for the patient; and yet there is danger from consecutive fever and kindred local affections; especially where inordinate dosing has been practiced, this holds true. It has been remarked, that when inebriates passed into a state of reaction following collapse, they were very apt to be attacked by *delirium tremens*, and were almost certain to die. I believe that about one half of all cholera patients in regular practice have perished with the disease.

Nature of Cholera.—The cholera is emphatically a disease of the mucous or lining membrane of the stomach and bowels. This internal *skin*, as it may be called, is much larger in extent than would at first be supposed. Beginning at the mouth and throat, descending, we have the œsophagus, stomach, duodenum or second stomach, the jejunum, illeum, the last three forming the small intestines; and the coecum, colon, and rectum, comprising the large intestine. This whole tract, upward of thirty feet in length, is lined with the mucous membrane, which is more than two thousand square inches, or about thirteen square feet in extent. It is upon

a thread. The aspect of the patient is hideous; the face very soon loses its fullness, and is contracted in a manner peculiar to these affections: but what causes the greatest astonishment, is the livid hue which spreads itself over the countenance as the disease advances. The extremities are cold; the tongue is usually pale, chill, broad, and flat; the breath cold, and the pulse feeble; the words are rather breathed than pronounced. The patient remains motionless, on the back; if you force them to lay upon the side, they cannot continue so long, but beg to be laid on their back, so that the breast may be raised. While the body thus remains still, they move the feet and hands, uncover the breast, complain of a fire within, and tear off the poultices and other warm applications placed on the stomach; they turn from one side to the other, but are not able to rise up. The color becomes darker and darker, and is soon livid. It varies, however, according to the natural complexion of the patient. Dark complexions become black or bluish; but those which are more transparent turn yellow, taking the color of bad gilding. This is followed by cessation of the pulse, which I shall call asphyxy. The pulse grows weak rapidly, and sometimes disappears in three hours, or even less. As soon as the pulse begins to grow feeble, the patient falls into the heaviness I have referred to: there are cases, however, in which he still preserves his strength when the pulse is extinct, and is even able to raise himself up, and go from one place to another; but this strength is soon lost, and the unhappy person falls powerless. After the cessation of the pulse, the black hue manifests itself with various rapidity, sometimes at the end of two or three hours, sometimes even in less; this depends upon the promptitude with which circulation ceases."

and through this great surface that the food is formed into chyme, afterward chyle, which last passes into the circulation and becomes blood. Effete and worn-out matters of the system are also thrown off in large quantities through the lower part of this surface. This extensive membrane is also supplied in all its parts, with myriads of nervous filaments, and through the ganglionic nervous system is brought into a very intimate connection with every part of the organism. Upon and through this membrane, the cholera manifests itself. There is congestion (stagnation of blood) in all of the abdominal organs; but if we are to regard the cholera a disease of any one particular part, it is the mucous membrane of the alimentary canal.

There are various theories among pathologists as to the true nature of cholera. Thus there is the nervous theory, so called—a theory implying that the nervous system, or the nervous fluid—of which so much is said and so little known—is wholly at fault. Another theory is that of congestion; and still another, that of acute inflammation. Whichever of these theories a practitioner may adopt, or whether he adopt no theory at all, he must treat the disease according to the SYMPTOMS as he finds them. All the most ingenious theorizing in the world will avail him nothing, when he comes to undertake the serious matter of treating the sick. I repeat, every judicious practitioner will treat cholera ACCORDING TO THE SYMPTOMS AS HE FINDS THEM AT THE TIME. Moreover, whether he be a theorizer or not, he must be, to a considerable extent, AN EXPERIMENTER, so difficult are many things in the medical art.

Orthodox Practice in Cholera.—Dr. Elliotson, of London, in "Principles and Practice of Medicine," says: "We are not in the least more informed as to the proper remedies, than we were when the first case of cholera occurred; we have not been instructed, in the least, by those who have had the disease to treat. Some say they have cured the disease by bleeding; others by calomel; others by opium; and others, again, say that opium does harm. No doubt many poor creatures have died uncomfortably, who would have died tranquilly if nothing had been done to them. Some were placed in hot water, or in hot air, and had opium and calomel, and other stimulants; which, altogether, were more than their systems would bear, and more than would have been borne if they had been so treated even in perfect health." And again

"I am sorry to say that, of the cases I had to treat, the patients nearly all died. I tried two or three sorts of treatment. Some had opium and calomel, in large and full doses; but they died. Hot air was applied externally; and I got two to BREATHE hot air. I had a tube passed through boiling water, so that they might inhale hot air. It was found vain to attempt to warm people by hot air applied EXTERNALLY. They were nearly as cold as before; we could not raise their temperature; and therefore I thought of making them breathe hot air; but both patients died about the period that death usually takes place. It was said that saline treatment was likely to be of use; and I accordingly tried it with some patients. At first I exhibited half a drachm of sesquicarbonate of soda every hour; and thinking that it might not be quite enough, I exhibited a drachm. In one patient, at St. Thomas's Hospital, I ordered an injection containing an ounce of the same remedy; but the greater part of it came away, and the patient died. Hot air was used in this case as well as the others." This quotation, from one of the most able as well as most candid of all medical authorities, exhibits truthfully the state of the old school as regards this dire disease.

Treatment of Cholera.—The diarrhœa which so generally precedes the real attack of cholera, should be treated like any other diarrhœa, on general principles. It would be better for the individual to practice entire fasting from all food—the *hunger-cure*—as the Germans call it—until the diarrhœa ceases. The human body, as I have said, is composed of about nine tenths water, in its best health; therefore it is that pure water alone will sustain it so wonderfully for days and even weeks. Barn-yard fowls, as before remarked, when kept without food, will not survive the ninth day if they have no water; but with water they will live more than twice as long—to the twentieth day. If you wish to cure a diarrhœa safely, effectually, and without harm to the constitution, practice fasting, and live on pure soft water until it ceases. Then begin taking food with extreme caution; at the regular meal-times only, and an exceedingly small quantity at first. Some will tell you that fasting produces disease, but physiology and pathology prove that neither fasting nor starvation causes any such result. The individual who is starved, having at the same time water to drink, dies of mere *inanition*, and not of *organic disease.*

According to the Graefenberg plan, the cold hip bath, cold water drinking, injections, pure fresh air, and the famous wet girdle of Priessnitz, are the means to be used; and these may be employed in connection with the fasting recommended.

The great thirst in cholera is one of the most troublesome symptoms, and, according to all experience, it is one of the most grateful things imaginable for the patient to be allowed all the cold water he desires. There is no disease in which thirst is so great—none in which so much cold water is drank. Some thought that cold water did harm in certain cases. So it might, if the water was hard and bad, or if the patient had been kept long from it, or, especially, if he had been over-drugged. In all cases of inward feverishness and thirst, it is of the greatest importance that the water be *pure* and *soft*. If people would take half the pains respecting water that they do in obtaining tea and coffee, they might have at least an abundance of filtered rain water, which is always a luxury, and remarkably favorable to health.

In 1831 and 1832, the practitioners of Europe and this country did not agree upon this matter; at least, not for a time at first. But at length the large majority came to believe in the free use of water and ice internally, to gratify the longings for drink. But there is a reason why some men might make a mistake in regard to their conclusion, as to whether the *ad libitum* use of water internally were safe in cholera; it is this: in certain states and conditions of the stomach and alimentary canal, *water appears to increase vomiting*. Thus I can conceive that a cholera patient would often be made to vomit worse on taking water, especially if it had been withheld from him. But we are not to infer from this that the water is necessarily bad. In poisoning, for instance, a patient may drink and vomit gallons of water, and yet when the offending cause is removed, the vomiting ceases. Causing a sedative effect upon the stomach—and water is one of the most effectual of all means possible by which to bring about this indication—is the best possible means of finally arresting vomiting from whatever cause. Give the patient, from the first, all the cold water he desires, and the stomach will take care of its own vomiting. Small pieces of ice held constantly in the mouth, and often swallowed, is believed by many the best mode of managing this symptom. The most judicious rule, I think, would be to consult the patient's inclination. I should not fear to let him drink all he desired; if the vomiting were increased at first, that would be no harm.

The drinking of water and the use of ice internally—any thing, in short, that produces a sedative effect upon the abdominal organs—will tend to arrest the vomiting and discharges from the bowels. Bathing also has the same effect, but more particularly the long-continued cold hip bath. This is Priessnitz's great means of arresting all unnatural discharges from the bowels. Meantime, also, cold injections are to be used. These cause a constringing effect, and act, also, as a tonic to the general system. All internal applications of cold water act by dilution as well as coolness, rendering morbid matters less acrid, and, by the water-purging, it also carries off these humors of disease. The wet girdle Priessnitz uses between the periods of the hip bath. This is, at least, three yards of good heavy linen toweling, one half its whole length wet, to come next the surface, and all well wrapped about the abdomen. It is a great tonic to the general system, as well as astringent to the stomach and bowels, in arresting the discharges.

Vomiting by water may be serviceable in cholera. Some practitioners have observed, strange as it may appear, that emetics serve to arrest vomiting in this disease. Vomiting by means of water—that is, vomiting caused by drinking quickly a large quantity of blood-warm water—a quart or more—is often very useful in derangements of the stomach and bowels. Spasms of the stomach I have known arrested immediately by this simple remedy. I am confident that a thorough cleansing of the stomach with lukewarm water in this way, would often be a most excellent remedy in the early stages of cholera. Vomiting thus practiced, acts partly by removing offensive matters from the stomach, partly by promoting a better circulation toward the surface, and partly by inducing a healthful perspiration upon the skin. This is a perfectly safe remedy, and is certain of doing some good. In fits of dyspepsia caused by surfeiting, the vomiting will be found most excellent. This advice may apply especially to those who cannot control their appetites, but would rather feast and gorge themselves, even at the expense of health.

All the internal applications, when properly made, do much good, by supplying serum for the blood. The great and copious discharges from the stomach and bowels rob the blood, with most fearful rapidity, of its watery part. Water, by drinking and by injections, as well as externally applied, goes directly to make up this deficiency; and hence the great benefit from the free use of water in this disease. It is to be remarked, also, that the greater the thirst, the more rapidly is water absorbed into the circulation by the mucous membrane of the stomach and bowels.

Experience proves—those tell us who have had the disease to treat—that heat externally applied, is productive of no benefit. It does no good to attempt to warm the patients. The general effect of heat is to debilitate; and the fact that cholera patients always dread hot air and hot baths, is proof enough why these should not be used; the constant desire in the active stages of the disease is for coolness, fresh air, and cold water to drink. I would not be understood as saying, that heat internally applied, by means of water, which produces at the same time various other effects than merely those of heat, can do no good. But the desire for coolness generally, in the active form of the disease, is, beyond doubt, the normal indication of nature, such as an animal would naturally seek to gratify.

Spasms in cholera are best relieved by the vigorous application of the rubbing wet sheet. Have a linen sheet of good weight (but cotton will answer), wring it only slightly out of cold water, and put it about the whole body, rubbing at the same time energetically, over the sheet and not with it. This is a famous application for bringing the blood to the surface, and of relieving spasms and cramps from whatever cause. In three or four minutes the sheet becomes warm, upon which it is again re-wet, and applied as before. Water by this application becomes a great antispasmodic.

It was found in the hospitals of Paris, that dry friction alone was often effectual in quieting spasms beyond any ordinary remedy; but wet friction is much the best.

The cold perspiration in cholera may be greatly relieved, if not wholly prevented, by ablutions. This is a symptom of debility, and the tonic effect of water to the skin is a sure preventive. In the night sweats of consumption, the same effects are caused by baths.

Priessnitz's treatment of Cholera.—In 1831, there was much cholera about Graefenberg, considering the number of inhabitants there. Priessnitz cured, he tells us, upward of twenty cases, being all that he had the opportunity of treating. He commenced in the first stages of the disease, and treated the patient as follows: they were subjected to a rubbing with a wet linen sheet, in which the whole body was wrapped, and all the parts of the surface were energetically rubbed with it—that is, over the sheet. To counteract the violent fits of nausea, much water was drank, so as to produce vomiting; after the rubbing, a cold water injection and a cold hip bath were employed, to counteract the diarrhœa; and while undergoing constant rubbing of the surface, the patients remained in the water till the sickness and diarrhœa subsided. After the hip bath and rubbing, a wet bandage or girdle was placed around the body, upon which the patients went to bed; after sleeping they were again put into a cold bath. Cold drinks and cold food only were taken during the convalescence; and by these means the disease was overcome.

This appears like a very simple treatment; but it may be made a most energetic one, as every physician acquainted with such applications can easily see. The dripping sheet, with the brisk rubbing upon its surface, is, as I have before said, a powerful means of relieving spasms, arising from whatever cause. The dry rubbing, which is not a tenth part as good as the wet, was found in Paris sufficient to render calm and quiet the poor sufferers, when the terrible spasms were upon them. The water drinking and vomiting in nausea cleanses the stomach, produces a tonic effect upon its internal surface, and thus forestalls the vomiting in cholera. It helps, moreover, to cleanse the bowels and prevent the diarrhœa. The deep, cold hip bath (for it is such that Priessnitz uses), has a very powerful effect in constringing the opening capillaries of the mucous membrane of the stomach, and alimentary canal generally, and in arresting the vomiting and discharges from the bowels. Each and all of these applications, if energetically persevered in, tend most powerfully to keep down the inordinate burning and thirst.

Priessnitz had not been in the habit of practicing warm water vomiting. I conversed much with him respecting all his modes of using water, during a stay of nearly two months at Graefenberg, last winter. To seek vomiting as an effect, seemed never to have been an object with him. Even by drinking cold water, vomiting sometimes comes on, but not often. If we wish to cause that symptom, as in cramps and distress arising from offending matters in the stomach or alimentary canal, blood-warm water is by far the most speedy and effectual in its action. In reference to this mode, Priessnitz remarked, that he would do no violence to the system. I told him I had practiced it in many instances, in cases of old and very feeble persons, and that the result was always apparently good. On reflection, he admitted that the remedy must be a good one. I will here remark, that if there is heat and thirst, the water should always be used cold, although the blood-warm will do much good even then.

Here let it be understood, I do not claim a great deal for Priessnitz's experience in cholera. He is a most candid man, and one that would not, for his right hand, mislead the world in so important a matter as treating the sick. He never fails to tell us that his cholera cases were taken in the very beginning of the disease. At the same time, however, he affirms that the water treatment is incomparably the best mode that can be adopted in all stages of the disease.

The Persian Treatment.—The Persian treatment of cholera, as given by Dr. Scouttetten, in some respects resembles that of Priessnitz. It is thus given:

"The following account will give an idea of the mode of treatment at Baku, which contains 12,000 Persians and 800 Russians. The treatment commenced at the moment of the attack. From the first symptoms the patients were undressed, even in the streets, and then cold affusions were applied. The extremities, the trunk, and particularly the chest and the shoulders, were rubbed and shampooed, and the contracted limbs were extended.

"These manipulations were performed for two or three hours by a dozen persons, on the same individual, while the affusion of cold water was continued. Having come home, he went to bed, and a warm tea was given him to produce perspiration; if this appeared, the patient was regarded as out of danger. A strict regimen was however enjoined for nine days; only light soups of rice and of tender meats were allowed, and he was recommended to take moderate exercise in the open air daily. Arrangements were made by the authorities so well, that vessels of water were placed at the corners of the streets, and even on the roads. No one passed the night alone. When a person was attacked with the cholera in the street, all the by-standers attended to him; every one ran to him with vessels of water in their hands, and when one was tired of rubbing another took his place. If a person was taken sick at his house, assistance was asked and immediately obtained."

All who are acquainted with the water-cure of Priessnitz, will see at once that the cold affusions often repeated, in connection with the friction and shampooing of the surface, would have a very powerful effect in bringing the blood toward that part, in relieving the spasms, preventing the internal heat and distress, arresting the vomiting and discharges, supporting the strength; in short, in warding off every symptom of the disease. The nine days' strict regimen, also, was most excellent; although soups, especially of flesh meat, are not the best in such cases. As to the warm drink, that is a small matter, even if not the best. One thing is certain, the Persian patients could not have longed much for cold water and fresh air while being subjected to so vigorous an out-door treatment with cold water.

Thus much I have considered necessary to say on cholera. Those who desire to peruse a much more detailed account of the disease, are referred to my lectures on the subject.

CHAPTER XX.

TREATMENT OF DISEASES CONCLUDED.

Hæmorrhages.—General Principles of Treatment.—Bleeding from the Lungs.—How to be Treated.—Bleeding from the Bowels.—Mode of Treatment.—Hæmorrhage from the Womb.—This is to be Treated on the same general Principles as all Hæmorrhages.—Nose Bleed.—Modes of Curing it.—Paronychia, Whitlow, and Felon.—Causes of the Disease, and Treatment.—Earache.—How to be Treated.—Toothache, and its Cure.

HÆMORRHAGES.

Hæmorrhages, or bleeding coming from the lungs, stomach, bowels, etc., are all to be treated on the same general principles. We cannot always tell from what part the blood issues; but we need not, for that reason, be at a loss how to proceed in the treatment.

BLEEDING FROM THE LUNGS

Is the most common form of internal hæmorrhage. The treatment may be conducted as follows: In a case that is at all alarming, the quick and thorough *chilling* of the system, and particularly the chest, should be practiced. The whole chest should, as quickly as possible, be covered with thick linen cloths, dripping wet in the very coldest water that can be obtained. Pounded ice, or snow, if these can be had, are more effectual. They should be placed immediately upon the skin. Thoroughly chilling the neck is good, at the same time. Professor Elliotson, of London, a man of very great experience, observes, that it is surprising how patients bear cold in this disease. He had never known a case to be injured in this way.

The patient must be kept as comfortable as possible, after the bleeding is arrested. Food must be very light. Drinking freely of the coldest water should be practiced at the first of the attack.

By physicians of the ordinary or old practice, bleeding is much relied upon, in cases that will bear it. But, generally, the symptom occurs in those of frail, weak systems. Such can poorly withstand this formidable means. Many are killed by it, and, in not a few cases, a severe relapse is caused by the so-called remedy.

HÆMORRHAGE FROM THE BOWELS.

The treatment here consists mainly of the same as in hæmorrhage from the lungs, except that the local applications are to be made over the bowels instead of the chest. Prolonged cold hip baths will here be very useful. The wet girdle should also be worn to invigorate the affected parts.

HÆMORRHAGE FROM THE WOMB.

This is to be treated on the same general principles as hæmorrhage from the bowels. In all these cases nothing is to be feared from the effects of cold. There is always too much heat in the part from which the blood escapes.

NOSE BLEED.

Every one knows the good effects of cold in this trifling, though sometimes dangerous affection. Placing a cold key in the neck will often arrest the hæmorrhage. A piece of ice, or pouring cold water in the neck, is still better. Cold water may be snuffed up the nostrils. Also, wash the face and neck, and the whole body, if need be, in cold water. The foot bath is very useful in this complaint.

PARONYCHIA, WHITLOW, OR FELON.

The word *paronychia* is derived from two Greek words, signifying "near" "the nail." This name was given anciently to an inflammation seated near this part, generally of the fingers, but sometimes of the toes. It may be seated quite near the surface, but is generally deeper, and often between the periosteum, or enveloping membrane of the bone, and the bone itself. The disease is generally known by the name of *whitlow,* or *felon,* the latter being the more common name, especially when it is severe.

Mechanical injuries appear sometimes to cause the disease. It comes on oftener, however, apparently without any exciting cause. As far as the writer's observation extends, the disease attacks only persons whose general health is not good. Such, at least, appears to be the general rule.

As this is one of the most painful affections to which we are subject, the treatment is no unimportant matter. There is an old woman's remedy which we will first mention,—one which is said sometimes to have effected a cure, especially if it is taken early. A vessel of weak lye is placed upon embers or a hot stove. The part affected is immersed in the liquid of a moderate temperature, which is gradually raised to as high a heat as can possibly be borne, so that the part is quite "par-boiled." We do not doubt but that such a mode will, in some cases, at once destroy the inflammation. Probably pure water, used without the lye, would be fully as good.

But, sometimes the inflammation may go on in spite of all ordinary means. What then is to be done? The mode, according to surgery, is freely to open the part. Lay it open for some distance beyond the tenderest part, deep down to the very bone. Thorough work must be made of it the first time, for patients never let us make the second attempt. In some instances, at the urgent request of patients, we have resorted to the knife, but we confess we would not allow it to be used upon ourselves; we should prefer keeping the part free from pain, and letting it take its course. We believe keeping it constantly immersed in ice-cold water would form the most effectual means of arresting the inflammation and preventing its raising to a head; and that this mode is certain to quell down the pain most effectually, every one who has the opportunity may test for himself. This is an affection in which we have a perfect demonstration of the great power of cold water to quell pain. Severe as it may be, we immerse the part in very cold water, when, all at once, the pain grows less and soon dies away. Keep it thus immersed, taking care to keep the water very cold, and the pain does not return. We lately had a case in which a physician's skill had been exhausted, and for days the patient could get no sleep. But by having a large bowl of cold water at his bed-side, and keeping his hand immediately therein, he could sleep as well as any one, and keeping the bad finger thus constantly cool, he soon got well.

EARACHE.

This disease, although considered a small affair, is not always free from danger, and is more liable to be attended with serious results than toothache. It has the same causes as inflammations in general.

Treatment.—As in all other aches, arising from inflammation, the patient should practice perfect and entire abstinence from all food (even though it should require days, although that would seldom be necessary), until all pain is gone. Water of course is to be drank as thirst demands. The great poultice, the wet sheet, is here good. Vapor baths and sweating are, in severe cases, likewise beneficial. The moist compress over the whole side of the head and neck is useful. Then having this covered by flannel, with a warm brick or bottle of water against it on going to rest, seems in many cases to be one of the best things that can be done, and sometimes better than the cold. Washing and rubbing the side of the face, neck, and back of the ear, violently, will be found serviceable. A general bath will often arrest this disease. While I was at Graefenberg the past winter (1847–8), a little fellow, about four years of age, undergoing the treatment, was attacked severely with the earache. For this Priessnitz ordered the head bath, to be taken on the side affected, the water to be slightly tepid, that is, to have the extreme chill taken off, it being very cold. This was to be taken as long and often as necessary. It very soon arrested the pain. The treatment was commenced near evening. Patient had no supper. He had for the night a wet bandage over the ear and side of the head, covered with a dry one; also a little wet lint within the ear. The little fellow slept well, and in the morning the ear broke and the matter exuded. In the afternoon again, the other ear commenced aching, and the same treatment was practiced, and with like success as before.

TOOTHACHE.

Cold water, taken in the mouth, every one knows, sometimes causes the toothache; especially with those who are in the habit of using hot and stimulating food and drinks. So, likewise, it is known that holding very cold water in the mouth for a continuance, changing it frequently, will often arrest the toothache, for the time at least.

Priessnitz's usual mode is as follows: Tepid water is held in the mouth until it begins to grow warm, when it is changed; at the same time the face, cheeks, neck, and parts behind the ears are rubbed violently with the hands, which are dipped frequently in very cold water. It is well also to rub the gums till they bleed smartly. Sometimes it is necessary to add cold shallow foot baths. Captain Claridge says, that while at Graefenberg he never saw toothache resist this treatment. Those who are accustomed to cold water, will find that a powerful douche, or any very cold general bath, will be very serviceable. Walking thinly clad in cold air is likewise a good means.

APPENDIX.

CHRONIC RHEUMATISM.—CASE OF COL. ROLPH.

"A single fact is worth a shipload of argument."

Something upward of two years ago, Col. J. R. Rolph, of Huntington, Long Island, wrote us as follows for publication in the Water-Cure Manual:

Huntington, February 3d, 1847.

Having been long afflicted with disease, and feeling that Hydropathy, with the blessing of God, has been the means of affording me more relief than any other mode of treatment to which I have ever resorted, I am induced to add to the multiplied cases of relief which the water-cure is effecting, my testimony as to its results in my own case.

For the last fifteen years I have been almost constantly dyspeptic, and being a farmer of slender frame but laborious habits, I was attacked four years since, after a season of uncommon toil and exposure, with rheumatism. This had been manifesting itself slightly for some months, but not so severely as to cause any alarm until mid-winter, when it became so severe that for several days I was hardly able to get from one room to another. This was from home. In about ten days I was able to get home. As I was slowly improving, no physician was called in. I continued to recover, so that in the spring I was able to resume my occupation. I soon found, however, that my rheumatic disease was manifesting itself in other parts of the system, and it continued to spread until I was unfit for labor; yet I did not yield to the dictates of prudence, but persevered, not merely in active exercise, but in hard labor, until by the close of the season, instead of exhibiting the sprightliness of a man of thirty years, I presented the decrepitude of approaching old age. I now made up my mind to rest from labor for a while, and try the effects of ease upon my complaint. For two years more I remained much as I had been for the year past, the enemy seeming to have complete possession of my joints, but sometimes showing himself by affecting only the muscles, and often my lameness would be manifested in the most distant and opposite parts at the same time, and often, as if by sympathy, the corresponding joints or parts of my limbs would be affected exactly alike at the same time. During this time I often conversed with, and frequently called in my family physician, a man whom I shall ever love for his candor and honesty of purpose in treating me. He having been long acquainted with my system and habits, was frank to admit his opinion as to the inefficacy of taking much medicine. I therefore confined myself principally to the application of domestic treatment, such as bathing the parts with warm lotions, wearing warm flannel, bandages, plasters, etc.; and occasionally, when my attacks were severe, with his advice, I applied blisters, which usually appeared to produce good effects. Upon the whole, my system appeared to be sinking. I was constantly dyspeptic, had an increasing sallowness of countenance, and my energies seemed to be on the decline. I have ever been slow to fall in with what so many stand ready to call the delusions of our day. I had heard and read of Priessnitz's new mode of treatment, and it appeared at first like a mere chimera; but feeling that ordinary medicine was not to give me relief, I gave the water treatment a little serious investigation, and after the strong recommendations of friends, and two or three consultations with yourself upon the subject, I concluded to make a trial of it, which I commenced at home. I almost immediately began to feel the good effects of it. But not believing that in this treatment every man might be his own doctor, I resolved to put myself under the care of some practitioner of the water-cure, and the time being in the extreme heat of mid-summer, when a residence in the cities is almost intolerable to countrymen, I resorted to an establishment in the country, where I remained five weeks under almost constant improvement of my lameness, and correction of my dyspeptic habits, after which I returned home, and have kept up the treatment with great success, following up the system of diet usually practiced at the establishments, which I consider an important aid to the treatment, and would go far toward preserving those who are already healthy from the need of medical treatment. Although I am almost entirely free from any symptoms of rheumatism, yet I do not consider myself well. I have some trouble yet from dyspepsia, increased perhaps by over-eating. My appetite is uniformly good, my strength is constantly increasing, and I think it must be said, to the praise of water treatment, I have not had the slightest cold this winter, although I have exposed myself to the weather every day without exception, and my clothing being much thinner than what I have ordinarily worn in winter. Since my return home, which is near six months, I have dismissed my cane, which had been my constant companion for months previous, and am happy to say that I have not once felt the need of its assistance. My treatment has consisted of sitz baths, the douche, the rubbing sheet, the wet sheet, wearing bandages constantly on the body and parts mostly affected, and the morning wash of my whole person never once omitted. The forms of crisis in my case have been various and repeated, and I have even at present one which water-cure patients hail as a harbinger of good. I cannot find terms to express the gratitude I feel for the confidence in the water treatment which I obtained from consultations with you, and for the strength of purpose which your advice has given me to persevere in it. J. R. R.

We will remark, that Col. Rolph commenced the treatment only a few months since. He is not one of those who are in the habit of exaggeration, but speaks the facts as they are. Although having received so great benefit, Mr. R. has but just entered upon the threshold of what he will yet experience.

We published the foregoing account by permission of our patient; and we now refer to the case as a very strong one for hydropathy. It was a very severe and obstinate one—one of the worst cases of chronic rheumatism we have ever known to be cured. Many persons with cases of scarce half the severity of Col. Rolph's, however, will fail of cure *for want of perseverance in the treatment.*

The colonel is none of your "half-way" men, in whatever he undertakes; and as to how large a share of credit his most estimable wife has in the matter, would not perhaps be easy to define. Getting up at 4 o'clock, morning after morning, through a whole tedious winter, and putting her crippled husband in a cold wet sheet, afterward giving him a cold bath, and then commencing the routine of household duties, all this to be followed by the forenoon, and afternoon, and evening treatment, would certainly test the patience of any devoted wife. The husband ought to be the wife's best nurse, and the wife the husband's; so it was in this case.

Col. Rolph is now well and strong. He has been so in fact for nearly the whole time since the above account was written. He has grown, month by month, more hardy, and is, as he says, as well, to all appearances, as he ever was in his life. He appears decidedly younger, and more healthful and enduring, than ever before, since we have known him, a period of nearly three years.

Chronic rheumatism, that has fixed itself deeply and firmly upon the system, be it remembered, is always a most difficult disease to cure. It requires more patience, self-denial, and perseverance than most men possess.—*Water-Cure Journal, May,* 1849.

HYGIENIC HABITS AND OPINIONS OF HOWARD, THE PHILANTHROPIST.

That Howard, the Philanthropist, was a great and pre-eminently good man, the world freely admits. A knowledge, therefore, of his hygienic habits and opinions concerning matters of health can but be interesting to every reflecting mind.

Howard lived at a time very different from the present. No temperance reformation had gone forth to shed its blessings upon millions of the degraded and suffering of humanity; the hygienic and medicinal virtues of cold water were comparatively unknown, and almost every notion in the popular mind concerning health was an erroneous one. Even at this day, in Howard's native country, it is believed by the many that alcoholic drinks, such as wine, porter, etc., are not only harmless but positively necessary, in order to enable the human body to withstand fatigue and exposure to cold, and to resist disease; and many pass through life without scarce ever tasting of pure cold water, much less to wash the body in that element; and in the construction of dwellings, and the habits of dress, the greatest pains are taken to avoid exposure to cold air, so injurious is it supposed to be. Howard, as we shall see, had the sagacity to detect many of these popular fallacies, and recommended his modes by example as well as precept.

Howard was exposed to the influence of pestilence and disease in its most malignant forms, probably more than any other human being who has ever lived. "This man," says one biographer, "visited all Europe, not to survey the sumptuousness of palaces, or the stateliness of temples; not to make accurate measurements of the remains of ancient grandeur, nor to form a scale of the curiosities of modern art; not to collect medals, or to collate manuscripts; but to dive into the depths of dungeons; to plunge into the infection of hospitals; to survey the mansions of sorrow and of pain; to take the gauge and dimensions of misery, depression, and contempt; to remember the forgotten; to attend to the neglected; to visit the forsaken; and to compare and collate the distresses of all men in all countries." "He traveled," says another, "between fifty and sixty thousand miles, for the sole purpose of relieving the distresses of the most wretched of the human race. The fatigue, the dangers, the privations he underwent or encountered for the good of others, were such as no one else was ever exposed to in such a cause, and such as few could have endured. He often traveled several days and nights in succession, without stopping—over roads almost impassable, in weather the most inclement, and with accommodations the meanest and most wretched. Summer and winter, heat and cold, rain and snow, in all their extremes, failed alike to stay him for a moment in his course: while plague, and pestilence, and famine, instead of being evils that he shunned, were those with which he was most familiar; and to many of whose horrors, he voluntarily exposed himself, visiting the foulest dungeons, filled with malignant infection—spending forty days in a filthy and infected lazaretto—plunging into military encampments where the plague was committing its most frightful ravages—and visiting where none of his conductors dared to accompany him."

Under such circumstances, the habits of Howard were very simple, rigid, and abstemious in the extreme. In all seasons he made it a point of the utmost importance to practice daily bathing. "Water," says Dr. Aiken, "was one of his principal necessaries, for he was a very Mussulman in his ablutions; and if nicety had place with him in any respect, it was in the perfect cleanliness of his whole person." "These ablutions," says another (Dr. Brown), "he regularly performed in the depth of the coldest winter, by plunging into a bath whenever he had the opportunity of doing so—and when he had not, he would frequently lay himself down for some considerable time between two sheets, wet for the express purpose of communicating to his body the desirable degree of cold." According to another author, "both on rising and going to bed, he often swathed himself in coarse towels, wet with the coldest water; in that state he remained half an hour, or more, and then threw them off, freshened and invigorated, as he said, beyond measure." He never used a great-coat, we are told, even when in the coldest countries. For many of the last years of his existence, he tasted neither flesh, fish, or fowl; and near the close of his life, he wrote in his diary, "I am firmly persuaded, as to the health of our bodies, that herbs and fruits will sustain nature, in every respect, far beyond the best flesh!" So prudent was he of time, that he strenuously avoided dining parties, nor would he sit when taking his simple meal of tea, milk, and rusks.

On becoming acquainted with these singular habits of Howard, one would naturally be led to suppose that his constitution must, from the first, have been a strong one, capable of enduring great exposures and fatigue. Such, however, is not the fact. He was, when young, as he himself tells us, of very feeble health.

Some of his peculiar habits and opinions appear in a quotation from Pratt's Gleanings (1796), as follows:

"Some days after his first return from an attempt to mitigate the plague at Constantinople, he favored me with a morning visit to London. The weather was so very terrific, that I had forgot his inveterate exactness, and had yielded up the hope of expecting him. Twelve at noon was the hour, and exactly as the clock struck, he entered my room; the wet—for it rained in torrents—dripping from every part of his dress, like water from a sheep just landed from its washing. He would not have attended to his situation, having sat himself down with the utmost composure, and begun conversation, had I not made an offer of dry clothes. 'Yes,' said he, smiling, 'I had my fears, as I knocked at your door, that we should go over the old business of apprehension about a little rain water, which, though it does not run off my back as it does from that of a duck, does me as little injury, and after a long drought is scarcely less refreshing. The coat that I have on has been as often wetted through as any duck's in the world, and indeed gets no other cleaning. I assure you, a good soaking shower is the best brush for broadcloth. You, like the rest of my friends, throw away your pity upon my supposed hardships with just as much reason as you commiserate the common beggars, who, being familiar with storms, necessity, and nakedness, are a thousand times (so forcible is habit) less to be compassioned than the sons and daughters of ease and luxury, who, accustomed to all the enfeebling refinements of feathers by night and fires by day, are taught to shiver at a breeze. All this is the work of art, my good friend; nature is intrepid, hardy, and adventurous; but it is a practice to spoil her with indulgences from the moment we come into the world. A soft dress and soft cradle begin our education in luxury, and we do not grow more manly the more we are gratified; on the contrary, our feet must tread upon carpets, breathe, as it were, in fire, and fear the least change in the weather. You smile,' said Mr. Howard, after a pause, 'but I am a living instance of the truths I insist on. A more puny youngster than myself was never seen. If I wet my feet I was sure to take cold. I could not put on my shirt without its being aired. To be serious, I am convinced *that what emasculates the body debilitates the mind,* and renders both unfit for those exertions which are of such use to us as social beings. I therefore entered upon a reform of my constitution, and have succeeded in such a degree that I have neither had a cough, cold, the vapors, nor any more alarming disorder, since I surmounted the seasoning. Formerly, mulled wines, and spirits, and great fires, were to comfort me, and to keep out the cold, as it is called; the perils of the day were to be baffled by something taken hot on going to bed; and before I pursued my journey the next morning, *a dram* was to be swallowed to fortify the stomach! Believe me,' said Mr. Howard, 'we are too apt to *invert the remedies which we ought to prescribe for ourselves.* Thus we are for ever giving *hot* things when we should administer *cold.* We bathe in hot instead of cold water, we use a dry bandage when we should use a wet one, and we increase our food and clothing when we should, by degrees, diminish both. If we should trust more to Nature, and suffer her to apply her own remedies to cure her own diseases, the formidable catalogue of maladies would be reduced to one half, at least, of their present number.' "

Concerning the treatment of certain diseases, and of the most fatal kind, which Howard's mode of life brought him much in contact with, his opinions were as singular, and as much opposed to the prevailing notions of the times in which he lived, as were those concerning the preservation of health. He had, moreover, as might well be expected from his great energy of character, remarkable success in his treatment of those diseases; and he was often called upon to prescribe in sickness, by those who knew him, in preference to regularly bred physicians; and, indeed, the malignant fever which terminated his existence, was caught while he was thus engaged in relieving the sick. From the best accounts we have, it appears his modes of treatment were very simple, and that he depended mainly upon the natural means of water, air, exercise, and diet. Respecting the best modes of preserving and invigorating the general health, amid the infection of hospitals prisons, etc., Howard remarked as follows:

"I have frequently been asked," says this distinguished philanthropist, "what precautions I used to preserve myself from infection in the prisons and hospitals which I visit. I here answer once for all, that next to the free goodness and mercy of the Author of my being, temperance and cleanliness are my preservatives. Trusting in Divine Providence, and believing myself in the way of my duty, I visit the most noxious cells, and while thus employed, I fear no evil. I never enter a hospital or a prison before breakfast, and in an infected room I seldom draw my breath deeply."

On his arrival at Scio, Howard visited a very convenient hospital for lepers, the only one he had ever seen; and with his usual attention to health and cleanliness, persuaded the vice-consul to recommend the directors to add a bath for each six persons.

Before he left England for the last time, Howard promised the much-lamented Dr. Currie that he would make more particular inquiries in regard to the empirical use of cold water in the plague, for in the raging frenzy attending this dire disease, some sailors at Constantinople had thrown themselves into the sea, and on being taken out, recovered—a happy temerity, as Dr. Currie says, not imitated by the regular practitioners.

Such were some of the hygienic habits and opinions of Howard, the Philanthropist. We do not contend that all his practices were the best that could be, but that, on the whole, he was far in advance of the age. His good sense and energy of character led him, in many respects, to practice in direct opposition to the opinions of the world. In the treatment of some of the most loathsome and intractable forms of disease, he was proverbially more successful than medical men. It is much to be regretted, however, that he erred in regard to the use of tea. He was led, no doubt, to believe, as thousands have done, *that the stimulation caused by the article was actual strength;* and thus his health was materially injured, and life shortened; but, on the whole, we can but admire much the good practical sense and habits of this truly great and good man.

HYDROPATHIC LACONICS.*

1. At all times and seasons hydropathy may be practiced with the most *certain advantage;* but Autumn, Winter, and Spring are the best seasons for carrying out the treatment most effectively.

2. It is *general disorder* which first produces *local disease*—and it is therefore the restoration of the *general health* which must constitute the first step toward the removal of *local disease.*

3. In treating chronic diseases, the effect of the hydropathic method is an exaltation of the general health and strength.

4 "Many persons of great experience practice well empirically (this is Priessnitz's case) without much brains or reasoning; but he who begins upon principle, and then profits by experience, must become a much more skilful practitioner."—*Billing's First Principles of Medicine.*

5. "The cure of all diseases must be effected by the *powers of the living system.* Remedies are merely to be employed with the view of placing the body under the most favorable circumstances for resisting disease."—*Dr. G. Gregory's Theory and Practice of Medicine.*

6. Pregnancy is no obstacle to the hydropathic treatment; on the contrary, by improving the health and strength, a modified employment of this treatment facilitates parturition, diminishes the severity and danger of labor, and prevents any great degree of subsequent weakness, and diseases consequent upon that weakness. Mrs. Priessnitz, a small, delicate woman, invariably practices it both immediately before and immediately after confinement, and occasionally during the whole term of gestation.

7. "In how few cases of indigestion is the stomach itself first diseased, though dyspepsia is a most convenient word, and the poor stomach is blamed for faults not its own!"—*Dr. Billing's*

* By Dr. Edward Johnson.

First Principles of Medicine. The fault consists in debility of the nervous system.

8. In some forms of disease enough of the hydropathic remedy may be carried out at the patient's own house—but in those cases which require the *full treatment,* with all its various adjuncts, it can only be carried out safely and *successfully* in the vicinity of a hydropathic establishment, where the patient is constantly under the eye of the practitioner.

9. There can be no danger in going into a cold bath while perspiring—first, because it has been practiced by Priessnitz on thousands of patients, for twenty years, and no single instance of mischief has ever been observed to arise from it. Secondly, it has been the habitual custom of the Russians since time immemorial, and no danger has been observed to attend it. Thirdly, the lower classes of society are constantly exposed to be drenched to the skin, almost daily, during the rainy months, while they are covered with perspiration, arising from their several out-of-doors employment, and no evil has been observed to accrue from it; on the contrary, *they suffer less from disease* than the classes above them.

10. "The physician, carrying his knowledge into the streets and highways of life, has labored assiduously (*the lancet in one hand and quinine in the other*) to arrest decay when hurrying forward with a too fatal precipitancy."—*Dr. Gregory.*

"The lancet in one hand," says Dr. Gregory, "and quinine in the other"—these being the two great engines of relief in acute and chronic diseases—the lancet, to *lower the pulse* in acute diseases, and quinine, to *strengthen the system* in chronic. Both these effects are produced by the right application of the hydropathic treatment. The *continued* application of cold in acute diseases, as by the cold bath or wet blanket or sheet, for *several hours, will lessen and lower the pulse even to a thread.* While the *occasional* use of the bath, accompanied by exercise, exposure to the air, simple diet, early hours, and all the other adjuncts of the treatment, will strengthen and harden the system to a degree infinitely beyond that which can be obtained by any other means whatever. Thus it supplies the place of the two grand engines of the old practice—viz., quinine and the lancet.

11. Physical man is an impressible mass of matter destined to perform certain actions (both internal and external) in obedience to the impressions made upon him by certain impressing causes.

When the impressing causes are right, the impressions will be right, and the actions performed in obedience to those impressions right also. This is health. When the impressing causes are wrong, the impressions will be wrong, and the actions resulting from those impressions wrong also. This is disease.

To substitute right *impressing causes* for wrong ones, therefore, is to substitute *right impressions* for wrong ones, and this is to substitute right actions for wrong ones—and this is to remove the causes of disease.

When wrong impressing causes have been removed, and right ones substituted, there is within the living body a restorative or curative principle, which will remove the wrong impressions made by the wrong impressing causes. To remove wrong impressing causes, therefore, and to substitute right ones, is to cure disease. But disease can never be cured while the wrong impressing causes which produced it are suffered to continue to operate.

12. A satisfactory explanation of the essential nature or proximate cause of a *common cold* has never been given. Liebig's theory of a mutual and equal resistance between the vital force and destructive force of oxygen explains it clearly. What are the symptoms of an ordinary cold? Defluxion from the nose—sore throat—hoarseness—cough—sneezing—and a sense of soreness over the whole surface of the body. What are the parts affected by these symptoms? The schneiderian membrane lining the nose—the parts of the throat near the root of the tongue—the air-passages leading to the lungs—and the skin. Why are these parts, in especial, first affected, when a man has taken cold, in preference to others? Because these are the parts of the body with which the oxygen of the air must necessarily come in contact before it can possibly enter the body so as to reach the internal organs. It happens thus: a continued stream of cold air, or continued exposure to wet, *while the body is inactive*—or excessive fatigue, or any other *debilitating cause*—first lowers the tone and diminishes the resistance of the vital force throughout the whole body, thus giving a preponderance to the action of oxygen over the resistance offered by the vital force. And as the oxygen must first come in contact with the skin, nostrils, throat, and air-passages leading to the lungs, before it can reach the internal organs (these being the inlets by which alone it can gain admission within the citadel), these are, therefore, precisely the parts on which, if Liebig's theory be

true, its destructive agency *ought* first to be exerted; and these *are* the parts on which it *is* first exerted—and inflammation of these parts *ought* to be the first manifestation of an undue intensity in the action of oxygen; and inflammation of these parts *is* the first manifestation of that undue intensity.

If the effect of the debilitating causes in lessening the resistance of the vital force have not been very great, then the vis medicatrix naturæ, or restorative principle, will restore the equilibrium between the resisting energy of the vital force and the destructive influence of oxygen, and thus remedy the mischief in a few days. But if the vital force have been greatly depressed, then the destructive agency of oxygen will be further manifested in the more internal organs, and fever, rheumatism, or inflammation of some deep-seated organ, will be the consequence, before the restorative principle has had time to perform its task of restoring the equilibrium. Nothing can more clearly illustrate Liebig's theory of disease than the phenomena of a common cold.

13. Nothing can be more self-evidently true than that the artificial is only another term for unnatural, since every thing which is not artificial must necessarily be natural, and every thing which is not natural must necessarily be artificial. There is no mean power between art and nature. Whatever does not result from the one must result from the other. It is allowed on all hands that the life of every highly cultivated society is highly *artificial.* It is therefore *unnatural.* But can that which is *unnatural* be possibly *proper?* Can art be considered a better judge of that which is fittest for man's welfare than nature? And is not the word nature, when thus used, obviously only another term for God himself? All the contrivances of art are the result of *human ingenuity:* the contrivances of nature are the result of *divine wisdom.*

Those several contrivances which we call comforts, and with which, in our polished condition, we surround ourselves, are the inventions and adaptations of *human ingenuity,* by which we administer, in an *undue degree, to sensual enjoyment.* What wonder they entail upon us disease and premature death! The influence of the weather, and all those various circumstances and impressions to which man is exposed in his primitive condition, are the institutions and adaptations of divine wisdom. What wonder that we should find them necessary to our health and well-being! What wonder that we should find it impossible to get rid of our diseases while we obstinately persevere in preferring the ordinances and contrivances of art to the manifest ordinances and contrivances of God himself!

But are we not to exercise and use the ingenuity wherewith God has endowed us? Certainly—to *use*, but not to *abuse* it. But how do we know that we are abusing God's gift of ingenuity or reason when we surround ourselves with all those appliances of pleasurable sensation which we call *comforts*, but which we *ought* to call luxurious indulgences? I answer: by the punishment of diseases and premature death, of which the evidence of our senses gives us daily proof. We know that they are wrong by the evil consequences which follow them. How do we know that intemperance is wrong? By the evil consequences which follow it. How do we know that poisons are injurious to the health? By the evil consequences which are observed to follow them. How do we know that it is wrong to indulge in the use of alcohol? By the evil consequences which follow its use. How then do we know that the domestic habits of a highly cultivated people are injurious? As in the former instances, by the evil consequences which are observed to follow them—by the multitudinous diseases and premature deaths which are every where observed to be inseparable from a highly cultivated condition of society, from which diseases and from which premature deaths a *primitive* condition of society is comparatively free.* Are there no other unwholesome and unnatural stimulants to the nervous system besides those of alcohol, wine, and beer? Thousands, and tens of thousands. All kinds of artificial stimulants do not elicit those peculiar phenomena called intoxication, but all operate injuriously upon the health—they all first excite, and finally exhaust, the nervous system. They all entail upon us the RETRIBUTE PLAGUE of numberless diseases and premature death. It is the punishment which God has awarded to the presuming pride of art, or the *abuse* of human reason. God did not create man for the purpose of getting money, nor of surrounding himself with all those multiform appliances of so-called comfort which *none but the rich can purchase;* and to prove that he did not, he has determined that none *shall* purchase them without purchasing disease and decrepitude along with them.

14. Hydropathy does but assert the supremacy of God.

* One half of civilized mankind die before the age of eight years.

15. Hydropathy, when taken with all its adjuncts, is an *artificial primitive condition* to which the sick man *temporarily* submits himself for a temporary purpose, viz., that of giving nature, assisted by art, a fair opportunity of healing his diseases.

16. But water, when used by the hydropathic physician as a remedy for disease, is a NATURAL INFLUENCE INTENSIFIED BY ART.

17. Total abstinence from every species of stimulating beverage is absolutely necessary to the success of the treatment.

18. Drinking large quantities of water, without some specific object (as, for instance, relaxing the bowels), is productive of no intelligible good, and proves injurious by distending the stomach, and over-stimulating the kidneys.

19. Every person in England who is cured of his disease by the hydropathic treatment, owes a large debt of gratitude to Captain Claridge, whose indefatigable exertions and indomitable courage, in spite of all opposition, have succeeded in planting hydropathy in this country—a soil in which, protected by humanity, and watered and pruned by science, it cannot fail to thrive, and grow, and flourish—a blessing to the people.

INDEX.

www.ingramcontent.com/pod-product-compliance
Lightning Source LLC
LaVergne TN
LVHW010152110826
845151LV00002B/494

* 9 7 8 1 4 2 5 5 3 8 6 2 0 *